Advances in Neonatal Neurology

Editors

PRAVEEN BALLABH
STEPHEN A. BACK

CLINICS IN PERINATOLOGY

www.perinatology.theclinics.com

Consulting Editor
LUCKY JAIN

March 2014 • Volume 41 • Number 1

ELSEVIER

1600 John F. Kennedy Boulevard • Suite 1800 • Philadelphia, Pennsylvania, 19103-2899

http://www.theclinics.com

CLINICS IN PERINATOLOGY Volume 41, Number 1
March 2014 ISSN 0095-5108, ISBN-13: 978-0-323-29620-5

Editor: Kerry Holland
Developmental Editor: Casey Jackson

Clinics in Perinatology (ISSN 0095-5108) is published quarterly by Elsevier Inc., 360 Park Avenue South, New York, NY 10010-1710. Months of issue are March, June, September, and December. Business and Editorial Offices: 1600 John F. Kennedy Blvd., Ste. 1800, Philadelphia, PA 19103-2899. Customer Service Office: 3251 Riverport Lane, Maryland Heights, MO 63043. Periodicals postage paid at New York, NY and additional mailing offices. Subscription prices are $285.00 per year (US individuals), $445.00 per year (US institutions), $340.00 per year (Canadian individuals), $545.00 per year (Canadian institutions), $420.00 per year (foreign individuals), $545.00 per year (foreign institutions), $135.00 per year (US students), and $195.00 per year (Canadian and foreign students). Foreign air speed delivery is included in all Clinics subscription prices. All prices are subject to change without notice. **POSTMASTER:** Send address changes to *Clinics in Perinatology*, Elsevier Health Sciences Division, Subscription Customer Service, 3251 Riverport Lane, Maryland Heights, MO 63043. **Customer Service: Telephone: 1-800-654-2452** (U.S. and Canada); **1-314-447-8871** (outside U.S. and Canada). **Fax: 1-314-447-8029. E-mail: journalscustomerservice-usa@elsevier.com** (for print support); **journalsonlinesupport-usa@elsevier.com** (for online support).

Reprints. For copies of 100 or more, of articles in this publication, please contact the Commercial Reprints Department, Elsevier Inc., 360 Park Avenue South, New York, NY 10010-1710. Tel. 212-633-3874; Fax: 212-633-3820; E-mail: reprints@elsevier.com.

Clinics in Perinatology is also pubilshed in Spanish by McGraw-Hill Interamericana Editores S.A., P.O. Box 5-237, 06500 Mexico D.F., Mexico.

Clinics in Perinatology is covered in *MEDLINE/PubMed (Index Medicus) Current Contents, Excepta Medica, BIOSIS and ISI/BIOMED.*

Printed and bound by CPI Group (UK) Ltd, Croydon, CR0 4YY

Contributors

CONSULTING EDITOR

LUCKY JAIN, MD, MBA
Richard W. Blumberg Professor and Executive Vice Chairman, Department of Pediatrics, Emory University School of Medicine; Executive Medical Director, Children's Physician Group, Emory Children's Center, Children's Healthcare of Atlanta, Atlanta, Georgia

EDITORS

PRAVEEN BALLABH, MD
Professor of Pediatrics and Cell Biology and Anatomy, Regional Neonatal Center, Maria Fareri Children's Hospital at Westchester Medical Center and New York Medical College, Valhalla, New York

STEPHEN A. BACK, MD, PhD
Professor of Pediatrics and Neurology, Oregon Health & Science University, Clyde and Elda Munson Professor of Pediatric Research, Director, Neuroscience Section, Papé Family Pediatric Research Institute, Portland, Oregon

AUTHORS

TOMOKI ARICHI, MBChB, MRCPCH, PhD
Centre for the Developing Brain, Department of Perinatal Imaging, St Thomas' Hospital, King's College London; Department of Bioengineering, Imperial College London, London, United Kingdom

STEPHEN A. BACK, MD, PhD
Professor of Pediatrics and Neurology, Oregon Health & Science University, Clyde and Elda Munson Professor of Pediatric Research, Director, Neuroscience Section, Papé Family Pediatric Research Institute, Portland, Oregon

PRAVEEN BALLABH, MD
Professor of Pediatrics and Cell Biology and Anatomy, Regional Neonatal Center, Maria Fareri Children's Hospital at Westchester Medical Center and New York Medical College, Valhalla, New York

OLIVIER BAUD, MD, PhD
Professor, University of Paris Diderot, Paris, France

MANON J.N.L. BENDERS, MD, PhD
Associate Professor in Neonatology, Department of Neonatology, Wilhelmina Children's Hospital, University Medical Center Utrecht, The Netherlands

LAURA BENNET, PhD
Professor of Physiology, Department of Physiology, University of Auckland, Auckland, New Zealand

VANN CHAU, MD
Division of Neurology, Department of Pediatrics, The Hospital for Sick Children; University of Toronto, Toronto, Ontario; Child & Family Research Institute, Vancouver, British Columbia, Canada

SERENA J. COUNSELL, PhD
Centre for the Developing Brain, Department of Perinatal Imaging, St Thomas' Hospital, King's College London, London, United Kingdom

LINDA S. DE VRIES, MD, PhD
Professor in Neonatal Neurology, Department of Neonatology, Wilhelmina Children's Hospital, University Medical Center Utrecht, The Netherlands

PAUL P. DRURY, BSc
Department of Physiology, University of Auckland, Auckland, New Zealand

A. DAVID EDWARDS, MBBS, FRCP, FRCPCH, FMedSci
Centre for the Developing Brain, Department of Perinatal Imaging, St Thomas' Hospital, King's College London; Department of Bioengineering, Imperial College London, London, United Kingdom

DONNA M. FERRIERO, MD, MS
Neonatal Brain Disorders Laboratory, University of California, San Francisco, San Francisco, California

BOBBI FLEISS, PhD
Senior Lecturer, University of Paris Diderot; PremUP, Paris, France; Centre for the Developing Brain, St Thomas' Campus, King's College, London, United Kingdom

HANNAH C. GLASS, MDCM, MAS
Associate Professor, Departments of Neurology and Pediatrics, Director, Neonatal Neurocritical Care Services, Neonatal Neurology Training Program Director, Benioff Children's Hospital University of California, San Francisco, California

PIERRE GRESSENS, MD, PhD
University of Paris Diderot; PremUP, Paris, France; Centre for the Developing Brain, St Thomas' Campus, King's College, London, United Kingdom

RUTH E. GRUNAU, PhD
Professor, University of British Columbia, Vancouver, British Columbia, Canada; Queens University Belfast, Belfast, Northern Ireland, United Kingdom

PASCALE V. GUILLOT, PhD
Institute of Reproductive and Developmental Biology, Imperial College London, London, United Kingdom

ALISTAIR J. GUNN, MBChB, PhD
Professor of Physiology and Paediatrics, Department of Physiology, Faculty of Medical and Health Sciences, University of Auckland; Paediatrician, Starship Children's Hospital, Grafton, Auckland, New Zealand

ELEANOR R. GUNN, MBChB
Department of Physiology, University of Auckland, Auckland, New Zealand

HENRIK HAGBERG, MD, PhD
Professor, Centre for the Developing Brain, St Thomas' Campus, King's College, London, United Kingdom; Departments of Clinical Sciences & Physiology and Neuroscience, Perinatal Center, Sahlgrenska Academy, Gothenburg University, Gothenburg, Sweden

PETRA S. HUPPI, MD, PhD
Chief Medical Officer, Department of Child and Adolescent, Service Development and Growth, University Hospital of Geneva, Geneva, Switzerland

SANDRA E. JUUL, MD, PhD
Department of Pediatrics, University of Washington, Seattle, Washington

KARINA J. KERSBERGEN, MD
PhD Student in Neonatal Neurology, Department of Neonatology, Wilhelmina Children's Hospital, University Medical Center Utrecht, The Netherlands

SOO HYUN KWON, MD
Department of Pediatrics, Yale University School of Medicine, New Haven, Connecticut

SHADI N. MALAEB, MD
Department of Pediatrics, St. Christopher's Hospital for Children, Drexel University College of Medicine, Philadelphia, Pennsylvania

DEBORAH E. MCFADDEN, MD
Child & Family Research Institute; Department of Pathology, BC Children's & Women's Health Center; University of British Columbia, Vancouver, British Columbia, Canada

CHRISTOPHER MCPHERSON, PharmD
Clinical Pharmacist, Neonatal Intensive Care, St. Louis Children's Hospital, St Louis, Missouri

LAURA R. MENT, MD
Departments of Pediatrics and Neurology, Yale University School of Medicine, New Haven, Connecticut

STEVEN P. MILLER, MDCM, MAS
Division of Neurology, Department of Pediatrics, The Hospital for Sick Children; Neurosciences and Mental Health Program, Research Institute, University of Toronto, Toronto, Ontario; Child & Family Research Institute, Vancouver, British Columbia, Canada

KENNETH J. POSKITT, MDCM
Child & Family Research Institute, University of British Columbia; Departments of Pediatrics and Radiology, BC Children's & Women's Health Center, Vancouver, British Columbia, Canada

NATALINA SALMASO, PhD
Associate Research Scientist, Child Study Center, Yale University, New Haven, Connecticut

SEETHA SHANKARAN, MD
Professor of Pediatrics, Wayne State University School of Medicine; Director, Division of Neonatal/Perinatal Medicine, Children's Hospital of Michigan and Hutzel Women's Hospital, Detroit, Michigan

BARBARA S. STONESTREET, MD
Professor of Pediatrics, Department of Pediatrics, Women & Infants Hospital of Rhode Island, The Alpert Medical School of Brown University, Providence, Rhode Island

SIDHARTHA TAN, MD
Clinical Professor, Department of Pediatrics, NorthShore University Health System, University Chicago Pritzker School of Medicine, Evanston, Illinois

LUIGI TITOMANLIO, MD, PhD
Professor, University of Paris Diderot, Paris, France

SIMONE TOMASI, MD, PhD
Post-Doctoral Associate, Child Study Center, Yale University, New Haven, Connecticut

NORA TUSOR, MD
Centre for the Developing Brain, Department of Perinatal Imaging, St Thomas' Hospital, King's College London, London, United Kingdom

FLORA M. VACCARINO, MD
Professor, Child Study Center, Yale University; Department of Neurobiology, Kavli Institute for Neuroscience, Yale University, New Haven, Connecticut

LANA VASUNG, MD, PhD
Department of Child and Adolescent, Service Development and Growth, University Hospital of Geneva, Geneva, Switzerland

BETTY R. VOHR, MD
Professor of Pediatrics, Alpert Medical School of Brown University; Director of Neonatal Follow-Up, Women and Infants Hospital, Providence, Rhode Island

Contents

> Increasing numbers of preterm neonates survive with motor and cognitive disabilities related to less destructive forms of cerebral injury that still result in reduced cerebral growth. White matter injury results in myelination disturbances related to aberrant responses to death of pre-myelinating oligodendrocytes (preOLs). PreOLs are rapidly regenerated but fail to mature to myelinating cells. Although immature projection neurons are more resistant to hypoxia-ischemia than preOLs, they display widespread disturbances in dendritic arbor maturation, which provides an explanation for impaired cerebral growth. Thus, large numbers of cells fail to fully mature during a critical window in development of neural circuitry. These recently recognized forms of cerebral gray and white matter dysmaturation suggest new therapeutic directions centered on reversal of the processes that promote dysmaturation.

> Infants who are born preterm have a high incidence of neurocognitive and neurobehavioral abnormalities, which may be associated with impaired brain development. Advanced magnetic resonance imaging (MRI) approaches, such as diffusion MRI (d-MRI) and functional MRI (fMRI), provide objective and reproducible measures of brain development. Indices derived from d-MRI can be used to provide quantitative measures of preterm brain injury. Although fMRI of the neonatal brain is currently a research tool, future studies combining d-MRI and fMRI have the potential to assess the structural and functional properties of the developing brain and its response to injury.

> Intraventricular hemorrhage (IVH) is a major neurologic complication of prematurity. Pathogenesis of IVH is attributed to intrinsic fragility of germinal matrix vasculature and to the fluctuation in the cerebral blood flow. Germinal matrix exhibits rapid angiogenesis orchestrating formation of immature

vessels. Prenatal glucocorticoid exposure remains the most effective means of preventing IVH. Therapies targeted to enhance the stability of the germinal matrix vasculature and minimize fluctuation in the cerebral blood flow might lead to more effective strategies in preventing IVH.

White matter injury and hemorrhage are common findings in extremely preterm infants. Large hemorrhages and extensive cystic lesions are identified with cranial ultrasound. MRI, which is more sensitive, is especially useful in the identification of small intraventricular hemorrhage; cerebellar hemorrhage; punctate lesion in the white matter and cerebellum; and diffuse, noncystic white matter injury. Imaging sequences such as diffusion-weighted, diffusion tensor, and susceptibility weighted imaging may improve recognition and prediction of outcome. These techniques improve understanding of the underlying pathophysiology of white matter injury and its effects on brain development and neurodevelopmental outcome.

Chorioamnionitis (or placental infection) is suspected to be a risk factor for brain injury in premature infants. The suggested association between chorioamnionitis and cystic periventricular leukomalacia and cerebral palsy is uncertain because of the variability of study designs and definitions of chorioamnionitis. Improvements in neonatal intensive care may have attenuated the impact of chorioamnionitis on brain health outcomes. Large multicenter studies using rigorous definitions of chorioamnionitis on placental pathologies and quantitative magnetic resonance techniques may offer the optimal way to clarify the complex role of chorioamnionitis in modifying brain health and long-term outcomes.

There is a certainty in malpractice cases that neurodevelopmental deficits are caused by preventable events at birth when the onset, nature, and timing of the insult in the antenatal and natal period are unknown. The biggest problem is determining timing. Electronic fetal monitoring is given excessive importance in legal cases. Before assigning fault on events at birth, a better understanding of developmental neurobiology and limitations of the present clinical biomarkers is warranted. The issues of single versus repeated episodes, timing of antenatal insults, pros and cons of legal arguments, interaction of various etiologic and anatomic factors are discussed.

This article explains the mechanisms underlying choices of pharmacotherapy for hypoxic-ischemic insults of both preterm and term babies. Some preclinical data are strong enough that clinical trials are now underway.

Challenges remain in deciding the best combination therapies for each age and insult.

This article introduces the basic concepts of modeling neonatal brain injury and provides background information regarding each of the commonly used types of stem cells. It summarizes the findings of preclinical research testing the therapeutic potential of stem cells in animal models of neonatal brain injury, reports briefly on the status of clinical trials, and discusses the important ongoing issues that need to be addressed before stem cell therapy is used to repair the injured brain.

This article examines the evidence regarding mortality and neurodevelopmental outcomes following hypothermia for neonatal hypoxic-ischemic encephalopathy. Data from randomized controlled trials regarding neurodevelopmental outcome at the end point of the major trials, and from 2 of the trials on childhood outcome following hypothermia for neonatal hypoxic-ischemic encephalopathy are presented. The predictors of outcome that can be evaluated in the neonatal period are also reviewed, as this information may assist in the counseling of families. Most trials of hypothermia have been performed in high-resource countries; published studies from the low- and middle-income countries are also reviewed.

Prolonged, moderate cerebral hypothermia initiated within a few hours after severe hypoxia-ischemia and continued until resolution of the acute phase of delayed cell death can reduce acute brain injury and improve long-term behavioral recovery in term infants and in adults after cardiac arrest. The specific mechanisms of hypothermic neuroprotection remain unclear, in part because hypothermia suppresses a broad range of potential injurious factors. This article examines proposed mechanisms in relation to the known window of opportunity for effective protection with hypothermia. Knowledge of the mechanisms of hypothermia will help guide the rational development of future combination treatments to augment neuroprotection with hypothermia and identify those most likely to benefit.

Seizures occur in approximately 1 to 5 per 1000 live births and are among the most common neurologic conditions managed by a neonatal neurocritical care service. There are several, age-specific factors that are particular to the developing brain, which influence excitability and seizure generation, response to medications, and impact of seizures on brain structure and function. Neonatal seizures are often associated with serious underlying brain injury such as hypoxia-ischemia, stroke, or hemorrhage. Conventional, prolonged, continuous video electroencephalogram is the gold standard for detecting seizures, whereas amplitude-integrated EEG is a convenient and useful bedside tool.

Deleterious effects result from both glucocorticoid insufficiency and excess glucocorticoid tissue exposure in the developing brain. Accumulating evidence suggests a net benefit of postnatal glucocorticoid therapy when administered shortly after the first week of life to premature infants with early and persistent pulmonary dysfunction, particularly in those with evidence of relative adrenal insufficiency. The decision to treat with steroids should ensure maximum respiratory benefit at the lowest possible neurologic risk, while avoiding serious systemic complications. Ongoing clinical trials must validate this approach.

Preclinical and clinical studies have demonstrated the adverse consequences of untreated pain and stress on brain development in the preterm infant. Sucrose has widely been implemented as standard therapy for minor procedural pain. Anesthetics are commonly utilized in preterm infants during major surgery. Pharmacologic agents (benzodiazepines and opioids) have been examined in clinical trials of preterm infants requiring invasive mechanical ventilation. Controversy exists regarding the safety and long-term impact of these interventions. Ongoing multidisciplinary research will help define the impact of these agents and identify potential alternative therapies.

The incidence of preterm birth is on the rise. The outcome of premature birth can vary widely, spanning completely normal development to severe neurologic deficits, with most children showing mild to moderate cognitive delay and increased incidence of neuropsychiatric conditions such as anxiety, attention deficit hyperactivity, and autism spectrum disorders. Several animal models have been employed to study the consequences of prematurity, one of the most promising being chronic perinatal hypoxia in mouse, which recapitulates the cognitive impairments, partial recovery over time and enhanced recovery with environmental enrichment.

Survival of extremely preterm infants has improved since 2000. Neurodevelopmental impairment rates remain high at the limits of viability. Although improved survival and neurodevelopmental impairment rates are associated with higher gestational age and more recent year of birth, significant variability in findings among geographic areas and networks is evident, and seems related to differences in population, management style, regional protocols, definitions, and outcome assessments. Outcome studies during adolescence and young adult age are needed to determine the long-term impact of extremely preterm birth.

Magnetic resonance imaging (MRI) is a safe and high-resolution neuroimaging modality that is increasingly used in the neonatal population to assess brain injury and its consequences on brain development. It is superior to cranial ultrasound for the definition of patterns of both white and gray matter maturation and injury and therefore has the potential to provide prognostic information on the neurodevelopmental outcomes of the preterm population. Furthermore, the development of sophisticated MRI strategies, including diffusion tensor imaging, resting state functional connectivity, and magnetic resonance spectroscopy, may increase the prognostic value, helping to guide parental counseling and allocate early intervention services.

PROGRAM OBJECTIVE

The goal of *Clinics in Perinatology* is to keep practicing perinatologists, neonatologists, obstetricians, practicing physicians and residents up to date with current clinical practice in perinatology by providing timely articles reviewing the state of the art in patient care.

TARGET AUDIENCE

Perinatologists, neonatologists, obstetricians, practicing physicians, residents and healthcare professionals who provide patient care utilizing findings from *Clinics in Perinatology.*

LEARNING OBJECTIVES

Upon completion of this activity, participants will be able to:
1. Review the pathophysiology and management of white and gray matter injury in newborns.
2. Discuss advances in mechanisms and management of neonatal seizures.
3. Review the role of neuroimaging in predicting neurodevelopmental outcomes of preterm neonates.

ACCREDITATION

The Elsevier Office of Continuing Medical Education (EOCME) is accredited by the Accreditation Council for Continuing Medical Education (ACCME) to provide continuing medical education for physicians.

The EOCME designates this enduring material for a maximum of 15 *AMA PRA Category 1 Credit*(s)™. Physicians should claim only the credit commensurate with the extent of their participation in the activity.

All other health care professionals requesting continuing education credit for this enduring material will be issued a certificate of participation.

DISCLOSURE OF CONFLICTS OF INTEREST

The EOCME assesses conflict of interest with its instructors, faculty, planners, and other individuals who are in a position to control the content of CME activities. All relevant conflicts of interest that are identified are thoroughly vetted by EOCME for fair balance, scientific objectivity, and patient care recommendations. EOCME is committed to providing its learners with CME activities that promote improvements or quality in healthcare and not a specific proprietary business or a commercial interest.

The planning committee, staff, authors and editors listed below have identified no financial relationships or relationships to products or devices they or their spouse/life partner have with commercial interest related to the content of this CME activity:
T. Arichi; Stephen Back, MD, PhD; Praveen Ballabh, MD; Olivier Baud; Manon JNL Benders; Laura Bennet, MBChB Student; Vann Chau; Serena Counsell, PhD; Linda Simone DeVries, MD, PhD; Paul P. Drury, BSc; David Edwards, MBBS, FRCP, FRCPCH, F.MedSci; Donna Ferriero, MD, MS; Bobbi Fleiss; Hannah Glass, MD; Pierre Gressens, MD, PhD; Ruth E. Grunau, PhD; Pascale V. Guillot; Alistair Gunn, MBChB, PhD; Eleanor R. Gunn, MBChB/PhD Student; Henrik Hagberg, MD, PhD; Kerry Holland; Brynne Hunter; Petra S. Hüppi, MD; Sandra E. Juul, MD, PhD; Karina Kersbergen, MD; Soo H. Kwon, MD; Sandy Lavery; Shadi N. Malaeb, MD; Deborah E. McFadden; Jill McNair; Christopher McPherson, Pharm.D; Laura R. Ment, MD; Steven P. Miller; Palani Murugesan, Lindsay Parnell; Kenneth J. Poskitt, MDCM; Natalina Salmaso; Seetha Shankaran, MD; Barbara Stonestreet, MD; Sidthartha Tan, MD; Luigi Titomanlio; Simone Tomasi; N. Tusor; Flora Vaccarino, MD; Lana Vasung, MD, PhD; Betty R. Vohr, MD.

The planning committee, staff, authors and editors listed below have identified financial relationships or relationships to products or devices they or their spouse/life partner have with commercial interest related to the content of this CME activity:

UNAPPROVED/OFF-LABEL USE DISCLOSURE

The EOCME requires CME faculty to disclose to the participants:
1. When products or procedures being discussed are off-label, unlabelled, experimental, and/or investigational (not US Food and Drug Administration (FDA) approved); and
2. Any limitations on the information presented, such as data that are preliminary or that represent ongoing research, interim analyses, and/or unsupported opinions. Faculty may discuss information about pharmaceutical agents that is outside of FDA-approved labelling. This information is intended solely for CME and is not intended to promote off-label use of these medications. If you have any questions, contact the medical affairs department of the manufacturer for the most recent prescribing information.

TO ENROLL

To enroll in the *Clinics in Perinatology* Continuing Medical Education program, call customer service at 1-800-654-2452 or sign up online at http://www.theclinics.com/home/cme. The CME program is available to subscribers for an additional annual fee of $235 USD.

METHOD OF PARTICIPATION

In order to claim credit, participants must complete the following:

1. Complete enrolment as indicated above.
2. Read the activity.
3. Complete the CME Test and Evaluation. Participants must achieve a score of 70% on the test. All CME Tests and Evaluations must be completed online.

CME INQUIRIES/SPECIAL NEEDS

For all CME inquiries or special needs, please contact elsevierCME@elsevier.com

CLINICS IN PERINATOLOGY

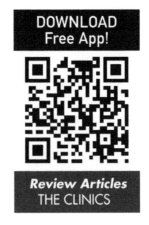

DOWNLOAD
Free App!

Review Articles
THE CLINICS

NOW AVAILABLE FOR YOUR iPhone and iPad

Foreword

Why the Human Fetus Has Such a Large Vulnerable Head And Why It Is Our Job to Protect It!

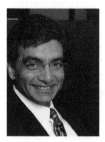

Lucky Jain, MD, MBA
Consulting Editor

Why does the human fetus have such a large head and why is the brain it seeks to protect so vulnerable? To answer this question, one has to address the bigger question: why is the human species so different from all other species and why did it evolve that way? In fact, the answer is embedded in the even more vexing question of what fundamentally makes us human!

As we look around, every species, it appears, is provided with some innate attribute that allows it to thrive in spite of the constant rivalry over resources and the big differences in size, strength, and aggressiveness. David Malouf,[1] in his book, "The Happy Life," talks about a special quality that each of the thriving creatures have that they use to protect themselves from the elements: the fur, feathers, and hide that protect them from cold; fangs and claws for protection against aggression; power of flight and swiftness; or sheer size when agility is lacking. What then is the distinguishing attribute that has allowed humans to not only thrive, but to dominate, the planet? It is the mind, the intellect, the cognitive ability. Thomas Suddendorf,[2] in his new book, "The Gap," believes that within the evolved brain, it is the ability to connect with other minds, "nested scenario building or mental time travel," that makes us unique. This dimension allows us to imagine situations without experiencing them and develop a mental picture of what another individual knows or is thinking. Suddendorf[2] contends that this unique attribute allows humans to navigate through complex social existence and participate in collective thinking. The emergence of *collective intelligence* nested in communities, rather than individuals, allowed for rapid interaction and collective behavior, which further accelerated the pace of progress.[3] And then there is the consciousness, "recursive awareness of their own awareness."

Clin Perinatol 41 (2014) xv–xvi
http://dx.doi.org/10.1016/j.clp.2013.12.001
0095-5108/14/$ – see front matter © 2014 Elsevier Inc. All rights reserved.

All of this leads us to the inevitable conclusion that our brain, unlike the speed, fangs, claws, and sheer size of other animals, is the defining attribute that has allowed humans to differentiate themselves from every other living being on this planet. This highly complex brain, however, comes with its challenges. The human fetus has a head size that is considerably larger in size when compared with the rest of its body; it is also much larger than the head size of its closest relatives, the great apes. Furthermore, it thrives on high-energy consumption and is not fully developed at birth. Anthropologists believe that the clash of the growing fetal head size with the size of maternal pelvis determines the need to be delivered early.[4] The consequent immaturity of the brain at birth, even in a full-term neonate, makes it vulnerable to injury from hypoxia, ischemia, infections, metabolic disorders, and other insults. Add to this the myriad of things we do in the NICU environment, some with dubious benefits, that can add insult to injury.

As Drs Ballabh and Back comment in their introduction to this issue, there has been remarkable progress in recent years in our understanding of the biologic underpinnings of neonatal brain injury and the efforts to reduce its long-term effect on the developing brain. In fact, introduction of cerebral hypothermia has revolutionized the way hypoxic ischemic encephalopathy is managed.[5] However, more needs to be done. Birth asphyxia and hypoxic ischemic encephalopathy are still frequent occurrences worldwide. In the tiniest preemies, intraventricular hemorrhage and periventricular white matter injury continue to be a cause of significant long-term morbidity.[6] The ill effects of many NICU practices including recurrent exposures to anesthetic agents and other neurotoxic drugs have yet to be fully understood.

I am delighted that Drs Ballabh and Back have put together a comprehensive review of advances in neonatal neurology in this edition of the *Clinics in Perinatology*. This issue is very timely and will serve as a wonderful update and reference guide. In addition to the authors, I would like to thank Kerry Holland and Elsevier for their support of this important topic.

Lucky Jain, MD, MBA
Department of Pediatrics
Emory Children's Center
Emory University School of Medicine
2015 Uppergate Drive
Atlanta, GA 30322, USA

E-mail address:
ljain@emory.edu

REFERENCES

1. Malouf D. The happy life: the search for contentment in the modern world. New York: Pantheon Books; 2011.
2. Suddendorf T. The gap: the science of what separates us from other animals. New York: Basic Books; 2013.
3. Ridley M. Humans: why they triumphed. The Wall Street Journal May 22, 2010.
4. Wittman AB, Wall LL. The evolutionary origins of obstructed labor: bipedalism, encephalization, and the human obstetric dilemma. Obstet Gynecol Surv 2007; 62:739–48.
5. Shankaran S, Pappas A, McDonald SA, et al. Childhood outcomes after hypothermia for neonatal encephalopathy. N Engl J Med 2012;366(22):2085–92.
6. Pavlova MA, Krägeloh-Mann I. Limitations on the developing preterm brain: impact of periventricular white matter lesions on brain connectivity and cognition. Brain 2013;136:998–1011.

Preface

Advances in Neonatal Neurology

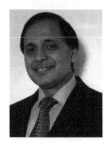 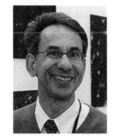

Praveen Ballabh, MD   Stephen A. Back, MD, PhD
Editors

We are extremely pleased to introduce this issue of *Clinics in Perinatology*, which focuses on "Advances in Neonatal Neurology." The last decade has witnessed remarkable progress in neonatal neurology that has come in part from major advances in neuroimaging, the introduction of cerebral hypothermia, and a wealth of basic science insights that have positioned us for sustained accelerated progress in the diagnosis and treatment of numerous disorders of preterm and term neonates. Our challenge in compiling this issue was, thus, to select from a wide spectrum of recent advances that span from bench to bedside. The 16 articles in this issue draw on the expertise of internationally recognized experts who have collectively provided cross-cutting reviews with a broad perspective on the current state of the field. We are very grateful to the authors for providing succinct, up-to-date clinical perspectives and for highlighting current controversies and future challenges. Thanks to them, we are able to offer you a cutting-edge compendium of this complex and fast-moving field. Throughout the issue, the reader is encouraged to acquire a more comprehensive perspective by drawing connections between earlier and later articles that are thematically grouped around issues dealing with pathogenesis, diagnosis, and therapy.

The issue begins by addressing two common problems in neonatal neurology from the perspectives of pathogenesis and neuroimaging: cerebral gray and white matter injury and intraventricular hemorrhage. The first article addresses the pathogenesis of cerebral injury in the premature infant. The considerable recent progress in the care of preterm infants has translated to substantial changes in the spectrum of cerebral injury sustained by these babies. The shift from predominantly destructive lesions to dysmature lesions has raised new challenges to define insults to the developing brain, which do not strictly adhere to our long-standing concepts about cerebral injury. Inherent in these challenges are complex issues related to disruption of the timing and progression of key neurodevelopmental events that progress rapidly in the last trimester of gestation. The first article is complemented by a second article

Clin Perinatol 41 (2014) xvii–xix
http://dx.doi.org/10.1016/j.clp.2013.11.002
perinatology.theclinics.com

by Dr Serena Counsell, Dr David Edwards, and their colleagues that provides a comprehensive review of the application of advanced MRI techniques to define the evolution of the events that underlie brain development in the preterm and term infants through diffusion and functional MRI. The application of these advanced neuroimaging techniques provides powerful noninvasive surrogate measures to define how perturbations in brain development affect cellular maturation and neuronal connectivity. This information also provides another avenue to accelerate progress toward improved preventive strategies and new directions in rehabilitation that will harness the intrinsic plasticity of the neonatal brain for regeneration and repair. Later in the issue, Dr Flora Vaccarino and her colleagues return to this exciting new direction to examine how prematurity and perinatal insults influence neurogenesis in the brain of premature infants and in experimental models with resultant microstructural and functional changes that translate to enduring changes in neurodevelopment.

In the third article on intraventricular hemorrhage, advances in the understanding of the pathogenesis and prevention of this common problem have been thoroughly reviewed. The article draws on a wealth of new insights into the complex developmental changes in the preterm vasculature as derived from both experimental models and human autopsy studies. This article is complemented by the fourth article by Dr Linda De Vries and her colleagues, which integrates the application of multiple neuroimaging modalities to define the progression of white matter injury and intraventricular hemorrhage. In the next article, Dr Steven Miller and his colleagues grapple with the on-going controversies and challenges to define the pathogenesis of white matter injury in terms of the relative contributions of maternal chorioamnionitis and postnatal infection.

Several authors were invited to address state-of-the-art diagnostic and neuroprotective strategies for the term neonate with hypoxic-ischemic encephalopathy. Dr Sidhartha Tan analyzes the application of clinical and MRI biomarkers for earlier detection of hypoxic-ischemic injury. Three articles address current advances in the prevention of hypoxic-ischemic injury to the term neonate by means of pharmacological strategies and cerebral hypothermia—a topic that Dr Donna Ferriero refreshingly refers to as cocktails and ice! Remarkably, as adult neurologists continue to struggle to develop viable therapies for stroke and other forms of hypoxic-ischemic brain injury, neonatal neurology is exploring new avenues to fine-tune the approach of combination therapies to augment the therapeutic efficacy of cerebral hypothermia with adjunctive pharmacological agents. Drs Sunny Juul and Donna Ferriero provide a highly current perspective on the most promising agents for neuroprotection. Dr Pierre Gressens and his coauthors have provided a comprehensive summary of the current status of both preclinical testing of stem cells in animal models and the current status of clinical trials with various forms of stem cell therapy. In her article, Dr Seetha Shankaran navigates through the outcome data on childhood hypoxic-ischemic encephalopathy to provide an up-to-date perspective on the current status of the efficacy and limitations of cerebral hypothermia. Dr Alistair Gunn and his colleagues have discussed molecular mechanisms of hypothermic neuroprotection, which may help clinicians to design effective combination therapies for hypothermia.

Three articles address timely and controversial issues related to management of preterm or term infants. Neonatal seizures frequently pose challenging diagnostic and management issues. Dr Hannah Glass has provided a valuable compendium of recent advances related to both the diagnosis and the management of neonatal seizures. Dr Barbara Stonestreet and her colleagues have extensively studied glucocorticoids and their impact on brain development and injury. They provide valuable insights into the physiological basis for the use of prenatal and postnatal glucocorticoids and discuss the risks and benefits of these agents in the preterm neonate. Drs Ruth Grunau and Christopher McPherson have contributed the article on neonatal pain control and the neurologic effects of anesthetics and sedatives in preterm infants. They assess the potential deleterious effects of analgesics and anesthetics for management of both acute and chronic pain in neonates in intensive care.

The issue concludes with two complementary articles that examine long-term outcomes in preterm and term neonates. Dr Betty Vohr has framed the problem with an outstanding article assessing the current status of neurodevelopmental outcomes of extremely preterm infants. Drs Petra Huppi, Laura Ment, and colleagues address the application of sophisticated MRI strategies, including diffusion tensor imaging, resting state functional connectivity, and magnetic resonance spectroscopy to better predict the prognosis for premature newborns and assist in early intervention services.

We are extremely grateful to Elsevier for the opportunity to serve as the guest editors for this issue that we expect will offer much valuable insight into the current management of the neurology problems of the preterm and term neonate. This issue underscores the vital importance of continued support to encourage and nurture collaboration among clinicians and scientists. We hope that this issue will serve as testimony to the passionate pursuit of progress achieved by our colleagues. We hope it will also inspire others to sustain the tremendous potential for further advances to optimize brain development for newborns in neonatal units throughout the world.

Praveen Ballabh, MD
Professor of Pediatrics and Cell Biology and Anatomy
Regional Neonatal Center
Maria Fareri Children's Hospital at Westchester Medical Center and
New York Medical College
Valhalla, New York 10595, USA

Stephen A. Back, MD, PhD
Professor of Pediatrics and Neurology
Oregon Health & Science University
Clyde and Elda Munson Professor of Pediatric Research
Director, Neuroscience Section, Papé Family Pediatric Research Institute
Mail Code: L481
Biomedical Research Building 317
3181 S.W. Sam Jackson Park Road, Portland, OR 97239-3098, USA

E-mail addresses:
pballabh@msn.com (P. Ballabh)
backs@ohsu.edu (S.A. Back)

Cerebral White and Gray Matter Injury in Newborns
New Insights into Pathophysiology and Management

Stephen A. Back, MD, PhD

KEYWORDS

- White matter • Gray matter • Cerebral • Newborns • Pathophysiology
- Management

KEY POINTS

- Contemporary cohorts of preterm infants commonly show less severe injury, which does not seem to involve pronounced neuronal or glial loss. These milder forms of injury are still associated with reduced cerebral growth.
- Myelination disturbances are one of the hallmarks of chronic white matter injury arising from hypoxia-ischemia.
- Although immature neurons seem to be more resistant to cell death from hypoxia-ischemia than glia, they show widespread disturbances in maturation of their dendritic arbors, which provides an explanation for impaired cerebral growth.
- Numerous immature neurons and preOLs fail to fully mature during a critical window in development of neural circuitry.

PRETERM SURVIVORS SHOW AN EVOLVING SPECTRUM OF BRAIN INJURY

Although major advances in the care of premature infants have resulted in striking improvements in the survival of very low birth weight (VLBW) infants (<1.5 kg), enhanced survival has been accompanied by a significant increase in the number of preterm survivors with long-term neurodevelopmental morbidity.[1,2] In the United States, the rate

This work was supported by the NIH (National Institutes of Neurologic Diseases and Stroke: 1R01NS054044, and R37NS045737-06S1/06S2, the National Institute of Aging: 1R01AG03189, the American Heart Association and the March of Dimes Birth Defects Foundation [S.A. Back]). The Neuroscience Imaging Center at Oregon Health & Science University is supported by NINDS grant P30NS061800.
Potential Conflicts of Interest: Nothing to report.
Neuroscience Section, Division of Pediatric Neuroscience, Department of Pediatrics, Pape' Family Pediatric Research Institute, Oregon Health & Science University, Mail Code: L481, Biomedical Research Building 317, 3181 Southwest Sam Jackson Park Road, Portland, OR 97239-3098, USA
E-mail address: backs@ohsu.edu

of preterm birth continues to increase, with prematurity complicating 1 in 8 deliveries, and VLBW infants comprise about 1.5% of the 4 million live births in the United States each year.[3]

Despite improved outcomes of children born preterm, there continues to be wide variation in functional disabilities, even among those born at the same gestational age.[4] Premature birth alone is associated with a greater risk for reduction in both cerebral white and gray matter volume, which is associated with poorer cognitive development.[5–12] In the setting of cerebral injury, 5% to 10% of preterm survivors sustain permanent major motor impairment, including cerebral palsy (CP), which ranges from mild motor dyspraxia to severe spastic motor deficits.[13–17] By school age, approximately half show a broad spectrum of cognitive dysfunction, which involves various aspects of learning, memory, language, vision, hearing, attention, and socialization.[14,18–32] Disabilities in multiple neurodevelopmental domains often co-occur[33] and persist to young adulthood.[24–26,34–37]

The diverse spectrum of cognitive and motor outcomes in preterm survivors has led to increasing recognition that widely distributed abnormalities in brain maturation occur. Until recently, preterm infants were at high risk for destructive brain lesions that resulted in cystic white matter injury (WMI) and secondary cortical and subcortical gray matter degeneration. These brain abnormalities lead to substantial deletion of axons and glia from necrotic white matter lesions and secondary loss of neurons in developing gray matter. However, the last decade has been accompanied by an increasing number of studies that support a shift to milder forms of chronic injury, in which tissue destruction is the minor component. Nevertheless, these milder forms of injury are also associated with reduced cerebral growth and adverse outcomes. As discussed later, recent human and experimental studies support that this impaired growth is related to distinctly different forms of disease, which involve aberrant responses to injury that disrupt the maturation of neurons and glial progenitors. These emerging findings suggest that brain injury in most preterm survivors involves a primary cerebral dysmaturation disorder, which may be amenable to a variety of rehabilitative strategies directed at promoting brain maturation and improved neurodevelopmental outcome.

WHAT DEFINES AN INSULT TO THE DEVELOPING BRAIN AND WHY DOES THIS MATTER?

Although the full impact of preterm cerebral insults is often not fully defined until a childhood neurodevelopmental assessment occurs, there is a critical need for improved means to identify insults closer to the time of occurrence in order to implement potential therapies to prevent early injury[38] or promote regeneration and repair of chronic lesions.[39] However, the critical windows for interventions remain poorly defined, because of our limited tools to define primary or secondary insults in terms of their timing/recurrence, severity, and progression. Identification of the timing of the early phase of insults remains challenging, because the approaches are limited for real-time monitoring of cerebral blood flow (CBF), central nervous system (CNS) tissue oxygenation, levels of CNS metabolites, and biomarkers of CNS injury. Such tools are vitally important to develop, because therapies are likely to have variable impact, depending on the timing of their implementation during the course of neonatal brain development. Human brain development is a moving target, which involves cellular activity-dependent events that coincide with multiple waves of neurogenesis, gliogenesis, glial and neuronal maturation, synaptogenesis, myelination, and the establishment of neural networks and connectivity. Hence, the timing of an insult to the developing brain, in a large measure, defines its potential impact on multiple key neurodevelopmental events that sculpt the complex neural substrates that define brain function in later life.

Definition of the severity of insults is an emerging challenge, which reflects the recent shift to milder forms of injury. Although magnetic resonance imaging (MRI) is the optimal imaging modality to define cerebral injury in preterm survivors,[40–43] the histopathologic features of MRI signal abnormalities have mostly been defined for WMI, in which more severe necrotic injury predominates.[44–49] More severe insults result in tissue destruction, which coincides with regional brain atrophy and signal abnormalities defined by MRI. More severe lesions also trigger glial barriers to regeneration and repair, which may, for example, impede the efficacy of neural stem cell therapy.[50] Despite the pronounced shift to milder forms of human cerebral injury, which have been defined by quantitative and diffusion-weighted MRI, the pathologic signatures of these MRI findings remain mostly undefined in the human infant. As discussed later, experimental studies have begun to bridge the gap between MRI-defined cerebral injury and the corresponding histopathologic features. Recent studies also support that the lack of tissue destruction or cell death also does not necessarily rule out the occurrence of a previous cerebral insult. As discussed later, we have recently identified that cerebral hypoxia-ischemia (H-I) can have a widespread impact on neuronal maturation in the absence of overt neuronal degeneration.

Lessening the impact of factors that modify injury progression represents an important direction to improve neurodevelopmental outcomes. It is increasingly appreciated that there are many genetic/epigenetic, systemic, or iatrogenic factors that adversely influence primary injury progression (eg, nutritional status, infection, endocrine status/ steroid exposure, peripheral organ dysfunction, and exposure to anesthetics, sedatives, or drugs of abuse) with potentially reversible or irreversible consequences. One recently identified factor associated with abnormal microstructural cortical growth in human preterm neonates is impaired somatic growth (weight, length, and head circumference), even after accounting for coexisting brain injuries on MRI and other aspects of systemic illness such as infection.[51] Procedural pain and stress have also been recently linked to altered brain maturation that involves gray and white matter structures, as well as impaired brain function.[52,53] Procedural pain in preterm neonates has also been associated with impaired postnatal growth,[54] a predictor of poor cortical development.[51]

In the remainder of this article, recent advances in our understanding of the role of H-I in the pathogenesis of preterm cerebral injury are reviewed, which begins to shed light on the mechanisms that underlie the shifting spectrum of cerebral injury in preterm survivors. The shift toward less severe injury seems to be related to changes in the timing, severity, and progression of H-I insults.

A MATURATION-DEPENDENT ROLE FOR H-I IN THE PATHOGENESIS OF CEREBRAL INJURY

Multiple lines of evidence support that cerebral ischemia is often the major factor that initiates cerebral injury in VLBW infants.[55–57] Given the limitations of human studies to directly link blood flow disturbances with injury, experimental studies in fetal sheep and other animal models have greatly strengthened our understanding of the contribution of cerebral H-I to gray matter injury and WMI. The timing of CBF disturbances during development is a critical factor that contributes to CNS susceptibility to H-I. For example, under conditions of prolonged global cerebral ischemia, acute injury to the cerebral cortex is low in the preterm fetal sheep, whereas severe panlaminar cortical necrosis occurs in the term animal.[58,59] In the near-term fetus, even brief severe global asphyxia, caused by a 10-minute occlusion of the umbilical cord, can result in prolonged hypoperfusion to cerebral gray and white matter.[60] Studies of global cerebral hypoperfusion found that the midgestation animal showed a predilection to periventricular and subcortical WMI, whereas the near-term animal showed predominantly parasagittal cortical neuronal injury.[58,59,61] In contrast to near-term animals with global cerebral hypoperfusion, near-term animals with severe umbilical cord occlusions showed more global cerebral injury. Systemic hypotension arising from intermittent or partial umbilical cord occlusion produced a variable degree of WMI in addition to primary damage to the cerebral cortex.[62-64]

The importance of cerebral ischemia is further supported by studies in which WMI was detected only infrequently in models of hypoxemia, in which a restriction in uteroplacental blood flow resulted in decreased oxygen delivery and mild acidemia to the fetus without systemic hypotension or cerebral hypoperfusion.[65-67] A model of fetal metabolic acidemia induced by maternal hypoxemia similarly produced mild to moderate injury in midgestation and near-term sheep.[68] By contrast, preterm ovine WMI was detected only after repeated systemic fetal endotoxin exposure, which triggered both transient hypoxemia and hypotension.[69,70] Hence, cerebral hypoperfusion in conjunction with hypoxia seems to be a critical factor to generate significant preterm WMI.

DO DISTURBANCES IN CEREBRAL AUTOREGULATION PLAY A ROLE IN THE PATHOGENESIS OF CEREBRAL INJURY FROM H-I?

A complex interplay of factors related to cerebrovascular immaturity predispose preterm cerebral white matter to injury from H-I. Central among these factors is a disturbance in cerebral autoregulation. Cerebral autoregulation refers to the maintenance of constant CBF over a range of changes in arterial blood pressure or cerebral perfusion pressure.[55,71,72] This autoregulatory range has both upper and lower limits; higher or lower than these limits, CBF does not remain constant but instead increases or decreases passively, along with changes in arterial blood pressure. Cerebral autoregulation has been reported in several species and across developmental stages. Although the mechanism remains elusive, it seems to involve an intrinsic property of arterial smooth muscle cells. Changes in transmural pressure modify muscle tone, by affecting the activation of potassium and calcium channels in smooth muscle cells, thereby affecting membrane potential.[73] Autoregulation is also mediated by a fine balance between endothelial cell–derived constricting and relaxing factors.[74] In adults, CBF remains constant over an autoregulatory range of mean blood pressures from 50 to 150 mm Hg.[72] In near-term fetal sheep, the range is lower and narrower (40–80 mm Hg), but normal blood pressure is no more than 5 to 10 mm Hg higher than the lower limit of the autoregulatory curve.[75] Preterm fetal lambs show even less autoregulatory capability.[76]

Impaired cerebral autoregulation in clinically unstable premature infants was initially studied by means of xenon clearance and Doppler and more recently by near infrared spectroscopy and spatially resolved spectroscopy.[55,77] Severe perinatal asphyxia, hypoxia, head trauma, and hypercapnic acidosis, even when mild, attenuate or even abolish autoregulation.[78-80] Nevertheless, considerable controversy remains regarding the role of pressure passivity in the pathogenesis of various forms of brain injury in the sick preterm neonate. This situation is shown, for example, by studies that failed to support a role for impaired autoregulation in the pathogenesis of intraventricular hemorrhage.[81,82] Hence, basic questions regarding cerebral autoregulation remain unanswered, including determining the optimal clinical practices for blood pressure regulation.[55]

DO VASCULAR END AND BORDER ZONES PLAY A ROLE IN THE PATHOGENESIS OF CEREBRAL INJURY FROM H-I?

Cerebral vascular development, particularly in the periventricular region, is clinically relevant, because of the propensity of the premature infant to both cerebral WMI and hemorrhage in the germinal matrix and ventricles.[83,84] The role of cerebral vascular immaturity in the pathogenesis of preterm WMI has been difficult to define in preterm infants. Analysis of the vascular supply to the periventricular white matter has yielded conflicting results. The periventricular white matter has 2 major blood supplies. Perforating arteries branch from leptomeningeal arteries, penetrate the cerebral cortex, and terminate as capillary beds adjacent to the ventricles. Branches of choroidal and striate arteries project toward the lateral ventricles and then deviate away from the ventricle toward their final termination in vascular capillary beds in the periventricular white matter. One early hypothesis proposed that these vascular beds collectively form vascular end zones and border zones, which render the periventricular white matter particularly susceptible to ischemia. However, the existence of these border zones remains controversial.[85–87] The presence of these vascular zones would provide a mechanism for WMI based on the notion that when periventricular white matter flow decreases lower than a critical threshold, this region would show greater susceptibility to WMI relative to a putatively better-perfused cerebral cortex.

To seek evidence for these vascular zones, we measured blood flow in histopathologically defined regions of injury in cerebral cortex and white matter in preterm fetal sheep.[88] Although white matter basal blood flows were lower than cerebral gray matter (**Fig. 1**A), there was no evidence for pathologically significant gradients of fetal blood flow within the periventricular white matter under conditions of global partial ischemia or reperfusion (see **Fig. 1**B, C). White matter lesions did not localize preferentially to regions susceptible to greater ischemia; nor did less vulnerable regions of cerebral white matter have greater flow during ischemia. An alternative explanation for the topography of cerebral white matter lesions is the distribution of susceptible cell types (see later discussion), particularly late oligodendrocyte progenitors (premyelinating oligodendrocytes [preOLs]), which are particularly susceptible to H-I.[59]

RELATIVE CONTRIBUTIONS OF H-I AND OLIGODENDROCYTE LINEAGE IMMATURITY TO WMI

The preterm fetal sheep (0.65 gestation) shows heterogeneous maturation of the oligodendrocyte (OL) lineage in periventricular white matter, which allowed us to define the relative contributions of OL maturation and vascular factors to acute WMI.[59] OL lineage maturation in medial cerebral white matter was similar to human (~23–28 weeks' gestation), in that preOLs were the major OL stage present. By contrast, lateral cerebral white matter was more differentiated and contained predominantly preOLs and early myelinating OLs. We found that moderate cerebral ischemia did not uniformly damage these adjacent regions of white matter. Rather, these adjacent regions sustained differing degrees of acute injury, even although they sustained a similar degree of low flow during prolonged ischemia-reperfusion. Hence, although global ischemia was necessary for WMI, no regional differences in blood flow were found within the white matter under basal or ischemic conditions to account for the differences in cell death between adjacent white matter regions. Rather, differences in the topography of WMI were closely correlated with the distribution of vulnerable preOLs. In regions of preOL degeneration, other neural cell types (astrocytes, microglia, and axons) were markedly more resistant to injury.[59,89,90]

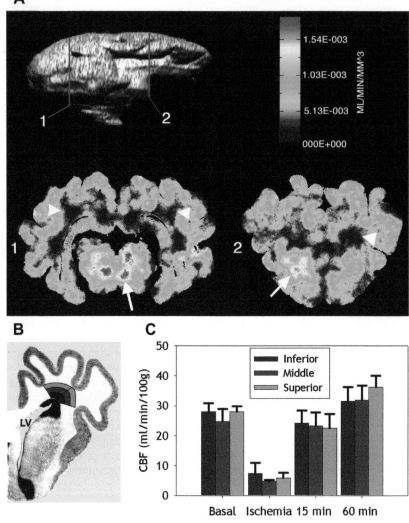

Fig. 1. Preterm fetal CBF does not show gradients of flow under basal or ischemia reperfusion conditions, which is consistent with vascular border zones or end zones. (*A*) Quantification of regional fetal CBF in vivo under conditions of basal flow. The top image in (*A*) represents a three-dimensional surface reconstruction of fluorescence images of a 0.65 gestation control ovine brain, which indicates the frontal and parietal levels to which the lower blood flow images correspond in (*1*) and (*2*). Representative pseudocolor scale basal flow images show higher blood flow (*arrows*) in the pons (*1*) and subcortical gray matter (*2*) and lower flow (*dark blue*) in the periventricular white matter (*arrowheads*). (*B*) The fetal cerebral white matter was segmented into medial and lateral sections, both of which were further segmented into inferior, middle, and superior regions. No differences were found between basal CBF values in medial and lateral white matter. (*C*) Basal CBF values (mean ± standard error of the mean) for the entire inferior, middle, and superior periventricular white matter. No differences in CBF were seen between superior and inferior regions of cerebral white matter, which supported a lack of gradients of CBF during basal or ischemia reperfusion conditions. (*Adapted from* Riddle A, Luo N, Manese M, et al. Spatial heterogeneity in oligodendrocyte lineage maturation and not cerebral blood flow predicts fetal ovine periventricular white matter injury. J Neurosci 2006;26:3045–55, with permission; and *From* McClure M, Riddle A, Manese M, et al. Cerebral blood flow heterogeneity in preterm sheep: lack of physiological support for vascular boundary zones in fetal cerebral white matter. J Cereb Blood Flow Metab 2008;28(5):995–1008, with permission.)

The timing of appearance of preOLs during white matter development also plays a major role in the severity of WMI. In a rabbit model of placental insufficiency, significant global fetal H-I caused minimal WMI at fetal day 22, but a similar insult 3 days later in gestation caused pronounced WMI.[91] The relative susceptibility of the white matter at these 2 developmental ages coincided with the timing of appearance of susceptible preOLs. Taken together, these findings suggest that perturbations in CBF are necessary but not sufficient for WMI. The developmental predilection for WMI seems to be related to both the timing of appearance and regional distribution of susceptible preOLs. These findings predict that some near-term infants with delayed OL differentiation and myelination might also be more susceptible to WMI. A variable degree of WMI was detected in near-term sheep after several insults.[61,62,64,67,68,92] Moreover, near-term and term infants with congenital heart disease are also at high risk for WMI.[93] Hence, the targeted death of preOLs from H-I could contribute to the pathogenesis of acute WMI across a broad range of gestational ages and regions of white matter.

Patterns of WMI in the immature brain thus result from selective vulnerability of pre-OLs, which are enriched in cerebral white matter during restricted windows in development.[94] The timing of appearance and spatial distribution of susceptible OL lineage cells coincides with the magnitude and distribution of acute ischemic injury in several experimental models of WMI. In particular, preOLs are highly susceptible to H-I and inflammation,[95] whereas earlier and later OL stages are markedly more resistant.[59,96,97] The enhanced susceptibility of preOLs is a cell intrinsic property, which is independent of the perinatal age of the animal or the location of these cells in the forebrain. The increasing developmental resistance of cerebral white matter to H-I is related to the onset of preOL differentiation to OLs, which show reduced susceptibility to H-I.[96]

THE CHANGING SPECTRUM OF HUMAN WMI

Cerebral WMI is the major form of brain injury recognized in survivors of premature birth.[98] The period of highest risk for WMI is ~23 to 32 weeks postconceptional age. Perinatal WMI, including periventricular leukomalacia (PVL), was the most common finding, seen in almost half (42.5%) of affected children.[99] MRI-defined WMI but not gray matter injury manifests in the first months of life as abnormal movements that are predictive of CP.[100–102]

The spectrum of white matter disease includes 3 major identifiable forms: focal cystic necrosis, focal microscopic necrosis, and diffuse nonnecrotic lesions. Cystic necrotic lesions are the most severe and have been widely appreciated since the classic descriptions of PVL by Banker and Larroche.[103–110] The cysts are typically larger than a millimeter in diameter and comprise degeneration of all cell types, including glia and axons.[90,111] In several series, focal cystic lesions were detected by MRI in less than 5% of cases.[112–117] Moreover, the overall burden of human necrotic WMI (cystic necrosis and microcysts), defined by pathology, was decreased by ~10-fold in contemporary cohorts relative to retrospective cases from earlier decades.[118]

Despite the pronounced reduction in cystic PVL, small foci of necrosis continue to be defined by neuropathologic examination of contemporary cases. These discrete foci of microscopic necrosis (microcysts) typically measure less than a millimeter.[119] Similar to cystic necrosis, microcysts evolve to lesions enriched in cellular debris, degenerating axons, and phagocytic macrophages.[118] In recent human autopsy cases from archival and contemporary cases,[118,119] microcysts were observed in at least 30% of cases. However, they comprised only ~1% to 5% of total lesion burden.[118] Hence, microscopic necrosis occurs with high incidence, but the burden often seems to be low.

Diffuse WMI is the characteristic pattern of brain injury most frequently observed in contemporary cohorts of premature newborns.[118] Recent human autopsy studies quantitatively analyzed the magnitude and distribution of diffuse WMI and found that these lesions are more extensive than previously appreciated from conventional neuropathologic approaches.[118] The hallmark of these lesions is a chronic diffuse reactive gliosis comprising activated astrocytes and microglia, which extend beyond foci of necrosis. Diffuse WMI targets the OL lineage with selective degeneration of pre-OLs, whereas axons are mostly spared, except in necrotic foci.[90,111] Human preOLs are particularly susceptible to oxidative damage,[120] which causes WMI with features consistent with H-I.[59,96]

CURRENT LIMITATIONS FOR NEUROIMAGING OF WMI

Although cranial ultrasonography is the preferred bedside imaging technique for diagnosing cystic necrotic WMI, it has limited sensitivity for diagnosing diffuse WMI.[112,115,116] MRI provides a noninvasive means for diagnosis of injury in the developing brain by conventional T1-weighted, T2-weighted, and diffusion-weighted images.[41,121] Nevertheless, there remains unexplained variability in the nature of lesions detected at different centers, which may reflect differences in clinical management, clinical acuity, or the modes of detection by MRI. On diagnostic MRI scans, WMI is indicated by discrete focal or more diffuse areas of magnetic resonance signal abnormalities. There are limitations to diagnostic MRI at regularly used clinical field strengths (eg, 1.5 or 3 T), which restrict its usefulness for diagnosis and prognosis. Chief among these limitations is the limited detection of microscopic necrosis. At a field strength of 3 T, MRI cannot resolve these lesions, which are typically a millimeter or less in diameter. The significance of microcysts, thus, remains an important but clinically inaccessible question. These lesions may be clinically silent or a significant contributor to motor disabilities, depending on the extent to which they localize to functionally important regions of white matter tracts. Microscopic necrosis may also contribute to the burden of cognitive dysfunction in preterm survivors, because gray matter injury was seen in association with microscopic necrosis, but not in cases in which diffuse WMI occurred in isolation.[119]

Microcysts can be visualized by MRI at ultrahigh magnetic field strength (12 T), as we recently showed in a global ischemia model of preterm WMI in fetal sheep (**Fig. 2**, upper panel).[89] This preparation generated a spectrum of WMI similar to that observed from human autopsy studies, as well as a reduction in cerebral white matter volume similar to that observed in preterm survivors.[41–43] We developed registration algorithms that defined the histopathologic features of 3 distinct forms of MRI-defined WMI (see **Fig. 2**).[89] Microcysts were not detected at 1 week after ischemia, but by 2 weeks, evolved to discrete lesions that were visualized by MRI at high field strength and confirmed by pathology.[89] Similar to the human autopsy studies discussed earlier,[118] microcysts were observed in 50% of animals and comprised only 1.5% of total lesion volume.[89,118] Hence, microscopic necrosis occurs with high incidence, but the amount of involved white matter seems to be low. The ability to resolve microcysts by MRI at clinical field strengths would be a significant advance to define the contribution of these lesions to neurodevelopmental disabilities in childhood survivors of prematurity.

Clinical MRI field strengths also may be a limiting factor to detect the full extent of diffuse WMI as the lesions become progressively more chronic. In particular, MRI may not fully define early diffuse lesions enriched in reactive astrocytes and microglia.[89] We recently analyzed diffuse WMI by ultrahigh-field MRI in our preterm fetal sheep model, in which animals survived for 1 or 2 weeks after global cerebral ischemia.

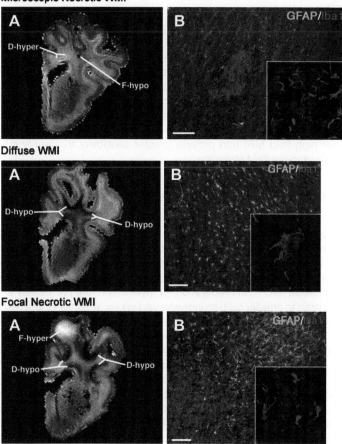

Fig. 2. Three forms of high-field MRI-defined perinatal WMI with corresponding histopathologic features that were generated in the 0.65 gestation fetal sheep brain at 1 or 2 weeks after global cerebral ischemia. (*Upper panel*) Microscopic necrotic WMI. (*A*) Representative appearance of a focal hypointense (*F-hypo*) lesion seen on a T2-weighted image at 2 weeks after injury. Note the substantial difference in the F-hypo lesion relative to a diffuse gliotic lesion at 2 weeks, which appears more hyperintense (*D-hyper*). (*B*) A typical microscopic necrotic lesion defined by a discrete focus of immunohistochemical staining for reactive microglia and macrophages with Iba1 (*red* and *inset*) and a paucity of staining for astrocytes with glial fibrillary acidic protein (*GFAP; green*). Nuclei in the inset are visualized with Hoechst 33,342 (*blue*). Bar in (*B*), 100 μm. (*Middle panel*) Diffuse WMI. (*A*) Representative appearance and distribution of diffuse hypointense (*D-hypo*) lesions seen on a T2-weighted image at 1 week after injury. (*B*) Diffuse WMI had pronounced astrogliosis defined by immunohistochemical staining of reactive astrocytes with glial fibrillary acidic protein (*GFAP; green*) and a lesser population of Iba1-labeled microglia/macrophages (*red*) with a reactive morphology (*inset*). Nuclei in the inset are visualized with Hoechst 33,342 (*blue*). Bar in (*B*), 100 μm. (*Lower panel*) Focal necrotic WMI. (*A*) Representative appearance from the largest focal hyperintense (*F-hyper*) lesion seen on a T2-weighted image at 1 week after injury. These lesions typically localized to subcortical white matter. Note the substantial difference in the F-hyper lesion relative to the diffuse gliotic lesions, which appears more hypointense (*D-hypo*). (*B*) A typical macroscopic necrotic lesion defined by diffuse dense staining for reactive microglia and macrophages with Iba1 (*red* and *inset*) and a paucity of GFAP-labeled astrocytes. Nuclei in the inset are visualized with Hoechst 33,342 (*blue*). Bar in (*B*), 100 μm. ([*Upper panel* (*A, B*)] *Adapted from* Riddle A, Dean J, Buser JR, et al. Histopathological correlates of magnetic resonance imaging-defined chronic perinatal white matter injury. Ann Neurol 2011;70(3):493–507; with permission.)

At 1 week after ischemia, high field MRI (12 T) identified a novel diffuse hypointense signal abnormality on T2-weighted images, with high sensitivity and specificity for lesions with astrogliosis (see **Fig. 2**, middle panel). These lesions showed MRI and histopathologic features that were distinctly different from the focal necrotic lesions typically seen in PVL (see **Fig. 2**, lower panel). These unexpected findings suggest that clinical MRI field strength may be a limiting factor to detect diffuse WMI, as well as microscopic necrosis. Additional clinical-pathologic studies are needed to determine whether high-field MRI can provide greater sensitivity to identify diffuse WMI than is feasible at lower field strengths.

DYSMATURATION OF GLIAL PROGENITORS IN CHRONIC WMI AND MYELINATION FAILURE

The propensity for myelination failure is a central feature of chronic diffuse WMI, the primary white matter lesion in preterm neonates.[118] The major cellular elements that contribute to myelination failure are the axon and the preOL. Recently, it was shown that axons also show maturation-dependent vulnerability to oxidative stress and H-I.[122] Larger caliber axons, in preparation for myelination, are particularly susceptible to injury, in contrast to smaller caliber unmyelinated axons, which are more resistant. The major sites of axonal degeneration are lesions that show cystic necrosis or microcysts, and premyelinating axons seem to be intact in diffuse WMI.[90] Hence, axonal degeneration does not seem to be a major component of diffuse WMI before active myelination.

Back and Volpe[123] initially proposed that myelination failure in chronic WMI arises from a persistent loss of preOLs, which are the precursors to myelinating OLs. Consistent with this hypothesis, preOLs were found to be markedly depleted in acute WMI in preterm human autopsy cases,[124] in perinatal rodents,[96] and fetal sheep.[59] In contrast to normal white matter (**Fig. 3**A), chronic WMI showed diffuse reactive astrogliosis and a striking loss of myelin (see **Fig. 3**B), which appeared consistent with the hypothesis that myelination failure resulted from preOL death. Although pronounced selective degeneration of preOLs occurs in acute WMI, a persistent loss of preOLs was not found in chronic lesions in a preterm-equivalent rat model of H-I.[97] This was the case even although pronounced preOL degeneration was observed for at least a week after H-I. This paradox was explained by the rapid onset of a glial proliferative response to acute WMI (see **Fig. 3**C). Within 24 hours after WMI, surviving preOLs rapidly increased in number to regenerate depleted preOLs.[97,125–127] This preOL expansion was driven mostly by early OL progenitors, which proliferated locally at the sites of WMI[97] or cortical injury[128] rather than from the subventricular zone, where less robust generation of OL lineage cells has been observed.[129–131]

Further analysis of the fate of the newly generated preOLs showed that they failed to mature to myelinating OLs within lesions enriched in reactive gliosis (astrocytes and microglia). Thus, regeneration of preOLs from the surviving preOL pool compensates for preOL death, but surviving preOLs show persistent arrested differentiation in chronic lesions (see **Fig. 3**C). More recently, arrested maturation of preOLs was also shown to contribute to myelination failure in diffuse WMI in both preterm fetal sheep and human.[89,118] In contrast to earlier studies,[132] a robust expansion of human preOLs was also recently defined in chronic lesions,[118] which was unexpected, given the significant loss of these cells during the acute phase of WMI.[120] Hence, chronic diffuse WMI is characterized by an aberrant response to acute injury, which involves a disrupted regeneration and repair process, in which preOLs are regenerated but they remain dysmature.

A role for arrested preOL maturation in chronic WMI is consistent with studies in adult animal models that have defined aberrant responses of the OL lineage in multiple

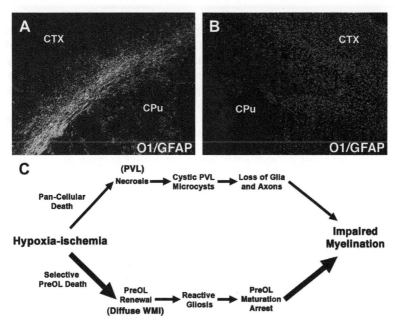

Fig. 3. Numerous late oligodendrocyte progenitors (preOLs) accumulate in chronic myelin-deficient perinatal white matter lesions. Lesions were generated in response to unilateral H-I in the postnatal day 3 (P3) rat, with the contralateral hemisphere serving as control.[97] (*A*) Normal early myelination (O1 antibody; *green*) in control subcortical white matter (corpus callosum/external capsule) at P10 is seen with low levels of GFAP-labeled astrocytes (*red*), mostly concentrated over the white matter. (*B*) Absence of myelin in the contralateral postischemic lesion coincided with a diffuse glial scar that stained for GFAP-labeled astrocytes. (*C*) Distinctly different pathogenetic mechanisms mediate impaired myelination in necrotic lesions (*PVL; upper pathway*) versus lesions with diffuse gliosis (diffuse WMI; *lower pathway*). H-I is shown as 1 potential trigger for WMI. More severe H-I triggers white matter necrosis (*upper pathway*) with pancellular degeneration, which depletes the white matter of glia and axons. Severe necrosis results in cystic PVL, whereas milder necrosis results in microcysts. Milder H-I (*lower pathway*) selectively triggers early preOL death. PreOLs are rapidly regenerated from a pool of early OL progenitors that are resistant to H-I. Chronic lesions are enriched in reactive glia (astrocytes and microglia/macrophages), which generate inhibitory signals that block preOL differentiation to mature myelinating OLs. Myelination failure in diffuse WMI thus results from preOL arrest rather than axonal degeneration. The molecular mechanisms that trigger preOL arrest are likely to be multifactorial and related to factors intrinsic and extrinsic to the preOLs. Note that the lower pathway is the dominant one in most contemporary preterm survivors, whereas the minor upper pathway reflects the declining burden of white matter necrosis, which has accompanied advances in neonatal intensive care.

sclerosis models of chronic demyelination. Myelination failure was also shown to involve a potentially reversible process linked to arrested preOL maturation. Reactive astrocyte-derived hyaluronic acid (HA), for example, accumulates in chronic WMI and reversibly inhibits preOL differentiation and myelination.[133] HA digestion by a CNS-enriched hyaluronidase, PH20, generates bioactive HA fragments that block OL differentiation in vitro and in vivo.[134,135] HA is also highly enriched in preterm diffuse WMI, as is its putative receptor, CD44,[118] which suggests a role for HA in blocking regeneration and repair of chronic WMI during development.

Although neuroimaging studies have defined impaired growth of central white matter pathways in preterm survivors, additional studies are needed to determine the temporal evolution and extent of impaired myelination in chronic lesions. It is critical to define the developmental window over which diffuse inflammation in the white matter generates inhibitory factors that sustain preOL arrest. Recent studies also support that viable OLs and myelination are critical for axon survival,[136] raising the possibility that preOL arrest could adversely affect the functional integrity of axons in chronic lesions. A wide variety of other inhibitory factors may also contribute to preOL arrest in chronic WMI.[137–140] Definition of these factors could also have important therapeutic relevance for a wide variety of other disorders of myelination failure in which preOL arrest is also implicated, including vascular dementias.[141]

CLINICAL IMPLICATIONS OF POTENTIAL ARRESTED WHITE MATTER DEVELOPMENT

As shown in **Fig. 3**C, the severity of an ischemic insult defines whether myelination failure arises primarily from necrotic WMI (upper pathway) or preOL maturation arrest (lower pathway). As discussed earlier, contemporary preterm survivors show less severe WMI, which coincides with preOL arrest. The potential for therapeutic interventions seems more promising for this form of injury than for WMI dominated by necrosis, in which essentially all cell types degenerate.

Chronic WMI thus coincides with an expanded developmental window over which preOL maturation arrest persists, which may enhance the risk for recurrent and potentially more severe brain injury in critically ill premature infants. As noted earlier, preOLs are selectively more vulnerable to H-I than are earlier or later stages of the OL lineage. The persistence of preOLs in chronic WMI suggests that these lesions would be more susceptible to recurrent H-I than more mature normal white matter that is enriched in OLs and myelin. In rat chronic lesions with preOL maturation arrest, the selective vulnerability of preOLs to acute H-I not only persisted but markedly increased.[97] A recurrent second episode of H-I triggered a massive selective degeneration of preOLs, which was more severe than that observed after the initial episode. Arrested preOLs showed a potentiated susceptibility to massive apoptotic degeneration, which rendered chronic white matter lesions susceptible to more severe injury. Taken together, these findings suggest that an initial insult, such as H-I or infection, may trigger WMI, which becomes progressively more severe with recurrent insults. Serial neuroimaging studies are thus needed to define the progression of WMI in preterm infants as well as term infants[40,142] who are at risk for recurrent insults. Such studies have identified clinical features that identify infants at risk for exacerbation of initial cerebral injury (eg, preterm newborns with postnatal sepsis). Recurrent and systemic illness is an important risk factor that may increase susceptibility to progressively more severe WMI.[143]

Future studies are needed in relevant experimental models and from human autopsy studies to define the evolution of cerebral white matter lesions over months to years. Such information is of critical importance to define the period over which the glial scar remodels in CP and to identify the responses of the cell types that persist during the process of myelination failure. These data also inform the therapeutic potential of strategies such as stem cell therapy[144,145] or therapies aimed at reversing preOL arrest to promote regeneration and repair of injured white matter in preterm survivors with CP or related neurologic disabilities.

AN EMERGING SPECTRUM OF GRAY MATTER INJURY AND NEURONAL DYSMATURATION

As proposed by Volpe[146] with the concept of an encephalopathy of prematurity, the cerebral gray matter of preterm survivors may involve both destructive and developmental disturbances.

Although several large human neuroimaging studies have identified significant reductions in the growth of cortical and subcortical gray matter structures, including the basal ganglia, thalamus, hippocampus, and cerebellum,[51,147–150] the relative contributions of destructive and developmental processes in contemporary preterm survivors are not yet clear. Significant neuronal loss has been reported in the human cortex, basal ganglia, thalamus, and cerebellum in association with necrotic WMI from archival autopsy cases.[119,151–153] In addition, subplate neurons, a transient cell population, required to establish thalamocortical connections, are vulnerable to perinatal H-I in rodents[154] and were found to be reduced in human autopsy cases, which were also diagnosed with necrotic WMI.[153]

However, neuroimaging studies of contemporary cohorts of preterm survivors support that premature newborns have more extensive gray matter abnormalities than injuries identified by signal abnormalities on conventional MRI. Moreover, children and adults born preterm with normal neurocognitive function express altered cortical activation and functional connectivity during language and visual processing.[155–159] Thalamocortical connections are also disrupted in preterm newborns with WMI, resulting in visual dysfunction.[160] Consistent with these structural studies, preterm newborns at term age also show reduced functional connectivity between the cortex and thalamus on functional connectivity MRI.[161] Altered functional connectivity in children and adolescents born preterm is now recognized as a critical risk factor for adverse neurocognitive outcomes.[156,157,162]

SUSCEPTIBILITY OF PRETERM CEREBRAL GRAY MATTER TO H-I

The susceptibility of the preterm gray matter to injury from H-I seems to be fundamentally different from that at term. Studies that used biomarkers of oxidative damage provide indirect support for preterm cerebral injury from H-I.[107,120] The magnitude of oxidative stress in preterm white matter was similar to that sustained by gray matter from H-I at term. Under these conditions of oxidative stress, we analyzed human autopsy cases with diffuse WMI and preOL degeneration and found that neither the preterm gray matter nor the white matter showed evidence of significant oxidative stress or cellular degeneration that involved neurons or axons.[120] The resistance of the preterm gray matter to neuronal degeneration from H-I is further shown by studies in preterm fetal sheep, in which the magnitude of global ischemia was similar in superficial cortex and deeper cerebral structures, including the caudate nucleus and periventricular white matter.[59,88] This similar degree of ischemia in gray and white matter resulted in diffuse WMI and significant preOL degeneration, but largely spared neurons in the gray and white matter.[59,88] Widespread neuronal degeneration was observed only under conditions of severe ischemia that caused severe white matter necrosis.[59] Significant neuronal loss was seen in the human cortex, basal ganglia, thalamus, and cerebellum in association with necrotic WMI,[119,151–153] but not in cases in which diffuse WMI occurred without significant necrosis.[119] Neuronal loss seems to principally arise from retrograde axonal degeneration in necrotic white matter lesions.[90,111] In the preterm gray matter, significant loss of neurons thus seems to be related to more severe ischemia, which causes destructive lesions.

IMPAIRED CEREBRAL GROWTH FROM PRETERM CEREBRAL H-I CAN OCCUR WITHOUT NEURONAL LOSS

H-I to the preterm brain also causes disturbances in growth of gray matter structures. This reduced growth of the cerebral cortex and the basal ganglia can also occur in response to conditions that disrupt neuronal maturation without neuronal or axonal loss. In response to cerebral ischemia, preterm fetal sheep acquired diffuse WMI, as well as a progressive reduction in cortical growth, which was not explained by neuronal loss.[163] The basis for this unexpected result was explained by detailed analysis of the maturation of the dendritic arbor of pyramidal neurons, the major population of cortical projections neurons. During normal development, pyramidal neurons are highly immature in the preterm cerebral cortex (**Fig. 4**A) but in near-term animals, the dendritic arbor becomes more complex (see **Fig. 4**B), which coincides with a marked increase in cortical volume and measures of neuronal arbor complexity (see **Fig. 4**C). In response to preterm ischemia, cortical growth impairment was accompanied by a significant reduction in the complexity of the dendritic arbor; consistent with

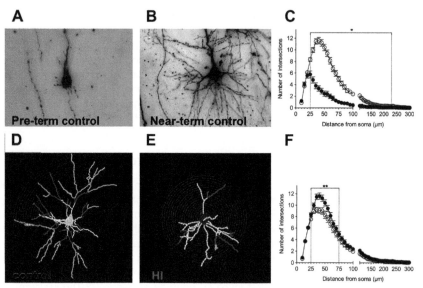

Fig. 4. The preterm brain is enriched in immature neurons that do not degenerate in response to ischemia, but are highly susceptible to impaired maturation that manifests as a less mature dendritic arbor with reduced spine density, as recently reported.[163] (*A*) A typical pyramidal neuron from the preterm cerebral cortex of a control fetal sheep. Note the paucity of processes in contrast to the highly complex dendritic arbor of a pyramidal neuron from a near-term animal (*B*). (*C*) A Sholl analysis compares the complexity of the dendritic arbor for a population of immature neurons at 0.65 gestation (*solid circles*) relative to near term animals (*open circles*) at ~0.85 gestation. Note the markedly greater complexity of the neurons from the near term animals, as indicated by a significantly higher number of intersections with the Sholl rings (*$P<.05$). (*D, E*) In response to preterm ischemia, cortical pyramidal neurons display disrupted maturation. Note that the typical control cell (*D*) is more highly arborized in contrast to the response to transient cerebral ischemia that resulted in a more simplified dendritic arbor (*E*). The relative complexity of the cells can be appreciated from the overlay of the red concentric Scholl rings, which illustrates that the processes of the dysmature neurons intersect less frequently with the rings. The yellow, white, pink, green and blue lines represent first-, second-, third-, fourth- and fifth-order branches, respectively, from the soma. Note the overall reduction in the size and complexity of the branching pattern in *E*. (*F*) A Sholl analysis compares the complexity of the dendritic arbor for a population of control neurons (*solid circles*) relative to neurons from animals that survived for 4 weeks after an ischemic insult at 0.65 gestation (*open circles*). Note the reduced complexity of the neurons from the ischemic animals, as indicated by a significantly higher number of intersections with the Sholl rings (*$P<.01$).

the notion that neuronal maturation was disrupted in the setting of cerebral ischemia. Compared with controls (see **Fig. 4**D), the ischemic animals showed neuronal dysmaturation (see **Fig. 4**E), which was reflected in a reduction in the total dendritic length as well as the number of branches, branch endings, and branch points. The dendritic arbor was most simplified closer to the cell body, where synaptic integration occurs (see **Fig. 4**F).

A role for neuronal dysmaturation in cognitive and behavioral disturbances in preterm survivors is suggested by analysis of dendritic spines,[163] the key sites for synaptic activity. We have observed reduced numbers of spines on the dysmature dendrites of projection neurons in both the cortex and caudate, which suggests that widespread disturbances in neuronal connectivity may contribute to the global disturbances in neurodevelopment seen in preterm survivors. Because disturbances in neuronal maturation occur at a critical window in the establishment of neuronal connections, even transient neuronal dysmaturation may have persistent global effects on the subsequent development of CNS circuitry.

Consistent with this notion, 2 recent studies found that the normal progressive loss of cortical fractional anisotropy (FA) was delayed in human preterm survivors with impaired postnatal growth[51] and with reduced cortical growth.[164] We made similar observations in preterm fetal sheep exposed in utero to global cerebral ischemia. Cortical FA was significantly higher in the ischemic animals relative to controls. To explain this observation, we developed a mathematical model to calculate FA based on the morphology of control and ischemic neurons and found that the FA values derived from MRI and neuronal morphology were similar.[163] Hence, despite a lack of overt gray matter injury, the cortex showed a delayed loss of cortical FA, which was related to widespread immaturity of the dendritic arbor of cortical projection neurons. One factor associated with abnormal microstructural cortical growth in human preterm neonates was impaired somatic growth (weight, length, and head circumference), even after accounting for coexisting brain injuries on MRI (eg, WMI) and other aspects of systemic illness (eg, infection).[51] Hence, multiple factors, including nutritional status and exposure to cerebral ischemia, may contribute to the pathogenesis of neuronal dysmaturation in preterm survivors.

SUMMARY

Our understanding of the pathogenesis of brain injury in the premature infant has recently undergone significant redefinition, which coincides with advances in neonatal care that have markedly reduced the overall severity and extent of the destructive processes associated with cerebral injury. Significant improvement in the care of premature neonates has also coincided with the emergence and application of improved brain imaging, which has provided better resolution of some of the key features of cerebral injury during the period of most rapid changes in brain growth and maturation. Nevertheless, further progress is needed to resolve important features of early and progressive WMI by MRI, particularly microscopic necrosis and diffuse WMI. Despite continued progress with many potentially promising therapies for the term neonate with H-I,[38,50] the development of a comparable therapeutic armamentarium for the preterm neonate has been limited by the greater fragility of these infants and the need for improved tools to identify the timing, distribution, severity, and evolution of preterm cerebral lesions in both white and gray matter.

Despite the reduced severity of brain injury for many babies, a lack of overt tissue destruction does not exclude a lack of insults to the developing brain. Subinjurious insults have been understudied, because the approaches required to identify cellular dysmaturation processes are laborious and time-consuming. Disruption in glial and neuronal maturation may have adverse consequences on multiple aspects of cerebral development, given that the timing of dysmaturation coincides with the period of most rapid brain growth and enhanced neuronal connectivity related to elaboration of the dendritic arbor and synaptogenesis, as well as myelination. The fact that preterm survivors commonly show disability in multiple neurodevelopmental domains suggests that widespread disturbances in neuronal dysmaturation may be involved. Thus a critical next step is to identify the disrupted neuronal networks that contribute to the widespread neurobehavioral impairments that commonly persist throughout life in preterm survivors.

These new findings raise the possibility that those chronic disabilities that arise primarily from diffuse cerebral dysmaturation may be amenable to strategies directed at promoting brain maturation and improved neurologic outcome. The activation of dysmaturation processes seems to coincide with disrupted regeneration and repair processes. Glial progenitors respond to WMI by partially but incompletely mounting a repair process that regenerates and expands the preOL pool, which is blocked from maturation. Similarly, some populations of immature projection neurons fail to normally mature. In contrast to mature neurons in the full-term neonate, which degenerate from H-I,[165] these immature neurons survive with a simplified dendritic arbor, which contributes to reduced cerebral growth.

The timing and nature of future interventions to prevent or reverse cellular dysmaturation may differ for gray and white matter. Factors such as improving infant nutrition, preventing infections, reducing neonatal stress, and implementing earlier behavioral interventions may all play a role in mitigating the impact of neuronal dysmaturation. Pharmacologic interventions aimed at blocking the inhibitory pathways that sustain preOL maturation arrest may reverse or prevent myelination failure with the potential for enhanced connectivity of CNS pathways. There is thus a wealth of potential new opportunities to promote enhanced brain maturation and growth, which were not feasible even a decade ago.

ACKNOWLEDGMENTS

We are grateful to Dr Steven Miller and Dr Evelyn McClendon for their many helpful suggestions in the preparation of the article.

REFERENCES

1. Synnes AR, Anson S, Arkesteijn A, et al. School entry age outcomes for infants with birth weight ≤ 800 grams. J Pediatr 2010;157(6):989–94.
2. Wilson-Costello D, Fridedman H, Minich N, et al. Improved survival rates with increased neurodevelopmental disability for extremely low birth weight infants in the 1990s. Pediatrics 2005;115(4):997–1003.
3. Available at: http://www.marchofdimes.com/mission/prematurity-campaign.aspx. Accessed December 19, 2013.
4. Stoll BJ, Hansen NI, Adams-Chapman I, et al. Neurodevelopmental and growth impairment among extremely low-birth-weight infants with neonatal infection. JAMA 2004;292(19):2357–65.
5. Peterson BS, Vohr B, Staib LH, et al. Regional brain volume abnormalities and long-term cognitive outcome in preterm infants. JAMA 2000;284(15):1939–47.
6. Kesler SR, Reiss AL, Vohr B, et al. Brain volume reductions within multiple cognitive systems in male preterm children at age twelve. J Pediatr 2008;152(4):513–20, 520.e1.

7. Soria-Pastor S, Padilla N, Zubiaurre-Elorza L, et al. Decreased regional brain volume and cognitive impairment in preterm children at low risk. Pediatrics 2009;124(6):e1161–70.
8. Aarnoudse-Moens CS, Weisglas-Kuperus N, van Goudoever JB, et al. Meta-analysis of neurobehavioral outcomes in very preterm and/or very low birth weight children. Pediatrics 2009;124(2):717–28.
9. Delobel-Ayoub M, Arnaud C, White-Koning M, et al. Behavioral problems and cognitive performance at 5 years of age after very preterm birth: the EPIPAGE Study. Pediatrics 2009;123(6):1485–92.
10. Anderson PJ, Doyle LW. Cognitive and educational deficits in children born extremely preterm. Semin Perinatol 2008;32(1):51–8.
11. Loeliger M, Inder T, Cain S, et al. Cerebral outcomes in a preterm baboon model of early versus delayed nasal continuous positive airway pressure. Pediatrics 2006;118(4):1640–53.
12. Scafidi J, Fagel DM, Ment LR, et al. Modeling premature brain injury and recovery. Int J Dev Neurosci 2009;27(8):863–71.
13. Hack M, Taylor H, Drotar D, et al. Chronic conditions, functional limitations, and special health care needs of school-aged children born with extremely low-birth-weight in the 1990's. JAMA 2005;294(3):318–25.
14. Miller SP, Ferriero DM, Leonard C, et al. Early brain injury in premature newborns detected with magnetic resonance imaging is associated with adverse early neurodevelopmental outcome. J Pediatr 2005;147(5):609–16.
15. Beaino G, Khoshnood B, Kaminski M, et al. Predictors of cerebral palsy in very preterm infants: the EPIPAGE prospective population-based cohort study. Dev Med Child Neurol 2010;52(6):e119–25.
16. Mercier CE, Dunn MS, Ferrelli KR, et al. Neurodevelopmental outcome of extremely low birth weight infants from the Vermont Oxford network: 1998-2003. Neonatology 2010;97(4):329–38.
17. Liu J, Li J, Qin GL, et al. Periventricular leukomalacia in premature infants in mainland China. Am J Perinatol 2008;25(9):535–40.
18. Vohr BR, Allan WC, Westerveld M, et al. School-age outcomes of very low birth weight infants in the indomethacin intraventricular hemorrhage prevention trial. Pediatrics 2003;111(4 Pt 1):e340–6.
19. Marlow N, Wolke D, Bracewell MA, et al. Neurologic and developmental disability at six years of age after extremely preterm birth. N Engl J Med 2005;352(1):9–19.
20. Bodeau-Livinec F, Marlow N, Ancel PY, et al. Impact of intensive care practices on short-term and long-term outcomes for extremely preterm infants: comparison between the British Isles and France. Pediatrics 2008;122(5):e1014–21.
21. Roberts G, Anderson PJ, Doyle LW. Neurosensory disabilities at school age in geographic cohorts of extremely low birth weight children born between the 1970s and the 1990s. J Pediatr 2009;154(6):829–34.e1.
22. Walsh MC, Hibbs AM, Martin CR, et al. Two-year neurodevelopmental outcomes of ventilated preterm infants treated with inhaled nitric oxide. J Pediatr 2010; 156(4):556–61.e1.
23. Roberts G, Anderson PJ, Doyle LW. The stability of the diagnosis of developmental disability between ages 2 and 8 in a geographic cohort of very preterm children born in 1997. Arch Dis Child 2010;95(10):786–90.
24. Grunau RE, Whitfield MF, Fay TB. Psychosocial and academic characteristics of extremely low birth weight (< or =800 g) adolescents who are free of major

impairment compared with term-born control subjects. Pediatrics 2004;114(6): e725–32.

25. Hack M, Flannery DJ, Schluchter M, et al. Outcomes in young adulthood for very-low-birth-weight infants. N Engl J Med 2002;346(3):149–57.

26. Lindstrom K, Winbladh B, Haglund B, et al. Preterm infants as young adults: a Swedish national cohort study. Pediatrics 2007;120(1):70–7.

27. Saigal S, den Ouden L, Wolke D, et al. School-age outcomes in children who were extremely low birth weight from four international population-based cohorts. Pediatrics 2003;112(4):943–50.

28. Litt J, Taylor H, Klein N, et al. Learning disabilities in children with very low birthweight: prevalence, neuropsychological correlates and educational interventions. J Learn Disabil 2005;8(2):130–41.

29. Jacobson LK, Dutton GN. Periventricular leukomalacia: an important cause of visual and ocular motility dysfunction in children. Surv Ophthalmol 2000;45(1):1–13.

30. Glass HC, Fujimoto S, Ceppi-Cozzio C, et al. White-matter injury is associated with impaired gaze in premature infants. Pediatr Neurol 2008;38(1):10–5.

31. Soria-Pastor S, Gimenez M, Narberhaus A, et al. Patterns of cerebral white matter damage and cognitive impairment in adolescents born very preterm. Int J Dev Neurosci 2008;26(7):647–54.

32. Anderson PJ, De Luca CR, Hutchinson E, et al. Attention problems in a representative sample of extremely preterm/extremely low birth weight children. Dev Neuropsychol 2011;36(1):57–73.

33. Marlow N, Rose AS, Rands CE, et al. Neuropsychological and educational problems at school age associated with neonatal encephalopathy. Arch Dis Child Fetal Neonatal Ed 2005;90(5):F380–7.

34. Nosarti C, Giouroukou E, Micali N, et al. Impaired executive functioning in young adults born very preterm. J Int Neuropsychol Soc 2007;13(4):571–81.

35. Taylor HG, Minich NM, Klein N, et al. Longitudinal outcomes of very low birth weight: neuropsychological findings. J Int Neuropsychol Soc 2004;10(2):149–63.

36. Curtis WJ, Lindeke LL, Georgieff MK, et al. Neurobehavioural functioning in neonatal intensive care unit graduates in late childhood and early adolescence. Brain 2002;125(Pt 7):1646–59.

37. Saavalainen P, Luoma L, Bowler D, et al. Spatial span in very prematurely born adolescents. Dev Neuropsychol 2007;32(3):769–85.

38. Robertson NJ, Tan S, Groenendaal F, et al. Which neuroprotective agents are ready for bench to bedside translation in the newborn infant? J Pediatr 2012; 160(4):544–52.e4.

39. Sherman L, Back S. A GAG reflex prevents repair of the damaged CNS. Trends Neurosci 2008;31(1):44–52.

40. Miller SP, Ferriero DM. From selective vulnerability to connectivity: insights from newborn brain imaging. Trends Neurosci 2009;32(9):496–505.

41. Ment LR, Hirtz D, Huppi PS. Imaging biomarkers of outcome in the developing preterm brain. Lancet Neurol 2009;8(11):1042–55.

42. Mathur AM, Neil JJ, Inder TE. Understanding brain injury and neurodevelopmental disabilities in the preterm infant: the evolving role of advanced magnetic resonance imaging. Semin Perinatol 2010;34(1):57–66.

43. Rutherford MA, Supramaniam V, Ederies A, et al. Magnetic resonance imaging of white matter diseases of prematurity. Neuroradiology 2010;52(6):505–21.

44. Hope PL, Gould SJ, Howard S, et al. Precision of ultrasound diagnosis of pathologically verified lesions in the brains of very preterm infants. Dev Med Child Neurol 1988;30(4):457–71.

45. Schouman-Claeys E, Henry-Feugeas MC, Roset F, et al. Periventricular leuko-malacia: correlation between MR imaging and autopsy findings during the first 2 months of life. Radiology 1993;189(1):59–64.

46. Felderhoff-Mueser U, Rutherford MA, Squier WV, et al. Relationship between MR imaging and histopathologic findings of the brain in extremely sick preterm infants. AJNR Am J Neuroradiol 1999;20(7):1349–57.

47. Inder TE, Neil JJ, Kroenke CD, et al. Investigation of cerebral development and injury in the prematurely born primate by magnetic resonance imaging and histopathology. Dev Neurosci 2005;27:100–11.

48. Childs AM, Cornette L, Ramenghi LA, et al. Magnetic resonance and cranial ultrasound characteristics of periventricular white matter abnormalities in newborn infants. Clin Radiol 2001;56(8):647–55.

49. Lodygensky G, West T, Moravec M, et al. Diffusion characteristics associated with neuronal injury and glial activation following hypoxia-ischemia in the immature brain. Magn Reson Med 2011;66(3):839–45.

50. Bennet L, Tan S, Van den Heuij L, et al. Cell therapy for neonatal hypoxia-ischemia and cerebral palsy. Ann Neurol 2012;71(5):589–600.

51. Vinall J, Grunau RE, Brant R, et al. Slower postnatal growth is associated with delayed cerebral cortical maturation in preterm newborns. Sci Transl Med 2013;5(168):168ra8.

52. Brummelte S, Grunau RE, Chau V, et al. Procedural pain and brain development in premature newborns. Ann Neurol 2012;71(3):385–96.

53. Smith GC, Gutovich J, Smyser C, et al. Neonatal intensive care unit stress is associated with brain development in preterm infants. Ann Neurol 2011;70(4):541–9.

54. Vinall J, Miller SP, Chau V, et al. Neonatal pain in relation to postnatal growth in infants born very preterm. Pain 2012;153(7):1374–81.

55. Greisen G. To autoregulate or not to autoregulate–that is no longer the question. Semin Pediatr Neurol 2009;16:207–15.

56. Tsuji M, Saul J, du Plessis A, et al. Cerebral intravascular oxygenation correlates with mean arterial pressure in critically ill premature infants. Pediatrics 2000;106(4):625–32.

57. Volpe JJ. Neurology of the newborn. Philadelphia: WB Saunders; 2008.

58. Reddy K, Mallard C, Guan J, et al. Maturational change in the cortical response to hypoperfusion injury in the fetal sheep. Pediatr Res 1998;43:674–82.

59. Riddle A, Luo N, Manese M, et al. Spatial heterogeneity in oligodendrocyte lineage maturation and not cerebral blood flow predicts fetal ovine periventricular white matter injury. J Neurosci 2006;26:3045–55.

60. Yan EB, Baburamani AA, Walker AM, et al. Changes in cerebral blood flow, cerebral metabolites, and breathing movements in the sheep fetus following asphyxia produced by occlusion of the umbilical cord. Am J Physiol Regul Integr Comp Physiol 2009;297(1):R60–9.

61. Raad RA, Tan WK, Bennet L, et al. Role of the cerebrovascular and metabolic responses in the delayed phases of injury after transient cerebral ischemia in fetal sheep. Stroke 1999;30(12):2735–41.

62. Clapp J III, Peress N, Wesley M, et al. Brain damage after intermittent partial cord occlusion in the chronically instrumented fetal lamb. Am J Obstet Gynecol 1988;159:504–9.

63. Ikeda T, Murata Y, Quilligan E, et al. Physiologic and histologic changes in near-term fetal lambs exposed to asphyxia by partial umbilical cord occlusion. Am J Obstet Gynecol 1998;178:24–32.

64. Ohyu J, Marumo G, Ozawa H, et al. Early axonal and glial pathology in fetal sheep brains with leukomalacia induced by repeated umbilical cord occlusion. Brain Dev 1999;21(4):248–52.

65. Rees S, Stringer M, Just Y, et al. The vulnerability of the fetal sheep brain to hypoxemia at mid-gestation. Brain Res Dev Brain Res 1997;103:103–18.

66. Rees S, Breen S, Loeliger M, et al. Hypoxemia near mid-gestation has long-term effects on fetal brain development. J Neuropathol Exp Neurol 1999;58(9):932–45.

67. Mallard E, Rees S, Stringer M, et al. Effects of chronic placental insufficiency on brain development in fetal sheep. Pediatr Res 1998;43(2):262–70.

68. Penning D, Grafe J, Hammond R, et al. Neuropathology of the near-term and midgestation ovine fetal brain after sustained in utero hypoxemia. Am J Obstet Gynecol 1994;170:1425–32.

69. Duncan J, Cock M, Scheerlinck J, et al. White matter injury after repeated endotoxin exposure in the preterm ovine fetus. Pediatr Res 2002;52(6):941–9.

70. Dalitz P, Harding R, Rees S, et al. Prolonged reductions in placental blood flow and cerebral oxygen delivery in preterm fetal sheep exposed to endotoxin: possible factors in white matter injury after acute infection. J Soc Gynecol Investig 2003;10(5):283–90.

71. Lassen N, Christensen M. Physiology of cerebral blood flow. Br J Anaesth 1976; 48:719–34.

72. Paulson O, Strandgaard S, Edvinsson L. Cerebral autoregulation. Cerebrovasc Brain Metab Rev 1990;2(2):161–92.

73. Greisen G. Autoregulation of cerebral blood flow in newborn babies. Early Hum Dev 2005;81:423–8.

74. Iadecola C, Nedergaard M. Glial regulation of the cerebral microvasculature. Nat Neurosci 2007;10:1369–76.

75. Papile L, Rudolph AM, Heymann M. Autoregulation of cerebral blood flow in the preterm fetal lamb. Pediatr Res 1985;19:159–61.

76. Helou S, Koehler RC, Gleason CA, et al. Cerebrovascular autoregulation during fetal development in sheep. Am J Physiol 1994;266(3):H1069–74.

77. du Plessis A. Cerebrovascular injury in premature infants: current understanding and challenges for future prevention. Clin Perinatol 2008;35:609–41.

78. Tweed A, Cote J, Lou H, et al. Impairment of cerebral blood flow autoregulation in the newborn lamb by hypoxia. Pediatr Res 1986;20:516.

79. Busija D, Heistad D. Factors involved in the physiological regulation of the cerebral circulation. Rev Physiol Biochem Pharmacol 1984;101:161.

80. Jones MD Jr, Sheldon RE, Peeters LL, et al. Regulation of cerebral blood flow in the ovine fetus. Am J Physiol 1978;235:H162–6.

81. Soul J, Hammer P, Tsuji M, et al. Fluctuating pressure-passivity is common in the cerebral circulation of sick premature infants. Pediatr Res 2007;61(4):467–73.

82. Wong F, Leung T, Austin T, et al. Impaired autoregulation in preterm infants identified by using spatially resolved spectroscopy. Pediatrics 2008;121(3):e604–11.

83. Takashima S, Tanaka K. Development of cerebrovascular architecture and its relationship to periventricular leukomalacia. Arch Neurol 1978;35:11–6.

84. Ballabh P. Intraventricular hemorrhage in premature infants: mechanism of disease. Pediatr Res 2010;67(1):1–8.

85. Nelson MD Jr, Gonzalez-Gomez I, Gilles FH. Dyke Award. The search for human telencephalic ventriculofugal arteries. AJNR Am J Neuroradiol 1991;12(2): 215–22.

86. Mayer PL, Kier EL. The controversy of the periventricular white matter circulation: a review of the anatomic literature. AJNR Am J Neuroradiol 1991;12(2):223–8.

87. Volpe JJ. The structure of blood vessels in the germinal matrix and the autoregulation of cerebral blood flow in premature infants [reply]. Pediatrics 2001; 108(4):1050.

88. McClure M, Riddle A, Manese M, et al. Cerebral blood flow heterogeneity in preterm sheep: lack of physiological support for vascular boundary zones in fetal cerebral white matter. J Cereb Blood Flow Metab 2008;28(5):995–1008.

89. Riddle A, Dean J, Buser JR, et al. Histopathological correlates of magnetic resonance imaging-defined chronic perinatal white matter injury. Ann Neurol 2011; 70(3):493–507.

90. Riddle A, Maire J, Gong X, et al. Differential susceptibility to axonopathy in necrotic and non-necrotic perinatal white matter injury. Stroke 2012;43(1):178–84.

91. Buser J, Segovia K, Dean J, et al. Timing of appearance of late oligodendrocyte progenitors coincides with enhanced susceptibility of preterm rabbit cerebral white matter to hypoxia-ischemia. J Cereb Blood Flow Metab 2010;30(5):1053–65.

92. Ikeda T, Choi BH, Yee S, et al. Oxidative stress, brain white matter damage and intrauterine asphyxia in fetal lambs. Int J Dev Neurosci 1999;17(1):1–14.

93. McQuillen P, Miller S. Congenital heart disease and brain development. Ann N Y Acad Sci 2010;1184:68–86.

94. Back SA, Luo NL, Borenstein NS, et al. Late oligodendrocyte progenitors coincide with the developmental window of vulnerability for human perinatal white matter injury. J Neurosci 2001;21(4):1302–12.

95. Favrais G, van de Looij Y, Fleiss B, et al. Systemic inflammation disrupts the developmental program of white matter. Ann Neurol 2011;70(4):550–65.

96. Back SA, Han BH, Luo NL, et al. Selective vulnerability of late oligodendrocyte progenitors to hypoxia-ischemia. J Neurosci 2002;22(2):455–63.

97. Segovia K, McClure M, Moravec M, et al. Arrested oligodendrocyte lineage maturation in chronic perinatal white matter injury. Ann Neurol 2008;63(4): 517–26.

98. Volpe JJ. Brain injury in premature infants: a complex amalgam of destructive and developmental disturbances. Lancet Neurol 2009;8(1):110–24.

99. Bax M, Tydeman C, Flodmark O. Clinical and MRI correlates of cerebral palsy: the European Cerebral Palsy Study. JAMA 2006;296(13):1602–8.

100. Constantinou JC, Adamson-Macedo EN, Mirmiran M, et al. Movement, imaging and neurobehavioral assessment as predictors of cerebral palsy in preterm infants. J Perinatol 2007;27(4):225–9.

101. Spittle AJ, Brown NC, Doyle LW, et al. Quality of general movements is related to white matter pathology in very preterm infants. Pediatrics 2008;121(5):e1184–9.

102. Spittle AJ, Boyd RN, Inder TE, et al. Predicting motor development in very preterm infants at 12 months' corrected age: the role of qualitative magnetic resonance imaging and general movements assessments. Pediatrics 2009;123(2): 512–7.

103. Banker B, Larroche J. Periventricular leukomalacia of infancy. A form of neonatal anoxic encephalopathy. Arch Neurol 1962;7:386–410.

104. DeReuck J, Chattha A, Richardson E. Pathogenesis and evolution of periventricular leukomalacia in infancy. Arch Neurol 1972;27:229–36.

105. Rorke LB. Pathology of perinatal brain injury. New York: Raven Press; 1982.

106. Leviton A, Gilles F. Acquired perinatal leukoencephalopathy. Ann Neurol 1984; 16:1–10.

107. Haynes RL, Folkerth RD, Keefe RJ, et al. Nitrosative and oxidative injury to premyelinating oligodendrocytes in periventricular leukomalacia. J Neuropathol Exp Neurol 2003;62(5):441–50.

108. Iida K, Takashima S, Ueda K. Immunohistochemical study of myelination and oligodendrocyte in infants with periventricular leukomalacia. Pediatr Neurol 1995;13:296–304.
109. Robinson S, Li Q, Dechant A, et al. Neonatal loss of gamma-aminobutyric acid pathway expression after human perinatal brain injury. J Neurosurg 2006; 104(Suppl 6):396–408.
110. Verney C, Monier A, Fallet-Bianco C, et al. Early microglial colonization of the human forebrain and possible involvement in periventricular white-matter injury of preterm infants. J Anat 2010;217(4):436–48.
111. Haynes RL, Billiards SS, Borenstein NS, et al. Diffuse axonal injury in periventricular leukomalacia as determined by apoptotic marker fractin. Pediatr Res 2008; 63(6):656–61.
112. Maalouf E, Duggan P, Counsell SJ, et al. Comparison of findings on cranial ultrasound and magnetic resonance imaging in preterm infants. Pediatrics 2001;107:719–27.
113. Hamrick S, Miller SP, Leonard C, et al. Trends in severe brain injury and neurodevelopmental outcome in premature newborn infants: the role of cystic periventricular leukomalacia. J Pediatr 2004;145(5):593–9.
114. Counsell S, Allsop J, Harrison M, et al. Diffusion-weighted imaging of the brain in preterm infants with focal and diffuse white matter abnormality. Pediatrics 2003; 112(1):176–80.
115. Inder TE, Anderson NJ, Spencer C, et al. White matter injury in the premature infant: a comparison between serial cranial sonographic and MR findings at term. AJNR Am J Neuroradiol 2003;24(5):805–9.
116. Miller SP, Cozzio CC, Goldstein RB, et al. Comparing the diagnosis of white matter injury in premature newborns with serial MR imaging and transfontanel ultrasonography findings. AJNR Am J Neuroradiol 2003;24:1661–9.
117. Groenendaal F, Termote JU, van der Heide-Jalving M, et al. Complications affecting preterm neonates from 1991 to 2006: what have we gained? Acta Paediatr 2010;99(3):354–8.
118. Buser J, Maire J, Riddle A, et al. Arrested pre-oligodendrocyte maturation contributes to myelination failure in premature infants. Ann Neurol 2012;71(1):93–109.
119. Pierson CR, Folkerth RD, Billiards SS, et al. Gray matter injury associated with periventricular leukomalacia in the premature infant. Acta Neuropathol 2007; 114(6):619–31.
120. Back SA, Luo NL, Mallinson RA, et al. Selective vulnerability of preterm white matter to oxidative damage defined by F2-isoprostanes. Ann Neurol 2005; 58(1):108–20.
121. Ment LR, Bada HS, Barnes P, et al. Practice parameter: neuroimaging of the neonate: report of the Quality Standards Subcommittee of the American Academy of Neurology and the Practice Committee of the Child Neurology Society. Neurology 2002;58(12):1726–38.
122. Alix JJ, Zammit C, Riddle A, et al. Central axons preparing to myelinate are highly sensitivity to ischemic injury. Ann Neurol 2012;72(6):936–51.
123. Back SA, Volpe JJ. Cellular and molecular pathogenesis of periventricular white matter injury. Ment Retard Dev Disabil Res Rev 1997;3:96–107.
124. Back SA, Luo NL, Mallinson RA, et al. Selective vulnerability of preterm white matter to oxidative damage defined by F2-isoprostanes. Ann Neurol 2005; 58(1):108–20.
125. Back SA, Han BH, Luo NL, et al. Selective vulnerability of late oligodendrocyte progenitors to hypoxia-ischemia. J Neurosci 2002;22(2):455–63.

126. Zhiheng H, Liu J, Cheung PY, et al. Long-term cognitive impairment and myelination deficiency in a rat model of perinatal hypoxic-ischemia brain injury. Brain Res 2009;1301:100–9.
127. Wright J, Zhang G, Yu TS, et al. Age-related changes in the oligodendrocyte progenitor pool influence brain remodeling after injury. Dev Neurosci 2010; 32(5–6):499–509.
128. Sizonenko SV, Camm EJ, Dayer A, et al. Glial responses to neonatal hypoxic-ischemic injury in the rat cerebral cortex. Int J Dev Neurosci 2008;26(1): 37–45.
129. Zaidi A, Bessert D, Ong J, et al. New oligodendrocytes are generated after neonatal hypoxic-ischemic brain injury in rodents. Glia 2004;46:380–90.
130. Felling RJ, Snyder MJ, Romanko MJ, et al. Neural stem/progenitor cells participate in the regenerative response to perinatal hypoxia/ischemia. J Neurosci 2006;26(16):4359–69.
131. Yang Z, Levison SW. Hypoxia/ischemia expands the regenerative capacity of progenitors in the perinatal subventricular zone. Neuroscience 2006;139(2): 555–64.
132. Billiards S, Haynes R, Folkerth R, et al. Myelin abnormalities without oligodendrocyte loss in periventricular leukomalacia. Brain Pathol 2008;18(2):153–63.
133. Back S, Tuohy T, Chen H, et al. Hyaluronan accumulates in demyelinated lesions and inhibits oligodendrocyte progenitor maturation. Nat Med 2005;9:966–72.
134. Sloane J, Batt C, Ma Y, et al. Hyaluronan blocks oligodendrocyte progenitor maturation and remyelination through TLR2. Proc Natl Acad Sci U S A 2010; 107(25):11555–60.
135. Preston M, Gong X, Su W, et al. Digestion products of the PH20 hyaluronidase inhibit remyelination. Ann Neurol 2013;73(2):266–80.
136. Lee Y, Morrison BM, Li Y, et al. Oligodendroglia metabolically support axons and contribute to neurodegeneration. Nature 2012;487(7408):443–8.
137. Kotter MR, Stadelmann C, Hartung HP. Enhancing remyelination in disease–can we wrap it up? Brain 2011;134(Pt 7):1882–900.
138. Fancy SP, Chan JR, Baranzini SE, et al. Myelin regeneration: a recapitulation of development? Annu Rev Neurosci 2011;34:21–43.
139. Fancy S, Harrington E, Yuen T, et al. Axin2 as regulatory and therapeutic target in newborn brain injury and remyelination. Nat Neurosci 2011;14(8):1009–16.
140. Ming X, Chew LJ, Gallo V. Transgenic overexpression of sox17 promotes oligodendrocyte development and attenuates demyelination. J Neurosci 2013; 33(30):12528–42.
141. Back S, Kroenke C, Sherman L, et al. White matter lesions defined by diffusion tensor imaging in older adults. Ann Neurol 2011;70(3):465–76.
142. Miller S, McQuillen P, Hamrick S, et al. Abnormal brain development in newborns with congenital heart disease. N Engl J Med 2007;357(19):1971–3.
143. Glass HC, Bonifacio SL, Chau V, et al. Recurrent postnatal infections are associated with progressive white matter injury in premature infants. Pediatrics 2008; 122(2):299–305.
144. Goldman SA, Schanz S, Windrem MS. Stem cell-based strategies for treating pediatric disorders of myelin. Hum Mol Genet 2008;17(R1):R76–83.
145. Webber DJ, van Blitterswijk M, Chandran S. Neuroprotective effect of oligodendrocyte precursor cell transplantation in a long-term model of periventricular leukomalacia. Am J Pathol 2009;175(6):2332–42.
146. Volpe JJ. Brain injury in premature infants: a complex amalgam of destructive and developmental disturbances. Lancet Neurol 2009;8(1):110–24.

147. Srinivasan L, Dutta R, Counsell SJ, et al. Quantification of deep gray matter in preterm infants at term-equivalent age using manual volumetry of 3-tesla magnetic resonance images. Pediatrics 2007;119(4):759–65.

148. Keunen K, Kersbergen KJ, Groenendaal F, et al. Brain tissue volumes in preterm infants: prematurity, perinatal risk factors and neurodevelopmental outcome: a systematic review. J Matern Fetal Neonatal Med 2012;25(Suppl 1):89–100.

149. Tam EW, Ferriero DM, Xu D, et al. Cerebellar development in the preterm neonate: effect of supratentorial brain injury. Pediatr Res 2009;66(1):102–6.

150. Nossin-Manor R, Chung AD, Whyte HE, et al. Deep gray matter maturation in very preterm neonates: regional variations and pathology-related age-dependent changes in magnetization transfer ratio. Radiology 2012;263(2): 510–7.

151. Andiman SE, Haynes RL, Trachtenberg FL, et al. The cerebral cortex overlying periventricular leukomalacia: analysis of pyramidal neurons. Brain Pathol 2010; 20(4):803–14.

152. Nagasunder AC, Kinney HC, Bluml S, et al. Abnormal microstructure of the atrophic thalamus in preterm survivors with periventricular leukomalacia. AJNR Am J Neuroradiol 2011;32(1):185–91.

153. Kinney H, Haynes R, Xu G, et al. Neuron deficit in the white matter and subplate in periventricular leukomalacia. Ann Neurol 2012;71(3):397–406.

154. McQuillen PS, Ferriero DM. Perinatal subplate neuron injury: implications for cortical development and plasticity. Brain Pathol 2005;15(3):250–60.

155. Doesburg SM, Ribary U, Herdman AT, et al. Altered long-range alpha-band synchronization during visual short-term memory retention in children born very preterm. Neuroimage 2011;54(3):2330–9.

156. Gozzo Y, Vohr B, Lacadie C, et al. Alterations in neural connectivity in preterm children at school age. Neuroimage 2009;48(2):458–63.

157. Schafer RJ, Lacadie C, Vohr B, et al. Alterations in functional connectivity for language in prematurely born adolescents. Brain 2009;132(Pt 3):661–70.

158. Narberhaus A, Lawrence E, Allin MP, et al. Neural substrates of visual paired associates in young adults with a history of very preterm birth: alterations in fronto-parieto-occipital networks and caudate nucleus. Neuroimage 2009;47(4): 1884–93.

159. Doesburg SM, Chau CM, Cheung TP, et al. Neonatal pain-related stress, functional cortical activity and visual-perceptual abilities in school-age children born at extremely low gestational age. Pain 2013;154(10):1946–52.

160. Counsell SJ, Dyet LE, Larkman DJ, et al. Thalamo-cortical connectivity in children born preterm mapped using probabilistic magnetic resonance tractography. Neuroimage 2007;34(3):896–904.

161. Smyser CD, Inder TE, Shimony JS, et al. Longitudinal analysis of neural network development in preterm infants. Cereb Cortex 2010;20(12):2852–62.

162. Mullen KM, Vohr BR, Katz KH, et al. Preterm birth results in alterations in neural connectivity at age 16 years. Neuroimage 2011;54(4):2563–70.

163. Dean J, McClendon E, Hansen K, et al. Prenatal cerebral ischemia disrupts MRI-defined cortical microstructure through disturbances in neuronal arborization. Sci Transl Med 2013;5(166–170):101–11.

164. Ball G, Srinivasan L, Aljabar P, et al. Development of cortical microstructure in the preterm human brain. Proc Natl Acad Sci U S A 2013;110(23):9541–6.

165. Ferriero DM. Neonatal brain injury. N Engl J Med 2004;351(19):1985–95.

Brain Development in Preterm Infants Assessed Using Advanced MRI Techniques

Nora Tusor, MD[a], Tomoki Arichi, MBChB, MRCPCH, PhD[a,b],
Serena J. Counsell, PhD[a],
A. David Edwards, MBBS, FRCP, FRCPCH, FMedSci[a,b,*]

KEYWORDS

- MRI • Diffusion-MRI • Functional MRI • Preterm • Brain

KEY POINTS

- Diffusion MRI (d-MRI) metrics change with maturation. These changes reflect, in white matter, alterations in water content, axonal caliber, oligodendrocyte proliferation, and myelination. In cortical gray matter changes in d-MRI measures represent increasing cellular density and maturing dendritic cytoarchitecture.
- White matter structure, as assessed by fractional anisotropy (FA), correlates with performance in specific neural systems. In addition, FA measures are negatively correlated with immaturity at birth and are reduced in comorbidities associated with preterm birth including acute and chronic respiratory disease and sepsis.
- Functional MRI (fMRI) allows the noninvasive assessment of functional brain activity and can study intrinsic neural activity (resting state fMRI) or the response to external stimulation (task-based fMRI) by sampling temporal changes in the blood oxygen level–dependent signal. Resting state networks demonstrate a network-specific rate of development, exhibiting different rates of coherent interhemispheric activity with advancing postmenstrual age, with the auditory system seemingly maturing before others.

INTRODUCTION

The incidence of preterm birth (delivery before 37 weeks' gestation) continues to increase, with an estimated 14.9 million infants (representing 11.1% of all births) delivered worldwide each year.[1] The importance of the preterm period (equivalent to the third trimester of gestation) for brain development is emphasized by a striking increase

The authors have no conflicts to disclose.
[a] Centre for the Developing Brain, Department of Perinatal Imaging, St Thomas' Hospital, King's College London, Westminster Bridge Road, London SE1 7EH, UK; [b] Department of Bioengineering, Imperial College London, South Kensington Campus, London SW7 2AZ, UK
* Corresponding author. Centre for the Developing Brain, King's College London, St Thomas' Hospital, Westminster Bridge Road, London SE1 7EH, UK.
E-mail address: ad.edwards@kcl.ac.uk

in the incidence of adverse neurodevelopmental outcome, with the spectrum of life-long dysfunction covering the motor, cognitive, and psychiatric domains.[2,3] In response, there has been an increase in the development of imaging techniques that can be used by both scientists and clinicians to characterize early brain development, to assess the response to perinatal brain injury, and as biomarkers for testing and monitoring the effects of potential interventional strategies.[4] Magnetic resonance imaging (MRI) during the neonatal period has become widely used to provide detailed images of the developing brain and define malformations, establish detailed patterns of brain injury, and provide prognostic information.[5–10] However, a significant proportion of preterm infants continue to suffer from cognitive impairment despite an apparently normal appearance to their MRI brain scan, suggesting that a more subtle but global insult underlies these difficulties.[11]

In addition to providing a highly detailed qualitative assessment of brain development, a major advantage of MRI lies in the quantifiable nature of the acquired signal and inherent flexibility of the technique, which can allow accurate measurement of diverse aspects of macroscopic brain tissue structure, integrity, composition, and even function. This review describes the principles underlying these advanced MRI techniques and the findings of studies that highlight their potential to understand early brain development, and in particular, characterize the pathophysiology of preterm brain injury. Due to spatial constraints, the review concentrates predominately on 2 exemplars that underline the ability of MRI to provide diverse yet detailed information about both brain tissue microstructure (diffusion weighted imaging [d-MRI]), and functional activity (blood oxygen level–dependent [BOLD] functional MRI [fMRI]).

NEONATAL BRAIN TEMPLATES AND ATLASES

To perform systematic MRI studies across populations of subjects, it is often necessary to normalize the data spatially by accurately aligning or "registering" each of the individual subject brain images to a common space (template).[12] Such templates can also allow alignment to standard brain "atlases", with which regions of the brain can be labeled by tissue type or anatomic location. Although in adult subjects this is relatively easily done using widely available standard space templates, this process is considerably more difficult when studying neonatal subjects because of the marked heterogeneity inherent to the developing brain, as its macroscopic structure proceeds along a dramatic, but highly structured sequence of maturation in the perinatal period and early infancy. To avoid significant bias, data should therefore be registered to an age-appropriate atlas, which accurately represents the dynamic changes occurring during early brain development (**Fig. 1**).[13,14] An important additional benefit of this process is that it is then possible to detect and quantify local tissue abnormalities by exact measurement of the variations in anatomy between an atlas and individual subjects.[15] Such atlases should be publically available resources, to allow for consistency and data sharing across the neonatal MRI community (www.brain-development.org).

D-MRI

Contrast in d-MRI is based on the random thermal motion of water molecules.[16] The travel of water molecules can be represented by a diffusion coefficient, which depends on several factors, including the temperature, molecular mass, viscosity, and microstructural features of the environment. The high sensitivity of the diffusion coefficient to the local microstructure in particular enables its use as a probe of the physical properties of biologic tissues. In the presence of a spatially varying magnetic field, the random motion of protons in diffusing water molecules results in dephasing of the

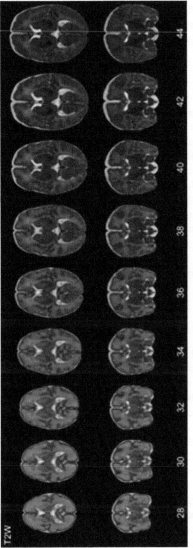

Fig. 1. A 4D atlas of the developing neonatal brain as visualized by T2-weighted MR images. Axial (top row) and coronal (bottom row) slices, with the postmenstrual age (in weeks) listed across the bottom of the figure. Such atlases are vital so that individual subject MRI data can be spatially normalized and allow population-wide studies. (*From* Serag A, Aljabar P, Ball G, et al. Construction of a consistent high-definition spatio-temporal atlas of the developing brain using adaptive kernel regression. Neuroimage 2012;59(3):2260; with permission.)

magnetic resonance signal, producing a reduction in its amplitude. Because spatially varying magnetic fields are used for slice selection and spatial encoding in all MRIs, water molecular diffusion leads to a reduction in signal intensity in all images, although the effect is normally quite small. However, by deliberately applying large magnetic field gradients in particular directions, diffusion can be made the dominant image contrast mechanism, and variations in diffusion properties can be visualized, including their directional dependence.[17]

In d-MRI, the diffusion coefficient is not measured directly; rather, it is inferred from observations of the molecular displacement over a given time. As the extent of diffusion in a given tissue depends on both the local microstructural environment and the choice of diffusion weighting, the diffusion coefficient estimated in a specific tissue is termed the apparent diffusion coefficient (ADC). To quantify diffusion, a minimum of 2 signal measurements are needed: one with diffusion weighting and one without diffusion weighting. The b value reflects the degree of diffusion weighting applied and in clinical settings its value ranges between 750 and 1500 s/mm^2.

The random motion of water molecules in a homogenous medium such as cerebrospinal fluid is equal in all directions (isotropic). If diffusing water molecules encounter any hindrance, the displacement per unit time will be lower than that observed in free water, and hence, the diffusion of water molecules in a tissue with ordered microstructure, such as white matter (WM), is directionally dependent (anisotropic).[18] Anisotropy is influenced by barriers to diffusion, which are both nonaxonal (such as the myelin sheath and neurofibrils) and axonal. Of particular salience to the unmyelinated WM found in the preterm brain, studies in both animals and human infants have shown the axonal membranes themselves are sufficient barriers to hinder water diffusion perpendicular to WM fibers (relative to diffusion along the fibers).[19-25] Moreover, genetically modified animal models of dysmyelination have shown that while myelin also modulates anisotropy, the effect is to a smaller degree than the axonal membranes.[26-30]

DIFFUSION TENSOR IMAGING

A mathematical tensor model (a "diffusion tensor") is commonly used to characterize diffusion in brain tissue, where water molecule displacement per unit time is unlikely to be equal in all directions. To examine diffusivity in a tissue with ordered microstructure, a minimum of 6 noncollinear directions of diffusion sensitization is required, in addition to one with no diffusion weighting. However, to construct the diffusion tensor accurately, frequently more than 30 directions are acquired. The diffusion tensor can be conceptualized as an ellipsoid, in which the long axis represents the direction with the highest diffusivity (termed axial diffusivity). Its magnitude is given by the major eigenvalue ($\lambda 1$) and its direction is given by the major eigenvector. Perpendicular to the major eigenvector are 2 short axes, with their respective eigenvalues ($\lambda 2$, $\lambda 3$), which are often averaged to produce a measure of radial diffusivity (**Fig. 2**).[17,31]

Averaged mean diffusivity can be calculated as one-third of the trace of the diffusion tensor that provides the overall magnitude of water diffusion. The most commonly used measure of diffusion is fractional anisotropy (FA), which is the fraction of the magnitude of diffusion that can be attributed to anisotropic diffusion. FA values range between 0 (diffusion that is equal in all directions) and 1 (**Fig. 3**).

D-MRI DATA ANALYSIS

The most frequently used and simplest technique for analyzing neonatal d-MRI data is to manually delineate regions of interest within which diffusion metrics are then

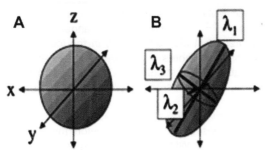

Fig. 2. The diffusion ellipsoid. (*A*) In an isotropic medium the diffusion is equal in all directions. (*B*) In an anisotropic medium the diffusion along one direction, termed the principal eigenvalue (λ1), is greater than the other 2 eigenvalues (λ2, λ3).

calculated. This form of analysis is particularly suited for studies that require quantitative assessment of tensor metrics in a clinically relevant timeframe for a single subject or assessment of a particular brain region.[32] However, it is time-consuming (especially when a large number of regions and/or subjects are assessed) and is prone to operator-dependent bias.[33]

Tract-based spatial statistics (TBSS) is a voxel-based whole brain technique for assessing FA in major WM tracts in an automated and operator-independent way.[34] The technique consists of 2 steps: first the individual subject FA images are registered into a common space; they are then projected onto a representation of the major WM tracts (the "mean FA skeleton") from which statistical inferences can then be made. Given maturational differences in brain structure and WM, the TBSS protocol is specifically optimized for use with neonatal data.[35] As TBBS can markedly improve the sensitivity, objectivity, and interpretability of analysis in multisubject diffusion imaging studies, it is particularly suitable for longitudinal studies of neonatal subjects, which require assessment of the whole brain WM and/or a large number of subjects.[36]

D-MRI OF BRAIN DEVELOPMENT

The neonatal brain contains more water than the brain of older children and adults, with a rapid reduction seen toward full term and during early infancy.[37] As a result, ADC values in both gray and WM are higher in the neonatal brain compared with adults and are higher in the WM than in gray matter.[25] Toward term, ADC values in the gray

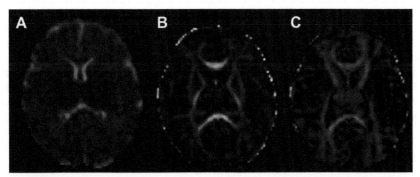

Fig. 3. Diffusion MR scalar maps: (*A*) mean diffusivity, (*B*) fractional anisotropy, and (*C*) color-coded fractional anisotropy maps of the brain in a healthy infant.

matter and hemispheric WM decrease and then continue to decrease further over the first 6 months post term.[23,24,38,39] These rapid changes in ADC represent not only changes in water content, but also differences in the localized restriction of water diffusion due to increasing numbers of oligodendrocytes and a gradual thickening of the water-impermeable myelin sheath. ADC values reach mature adult levels by about 2 years of age, although small decreases may still be found until early adulthood.[23,39]

FA increases with WM maturation and decreases with cortical maturation. This increase takes place in 2 stages: the first occurring before myelin is evident histologically and is attributed to changes in WM structure, which accompany the premyelinating state, including an increase in axonal membrane maturation, microtubule-associated proteins, a change in axon caliber, and an increase in oligodendrocyte number.[24,25,40] At this stage, the highest FA values are seen in the unmyelinated but highly organized commissural fibers in the splenium and genu of the corpus callosum. The second stage is associated with the histologic appearance of myelin and subsequent maturation, with the earliest signs observed in the projection fibers of the posterior limb of the internal capsule around term.[41]

D-MRI OF THE PRETERM BRAIN

Diffusion characteristics of WM in the developing preterm brain have been well described.[24,42–47] FA values in the WM of preterm infants at term-equivalent age are significantly lower in comparison to term-born controls in several regions, suggesting widespread microstructural abnormalities, even in absence of major focal lesions.[46,48,49] This decreased FA may reflect underlying reductions in myelination or decreased fiber coherence. Preterm birth–associated comorbidities, including acute and chronic lung disease (**Fig. 4**), punctate lesions, sepsis, and infants who are small for gestational age, have all been found to be associated with altered WM microstructure, including increased radial diffusivity and reduced FA.[35,47,50–52]

d-MRI techniques are also particularly useful for visualizing ischemic WM lesions, which demonstrate restricted diffusion and a corresponding low ADC during the acute phase, thought to be related to cytotoxic edema.[53,54] Of importance, these changes can be seen on d-MRI before they are evident on conventional MRI.[53] In infants with cystic periventricular leukomalacia, altered WM microstructure is seen in areas distant from the focal cystic lesions[48] at term-equivalent age and in more diffuse WM injury, ADC values are elevated in both the periventricular and the subcortical WM.[48,55]

d-MRI measures correlate with subsequent neurodevelopmental performance. Increased ADC values in the WM at term-equivalent age are predictive of adverse neurodevelopmental outcome,[56] and FA, assessed using TBSS, correlates with neurodevelopmental outcome at 2 years (**Fig. 5**).[57,58] d-MRI can be used to assess specific neural systems, for example, FA in the optic radiation delineated with probabilistic tractography, correlate with visual performance at term-equivalent age.[45,59] In a longitudinal study of preterm infants, visual performance correlated with FA in the optic radiation at term-equivalent age but not during the preterm period, suggesting that WM injury occurs between birth and term and that there may be a window of opportunity for therapeutic intervention aimed at reducing preterm WM injury.[60]

CHARACTERIZING CORTICAL MATURITY AND THALAMOCORTICAL CONNECTIVITY WITH D-MRI

In addition to studying WM, cortical maturation can be studied with d-MRI. Less than 32 weeks' gestation, the cortex is dominated by perpendicular radial glia and apical

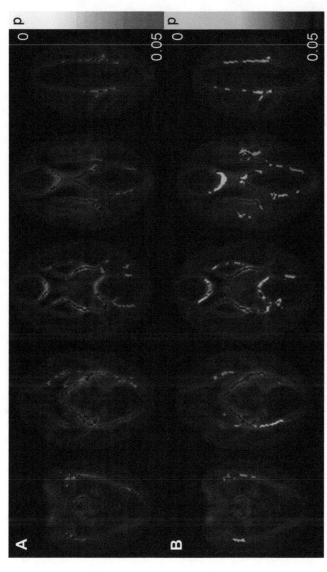

Fig. 4. Respiratory morbidity is associated with altered WM microstructure in preterm neonates. Using TBSS, chronic lung disease was found to be associated with significantly increased radial diffusivity (A) and decreased FA (B) but not axial diffusivity independent of both gestational age at birth and postmenstrual age at scan (FWE-corrected, $P<.05$; color bars indicate P value). The mean FA skeleton is shown in dark green. (*From* Ball G, Counsell SJ, Anjari M, et al. An optimised tract-based spatial statistics protocol for neonates: applications to prematurity and chronic lung disease. Neuroimage 2010;53(1):99; with permission.)

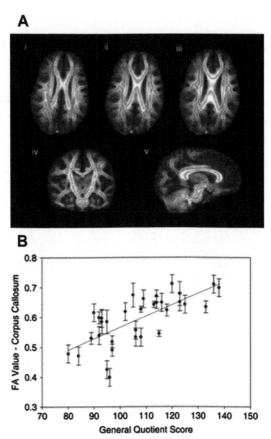

Fig. 5. Correlation between FA and neurodevelopmental performance at 2 years. (*A*) Mean fractional anisotropy (FA) skeleton (green) overlaid on mean FA map in the axial (i–iii), coronal (iv), and sagittal (v) planes. Voxels showing a significant correlation (*P*<.01) between FA and developmental assessment score are shown in blue and include the body and isthmus of the corpus callosum. (*B*) Graph showing the relationship between FA and developmental assessment score. (*From* Counsell SJ, Edwards AD, Chew AT, et al. Specific relations between neurodevelopmental abilities and white matter microstructure in children born preterm. Brain 2008;131(Pt 12):3204; with permission.)

dendrites, resulting in nonzero anisotropy,[61] and is accompanied by decreases in both averaged mean diffusivity and FA due to increasing cellular density, complexity, neurite overgrowth, and maturing dendritic cytoarchitecture.[25,61–63] Cortical FA declines until 38 weeks, with higher initial values and rate of change in the frontal and temporal poles, and parietal cortex, and lower initial values in the perirolandic, and medial occipital cortices, suggesting that elongation and branching of dendrites orthogonal to cortical columns happen later in the association cortex.[63] Elegant studies in a fetal sheep model suggest alterations in cortical FA observed in preterm brain injury are related to disturbances in dendritic arborization and synapse formation.[64] Cortical development, as assessed by d-MRI, is impaired in preterm infants who have slower postnatal growth.[65] Moreover, the rate of microstructural maturation correlates not only with local cortical growth but also importantly with neurodevelopmental performance at 2 years of age.[63]

A vital process in the establishment of the mature cortex and its underlying framework of structural and functional connectivity is thought to be the complex interplay between the cortex itself and a network of connections with the thalamus. Fundamental to the development of thalamo-cortical connectivity during the second and third trimester of human gestation is a cell-sparse but highly functional transient layer known as the subplate, which is thought to act as a "waiting area" for axons before they reach their cortical destination.[66,67] This period may represent a critical window of vulnerability following preterm birth, where disruption of the key transient developmental processes that underlie thalamo-cortical connectivity may result in complex and life-long cerebral abnormalities.[11,67,68]

Morphologic studies of the developing preterm brain have demonstrated complex white and gray matter abnormalities suggestive of disruption to the thalamo-cortical system.[11,69–71] The thalamus appears to be particularly vulnerable following preterm birth, with several studies demonstrating a reduction in volume, which correlates with adverse neurodevelopmental outcome later in infancy.[70,72–75] At term-equivalent age, thalamo-cortical connectivity is sufficiently established such that the connections to and from different cortical regions to thalamic nuclei can be delineated with probabilistic tractography. Preterm birth results in diminished thalamo-cortical connectivity, with the frontal, supplementary motor, occipital, and temporal regions particularly affected (**Fig. 6**).[76]

FMRI

fMRI allows the noninvasive assessment of functional brain activity through sampling temporal changes in the BOLD signal.[77–79] The underlying basic premise is that the magnetic properties of hemoglobin are altered by oxygen binding, and that neural activity triggers a neurovascular coupling cascade, which results in increased local cerebral blood flow and an increase in oxyhemoglobin, which can be detected by an appropriately sensitized T2*-weighted MRI sequence.[77] Such changes are typically localized within 2 to 3 mm of the neural activity, thereby allowing for relatively good, whole brain spatial localization. fMRI has become widely applied across the neuroscience community, with studies typically motivated by 2 contrasting views of brain function.[80] The first posits that the brain is primarily reflexive and is driven by momentary demands related to the environment, which has therefore motivated studies to measure brain responses to specific forms of external stimulation. In contrast, it has also been proposed that the brain's activity is predominately intrinsic in origin, leading to detailed studies of correlations in resting brain activity ("resting state networks" [RSN]).[81,82]

In addition to general issues that may affect all MRI of the neonatal brain, such as a smaller brain size, a shorter neck, and uncontrolled head motion, there are also several factors that can also specifically influence the BOLD fMRI signal.[83,84] These factors include higher heart and respiratory rates leading to a more dynamic cardiorespiratory cycle and greater pulsatility transmitted to the cortex,[85] fetal hemoglobin leading to differences in the oxygen carrying capacity of blood,[86–88] and more diffuse and less efficient synaptic connections.[84] Although the relationship between structural immaturity and the physiology of the BOLD signal is not precisely known, it likely diminishes the magnitude of responses and limits detection.[83]

TASK-BASED FMRI

In a typical task-based fMRI experiment, a series of BOLD contrast images are rapidly acquired while a subject is presented with an external stimulus (or performs a task)

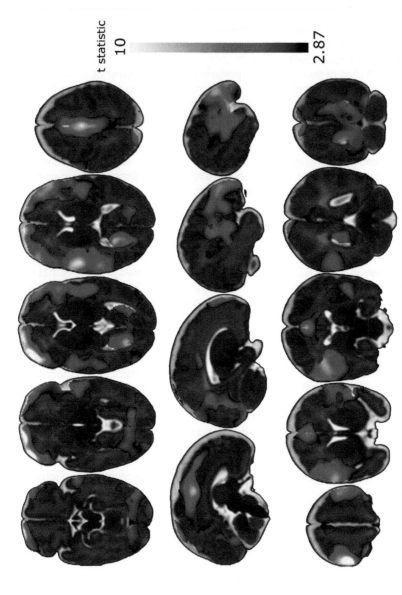

Fig. 6. Thalamo-cortical connectivity in the preterm brain. Regions of significantly lower thalamo-cortical connectivity in preterm infants compared with term-born controls, are shown in orange-yellow. Statistical images are displayed on a population-based T2-weighted template. (*From* Ball G, Boardman JP, Aljabar P, et al. The influence of preterm birth on the developing thalamocortical connectome. Cortex 2013;49(6):1715; with permission.)

alternating with periods of rest. Areas of activity are then subsequently statistically identified by locating areas where the BOLD signal has changed from baseline, corresponding to the time of stimulus presentation or task. There is now a small but growing body of literature in which fMRI responses in localized brain regions have been identified with a variety of stimulus paradigms in neonatal subjects. Most early studies (including the first described by Born and colleagues in 1996[88–90]) used a visual stimulus to identify brain activity in the primary visual areas of the occipital cortex.[91–95] A counterintuitive decrease in the BOLD signal following stimulation (termed "negative BOLD") was prominently seen in these early studies, leading the authors to suggest that such responses occur during early life (after 8 weeks) as a normal developmental stage in early infancy. Localized and predominately positive BOLD responses have since been described with auditory stimulation paradigms,[96–100] simple somatosensory stimulation,[101–104] and olfactory stimulation.[105] Therefore, the discrepancy in BOLD response amplitude is predominately seen only following visual stimulation, which may support a differing developmental trajectory specific to the visual system and occipital lobes, with early vision supported by the subcortical extrageniculate system.[106] The ability to identify positive BOLD responses is also further enhanced by using an age-appropriate hemodynamic response function in the analysis (which takes into account the physiologic delay in the vascular response to neural activity) and has been shown to display a clear maturational trend (with faster and higher amplitude responses with increasing maturity) in both neonatal rodents and humans (**Fig. 7**).[103,107]

RESTING STATE FMRI

Even at rest, the brain is known to be spontaneously active and shows rich intrinsic dynamics, which can be modulated by external stimuli. This intrinsic neural activity can be detected as localized and continuous low-frequency fluctuations of the BOLD signal, by acquiring a series of images using an fMRI sequence while the subject lies "resting" in the MRI scanner.[82] Specific RSNs can be readily identified that spatially replicate functional networks exhibited by the brain over its range of possible tasks.[108] Furthermore, RSNs transcend levels of consciousness and are robustly reproducible across subjects.[109–113] They encompass distinct neural systems, including medial, lateral, and dorsal visual, auditory, somatomotor, executive control, and default mode networks.[114,115] The term "functional connectivity" describes correlation between the BOLD signal time series in these distinct brain regions and is therefore interpreted as representative of the level of functional communication between regions.[116–118] Of importance, although RSNs respect patterns of anatomic connectivity, they are not constrained by such connections.[110,119–121]

The simplicity of resting state fMRI acquisition and the possibility of powerful segregation of several networks in the same acquisition make the technique intrinsically attractive to study functional brain organization of the brain in both healthy infants and those with brain injury.[122] A repertoire of RSNs have been identified in healthy full-term infants within 2 weeks of birth, in the occipital, sensorimotor, temporal, parietal, prefrontal cortices, and basal ganglia.[123] Similarly, RSNs are also readily identified in infants born preterm at term-equivalent age, with bilateral networks suggestive of strong interhemispheric connections in the occipital, somatomotor, temporal, parietal, and anterior prefrontal cortices.[124–126] In longitudinal analyses of RSNs in preterm infants up to term-equivalent age, functional connections between spatially distant regions do not to seem to be present until late in the equivalent of the third trimester. In addition, RSNs demonstrate a network-specific rate of development,

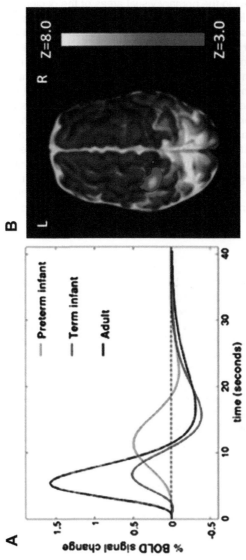

Fig. 7. BOLD hemodynamic response function. (*A*) Faster and higher amplitude responses are seen with increasing maturity. Taking these differences into account makes a significant difference in the ability of the analysis to identify functional activity, particularly in preterm infants. (*B*) In this 32+4 weeks' postmenstrual age infant, a well-localized cluster of positive BOLD functional activation can be seen in the contralateral (left) primary somatosensory cortex following passive movement of the right wrist. (*From* Arichi T, Fagiolo G, Varela M, et al. Development of BOLD signal hemodynamic responses in the human brain. Neuroimage 2012;63(2):668; with permission.)

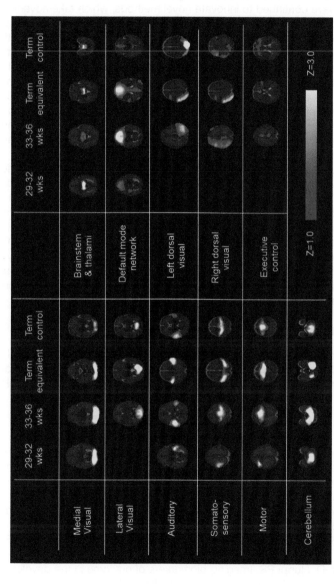

Fig. 8. Spontaneous functional activity patterns in preterm infants at 29 to 32 weeks' postmenstrual age (PMA) (first column); 33 to 36 weeks PMA (second column); at term-equivalent PMA (third column); and in healthy infants born at full-term gestation (fourth column). RSNs identified with probabilistic independent component analysis have been overloaded onto axial slices from age-specific templates. A maturational trend in the spatial distribution of networks can be seen, with a tendency toward increasing long-range and interhemispheric connectivity toward term-equivalent PMA. (*Adapted from* Doria V, Beckmann CF, Arichi T, et al. Emergence of resting state networks in the preterm human brain. Proc Natl Acad Sci U S A 2010;107(46):20016; with permission.)

exhibiting different rates of coherent interhemispheric activity with advancing PMA, with the auditory system seemingly maturing before others **(Fig. 8)**.[125]

FUTURE DIRECTIONS

Researchers in MRI have been constantly pushing the boundaries of the capabilities of the technique and have continued to innovate novel methods, which take advantage of the quantifiable data it provides and the flexibility of image acquisition. Recent advances in d-MRI can offer more specific markers of microstructural complexity in the WM, by moving beyond the diffusion tensor model, which is potentially limited by the assumption that within each voxel there is a single diffusing process. Indeed, at higher b values studies have suggested that the diffusion signal from a single voxel may reflect the contribution of several tissue compartments, and that a voxel's diffusion profile can be more accurately measured by acquiring data with high angular resolution diffusion imaging.[127] In addition, more complex indices, such as constrained spherical deconvolution, can allow more precise estimation of multiple crossing and interdigitating fibers of the neonatal brain.[127]

An area of particular interest in the neuroimaging community is the characterization of the human brain "connectome" using the advanced MRI techniques described in this review.[128,129] The emphasis of such projects is to use cutting-edge methods to map all of the structural and functional connections accurately, which exist in the brain across a large population of subjects. Although undertaking such a challenge in the developing neonatal brain is clearly daunting, the possibility of deciphering how the brain establishes patterns of long-distance structural and functional connectivity is extremely compelling. In addition, one might envisage that such a process would shed dramatic and important new insights onto the underlying pathophysiology of premature and acquired neonatal brain injury.

ACKNOWLEDGMENTS

We are grateful for the support of the Medical Research Council (UK) and the NIHR Comprehensive Biomedical Research Centre at Guy's and St Thomas' NHS Foundation Trust in partnership with King's College London and King's College Hospital NHS Foundation Trust.

REFERENCES

1. Blencowe H, Cousens S, Oestergaard MZ, et al. National, regional, and worldwide estimates of preterm birth rates in the year 2010 with time trends since 1990 for selected countries: a systematic analysis and implications. Lancet 2012;379(9832):2162–72.
2. Doyle LW, Anderson PJ. Adult outcome of extremely preterm infants. Pediatrics 2010;126(2):342–51.
3. Johnson S, Marlow N. Preterm birth and childhood psychiatric disorders. Pediatr Res 2011;69(5 Pt 2):11R–8R.
4. Ment LR, Hirtz D, Huppi PS. Imaging biomarkers of outcome in the developing preterm brain. Lancet Neurol 2009;8(11):1042–55.
5. Barkovich AJ. MR and CT evaluation of profound neonatal and infantile asphyxia. AJNR Am J Neuroradiol 1992;13(3):959–72 [discussion: 973–5].
6. Kuenzle C, Baenziger O, Martin E, et al. Prognostic value of early MR imaging in term infants with severe perinatal asphyxia. Neuropediatrics 1994;25(4): 191–200.

7. Mercuri E, Rutherford M, Cowan F, et al. Early prognostic indicators of outcome in infants with neonatal cerebral infarction: a clinical, electroencephalogram, and magnetic resonance imaging study. Pediatrics 1999;103(1):39–46.
8. Rutherford M, Srinivasan L, Dyet L, et al. Magnetic resonance imaging in perinatal brain injury: clinical presentation, lesions and outcome. Pediatr Radiol 2006;36(7):582–92.
9. Woodward LJ, Anderson PJ, Austin NC, et al. Neonatal MRI to predict neurodevelopmental outcomes in preterm infants. N Engl J Med 2006;355(7):685–94.
10. Nongena P, Ederies A, Azzopardi DV, et al. Confidence in the prediction of neurodevelopmental outcome by cranial ultrasound and MRI in preterm infants. Arch Dis Child Fetal Neonatal Ed 2010;95(6):F388–90.
11. Volpe JJ. Brain injury in premature infants: a complex amalgam of destructive and developmental disturbances. Lancet Neurol 2009;8(1):110–24.
12. Jenkinson M. Registration, atlases and cortical flattening. In: Jezzard P, Matthews PM, Smith SM, editors. Functional Magnetic Resonance Imaging. An introduction to methods. New York: Oxford University Press; 2001. p. 271–93.
13. Kuklisova-Murgasova M, Aljabar P, Srinivasan L, et al. A dynamic 4D probabilistic atlas of the developing brain. Neuroimage 2011;54(4):2750–63.
14. Serag A, Aljabar P, Ball G, et al. Construction of a consistent high-definition spatio-temporal atlas of the developing brain using adaptive kernel regression. Neuroimage 2012;59(3):2255–65.
15. Aljabar P, Bhatia KK, Murgasova M, et al. Assessment of brain growth in early childhood using deformation-based morphometry. Neuroimage 2008;39(1):348–58.
16. Le Bihan D, Breton E, Lallemand D, et al. MR imaging of intravoxel incoherent motions: application to diffusion and perfusion in neurologic disorders. Radiology 1986;161(2):401–7.
17. Le Bihan D, Mangin JF, Poupon C, et al. Diffusion tensor imaging: concepts and applications. J Magn Reson Imaging 2001;13(4):534–46.
18. Moseley ME, Cohen Y, Kucharczyk J, et al. Diffusion-weighted MR imaging of anisotropic water diffusion in cat central nervous system. Radiology 1990;176(2):439–45.
19. Beaulieu C, Allen PS. Determinants of anisotropic water diffusion in nerves. Magn Reson Med 1994;31(4):394–400.
20. Beaulieu C, Allen PS. Water diffusion in the giant axon of the squid: implications for diffusion-weighted MRI of the nervous system. Magn Reson Med 1994;32(5):579–83.
21. Beaulieu C, Allen PS. An in vitro evaluation of the effects of local magnetic-susceptibility-induced gradients on anisotropic water diffusion in nerve. Magn Reson Med 1996;36(1):39–44.
22. Beaulieu C, Fenrich FR, Allen PS. Multicomponent water proton transverse relaxation and T2-discriminated water diffusion in myelinated and nonmyelinated nerve. Magn Reson Imaging 1998;16(10):1201–10.
23. Toft PB, Leth H, Peitersen B, et al. The apparent diffusion coefficient of water in gray and white matter of the infant brain. J Comput Assist Tomogr 1996;20(6):1006–11.
24. Huppi PS, Maier SE, Peled S, et al. Microstructural development of human newborn cerebral white matter assessed in vivo by diffusion tensor magnetic resonance imaging. Pediatr Res 1998;44(4):584–90.
25. Neil JJ, Shiran SI, McKinstry RC, et al. Normal brain in human newborns: apparent diffusion coefficient and diffusion anisotropy measured by using diffusion tensor MR imaging. Radiology 1998;209(1):57–66.

26. Ono J, Harada K, Mano T, et al. Differentiation of dys- and demyelination using diffusional anisotropy. Pediatr Neurol 1997;16(1):63–6.

27. Gulani V, Iwamoto GA, Lauterbur PC. Apparent water diffusion measurements in electrically stimulated neural tissue. Magn Reson Med 1999;41(2):241–6.

28. Beaulieu C. The basis of anisotropic water diffusion in the nervous system—a technical review. NMR Biomed 2002;15(7–8):435–55.

29. Song SK, Sun SW, Ramsbottom MJ, et al. Dysmyelination revealed through MRI as increased radial (but unchanged axial) diffusion of water. Neuroimage 2002; 17(3):1429–36.

30. Nair G, Tanahashi Y, Low HP, et al. Myelination and long diffusion times alter diffusion-tensor-imaging contrast in myelin-deficient shiverer mice. Neuroimage 2005;28(1):165–74.

31. Mori S, Zhang J. Principles of diffusion tensor imaging and its applications to basic neuroscience research. Neuron 2006;51(5):527–39.

32. Seo Y, Wang ZJ, Morriss MC, et al. Minimum SNR and acquisition for bias-free estimation of fractional anisotropy in diffusion tensor imaging - a comparison of two analytical techniques and field strengths. Magn Reson Imaging 2012;30(8): 1123–33.

33. Pannek K, Guzzetta A, Colditz PB, et al. Diffusion MRI of the neonate brain: acquisition, processing and analysis techniques. Pediatr Radiol 2012;42(10): 1169–82.

34. Smith SM, Jenkinson M, Johansen-Berg H, et al. Tract-based spatial statistics: voxelwise analysis of multi-subject diffusion data. Neuroimage 2006;31(4): 1487–505.

35. Ball G, Counsell SJ, Anjari M, et al. An optimised tract-based spatial statistics protocol for neonates: applications to prematurity and chronic lung disease. Neuroimage 2010;53(1):94–102.

36. Ball G, Boardman JP, Arichi T, et al. Testing the sensitivity of tract-based spatial statistics to simulated treatment effects in preterm neonates. PLoS One 2013; 8(7):e67706.

37. Dobbing J, Sands J. Quantitative growth and development of human brain. Arch Dis Child 1973;48(10):757–67.

38. Nomura Y, Sakuma H, Takeda K, et al. Diffusional anisotropy of the human brain assessed with diffusion-weighted MR: relation with normal brain development and aging. AJNR Am J Neuroradiol 1994;15(2):231–8.

39. Morriss MC, Zimmerman RA, Bilaniuk LT, et al. Changes in brain water diffusion during childhood. Neuroradiology 1999;41(12):929–34.

40. Wimberger DM, Roberts TP, Barkovich AJ, et al. Identification of "premyelination" by diffusion-weighted MRI. J Comput Assist Tomogr 1995;19(1):28–33.

41. Kinney HC, Brody BA, Kloman AS, et al. Sequence of central nervous system myelination in human infancy. II. Patterns of myelination in autopsied infants. J Neuropathol Exp Neurol 1988;47(3):217–34.

42. Miller SP, Vigneron DB, Henry RG, et al. Serial quantitative diffusion tensor MRI of the premature brain: development in newborns with and without injury. J Magn Reson Imaging 2002;16(6):621–32.

43. Ling X, Tang W, Liu G, et al. Assessment of brain maturation in the preterm infants using diffusion tensor imaging (DTI) and enhanced T2 star weighted angiography (ESWAN). Eur J Radiol 2013;82:e476–83.

44. Partridge SC, Mukherjee P, Henry RG, et al. Diffusion tensor imaging: serial quantitation of white matter tract maturity in premature newborns. Neuroimage 2004;22(3):1302–14.

45. Berman JI, Glass HC, Miller SP, et al. Quantitative fiber tracking analysis of the optic radiation correlated with visual performance in premature newborns. AJNR Am J Neuroradiol 2009;30(1):120–4.

46. Anjari M, Srinivasan L, Allsop JM, et al. Diffusion tensor imaging with tract-based spatial statistics reveals local white matter abnormalities in preterm infants. Neuroimage 2007;35(3):1021–7.

47. Anjari M, Counsell SJ, Srinivasan L, et al. The association of lung disease with cerebral white matter abnormalities in preterm infants. Pediatrics 2009;124(1): 268–76.

48. Counsell SJ, Allsop JM, Harrison MC, et al. Diffusion-weighted imaging of the brain in preterm infants with focal and diffuse white matter abnormality. Pediatrics 2003;112(1 Pt 1):1–7.

49. Wang S, Fan G, Xu K, et al. Potential of diffusion tensor MR imaging in the assessment of cognitive impairments in children with periventricular leukomalacia born preterm. Eur J Radiol 2013;82(1):158–64.

50. Bassi L, Chew A, Merchant N, et al. Diffusion tensor imaging in preterm infants with punctate white matter lesions. Pediatr Res 2011;69(6):561–6.

51. Lepomaki V, Matomaki J, Lapinleimu H, et al. Effect of antenatal growth on brain white matter maturation in preterm infants at term using tract-based spatial statistics. Pediatr Radiol 2013;43(1):80–5.

52. Chau V, Brant R, Poskitt KJ, et al. Postnatal infection is associated with widespread abnormalities of brain development in premature newborns. Pediatr Res 2012;71(3):274–9.

53. Inder T, Huppi PS, Zientara GP, et al. Early detection of periventricular leukomalacia by diffusion-weighted magnetic resonance imaging techniques. J Pediatr 1999;134(5):631–4.

54. Roelants-van Rijn AM, Nikkels PG, Groenendaal F, et al. Neonatal diffusion-weighted MR imaging: relation with histopathology or follow-up MR examination. Neuropediatrics 2001;32(6):286–94.

55. Miller SP, Ferriero DM, Leonard C, et al. Early brain injury in premature newborns detected with magnetic resonance imaging is associated with adverse early neurodevelopmental outcome. J Pediatr 2005;147(5):609–16.

56. Krishnan ML, Dyet LE, Boardman JP, et al. Relationship between white matter apparent diffusion coefficients in preterm infants at term-equivalent age and developmental outcome at 2 years. Pediatrics 2007;120(3):e604–9.

57. Counsell SJ, Edwards AD, Chew AT, et al. Specific relations between neurodevelopmental abilities and white matter microstructure in children born preterm. Brain 2008;131(Pt 12):3201–8.

58. van Kooij BJ, de Vries LS, Ball G, et al. Neonatal tract-based spatial statistics findings and outcome in preterm infants. AJNR Am J Neuroradiol 2012;33(1):188–94.

59. Bassi L, Ricci D, Volzone A, et al. Probabilistic diffusion tractography of the optic radiations and visual function in preterm infants at term equivalent age. Brain 2008;131(Pt 2):573–82.

60. Groppo M, Ricci D, Bassi L, et al. Development of the optic radiations and visual function after premature birth. Cortex 2012. [Epub ahead of print]. http://dx.doi.org/10.1016/j.cortex.2012.02.008.

61. McKinstry RC, Miller JH, Snyder AZ, et al. A prospective, longitudinal diffusion tensor imaging study of brain injury in newborns. Neurology 2002;59(6):824–33.

62. Mukherjee P, Miller JH, Shimony JS, et al. Diffusion-tensor MR imaging of gray and white matter development during normal human brain maturation. AJNR Am J Neuroradiol 2002;23(9):1445–56.

63. Ball G, Srinivasan L, Aljabar P, et al. Development of cortical microstructure in the preterm human brain. Proc Natl Acad Sci U S A 2013;110(23):9541–6.

64. Dean JM, McClendon E, Hansen K, et al. Prenatal cerebral ischemia disrupts MRI-defined cortical microstructure through disturbances in neuronal arborization. Sci Transl Med 2013;5(168):168ra7.

65. Vinall J, Grunau RE, Brant R, et al. Slower postnatal growth is associated with delayed cerebral cortical maturation in preterm newborns. Sci Transl Med 2013;5(168):168ra8.

66. Molnar Z, Higashi S, Lopez-Bendito G. Choreography of early thalamocortical development. Cereb Cortex 2003;13(6):661–9.

67. Kostovic I, Judas M. The development of the subplate and thalamocortical connections in the human foetal brain. Acta Paediatr 2010;99(8):1119–27.

68. Allendoerfer KL, Shatz CJ. The subplate, a transient neocortical structure: its role in the development of connections between thalamus and cortex. Annu Rev Neurosci 1994;17:185–218.

69. Ajayi-Obe M, Saeed N, Cowan FM, et al. Reduced development of cerebral cortex in extremely preterm infants. Lancet 2000;356:1162–3.

70. Inder T, Neil J, Kroenke C, et al. Investigation of cerebral development and injury in the prematurely born primate by magnetic resonance imaging and histopathology. Dev Neurosci 2005;27(2–4):100–11.

71. Kapellou O, Counsell SJ, Kennea N, et al. Abnormal cortical development after premature birth shown by altered allometric scaling of brain growth. PLoS Med 2006;3(8):e265.

72. Boardman JP, Counsell SJ, Rueckert D, et al. Abnormal deep grey matter development following preterm birth detected using deformation-based morphometry. Neuroimage 2006;32(1):70–8.

73. Srinivasan L, Dutta R, Counsell SJ, et al. Quantification of deep gray matter in preterm infants at term-equivalent age using manual volumetry of 3-tesla magnetic resonance images. Pediatrics 2007;119(4):759–65.

74. Boardman JP, Craven C, Valappil S, et al. A common neonatal image phenotype predicts adverse neurodevelopmental outcome in children born preterm. Neuroimage 2010;52(2):409–14.

75. Ball G, Boardman JP, Rueckert D, et al. The effect of preterm birth on thalamic and cortical development. Cereb Cortex 2012;22(5):1016–24.

76. Ball G, Boardman JP, Aljabar P, et al. The influence of preterm birth on the developing thalamocortical connectome. Cortex 2013;49(6):1711–21.

77. Ogawa S, Lee TM, Kay AR, et al. Brain magnetic resonance imaging with contrast dependent on blood oxygenation. Proc Natl Acad Sci U S A 1990;87(24):9868–72.

78. Ogawa S, Tank DW, Menon R, et al. Intrinsic signal changes accompanying sensory stimulation: functional brain mapping with magnetic resonance imaging. Proc Natl Acad Sci U S A 1992;89(13):5951–5.

79. Kwong KK, Belliveau JW, Chesler DA, et al. Dynamic magnetic resonance imaging of human brain activity during primary sensory stimulation. Proc Natl Acad Sci U S A 1992;89(12):5675–9.

80. Llinas R, Ribary U. Consciousness and the brain. The thalamocortical dialogue in health and disease. Ann N Y Acad Sci 2001;929:166–75.

81. Brown TG. On the nature of the fundamental activity of the nervous centres; together with an analysis of the conditioning of rhythmic activity in progression, and a theory of the evolution of function in the nervous system. J Physiol 1914;48(1):18–46.

82. Biswal B, Yetkin FZ, Haughton VM, et al. Functional connectivity in the motor cortex of resting human brain using echo-planar MRI. Magn Reson Med 1995; 34(4):537–41.
83. Gaillard WD, Grandin CB, Xu B. Developmental aspects of pediatric fMRI: considerations for image acquisition, analysis, and interpretation. Neuroimage 2001;13(2):239–49.
84. Harris JJ, Reynell C, Attwell D. The physiology of developmental changes in BOLD functional imaging signals. Dev Cogn Neurosci 2011;1(3):199–216.
85. Poncelet BP, Wedeen VJ, Weisskoff RM, et al. Brain parenchyma motion: measurement with cine echo-planar MR imaging. Radiology 1992;185(3):645–51.
86. Garby L, Vuille JC. Studies on erythro-kinetics in infancy. I. A modified one-minute alkali denaturation-precipitation method for haemoglobin F determination: agreement with spectrophotometric method. Acta Paediatr 1962;51: 197–200.
87. Garby L, Sjolin S, Vuille JC. Studies on erythro-kinetics in infancy. II. The relative rate of synthesis of haemoglobin F and haemoglobin A during the first months of life. Acta Paediatr 1962;51:245–54.
88. Born P, Rostrup E, Leth H, et al. Change of visually induced cortical activation patterns during development. Lancet 1996;347(9000):543.
89. Born P, Leth H, Miranda MJ, et al. Visual activation in infants and young children studied by functional magnetic resonance imaging. Pediatr Res 1998;44(4): 578–83.
90. Born AP, Miranda MJ, Rostrup E, et al. Functional magnetic resonance imaging of the normal and abnormal visual system in early life. Neuropediatrics 2000; 31(1):24–32.
91. Yamada H. Brain functional MRI of the visual cortex with echo planar imaging. Nihon Rinsho 1997;55(7):1684–7 [in Japanese].
92. Morita T, Kochiyama T, Yamada H, et al. Difference in the metabolic response to photic stimulation of the lateral geniculate nucleus and the primary visual cortex of infants: a fMRI study. Neurosci Res 2000;38(1):63–70.
93. Muramoto S, Yamada H, Sadato N, et al. Age-dependent change in metabolic response to photic stimulation of the primary visual cortex in infants: functional magnetic resonance imaging study. J Comput Assist Tomogr 2002;26(6): 894–901.
94. Lee W, Donner EJ, Nossin-Manor R, et al. Visual functional magnetic resonance imaging of preterm infants. Dev Med Child Neurol 2012;54(8):724–9.
95. Konishi Y, Taga G, Yamada H, et al. Functional brain imaging using fMRI and optical topography in infancy. Sleep Med 2002;3(Suppl 2):S41–3.
96. Altman NR, Bernal B. Brain activation in sedated children: auditory and visual functional MR imaging. Radiology 2001;221(1):56–63.
97. Anderson AW, Marois R, Colson ER, et al. Neonatal auditory activation detected by functional magnetic resonance imaging. Magn Reson Imaging 2001;19(1):1–5.
98. Dehaene-Lambertz G, Dehaene S, Hertz-Pannier L. Functional neuroimaging of speech perception in infants. Science 2002;298(5600):2013–5.
99. Perani D, Saccuman MC, Scifo P, et al. Functional specializations for music processing in the human newborn brain. Proc Natl Acad Sci U S A 2010;107(10): 4758–63.
100. Perani D, Saccuman MC, Scifo P, et al. Neural language networks at birth. Proc Natl Acad Sci U S A 2011;108(38):16056–61.
101. Erberich SG, Panigrahy A, Friedlich P, et al. Somatosensory lateralization in the newborn brain. Neuroimage 2006;29(1):155–61.

102. Arichi T, Moraux A, Melendez A, et al. Somatosensory cortical activation identified by functional MRI in preterm and term infants. Neuroimage 2010;49(3): 2063–71.

103. Arichi T, Fagiolo G, Varela M, et al. Development of BOLD signal hemodynamic responses in the human brain. Neuroimage 2012;63(2):663–73.

104. Allievi AG, Melendez-Calderon A, Arichi T, et al. An fMRI compatible wrist robotic interface to study brain development in neonates. Ann Biomed Eng 2013;41(6):1181–92.

105. Arichi T, Gordon-Williams R, Allievi A, et al. Computer-controlled stimulation for functional magnetic resonance imaging studies of the neonatal olfactory system. Acta Paediatr 2013;102:868–75.

106. Johnson M. Cortical maturation and the development of visual attention in early infancy. J Cogn Neurosci 1990;2(2):81–95.

107. Colonnese MT, Phillips MA, Constantine-Paton M, et al. Development of hemodynamic responses and functional connectivity in rat somatosensory cortex. Nat Neurosci 2008;11(1):72–9.

108. Smith SM, Fox PT, Miller KL, et al. Correspondence of the brain's functional architecture during activation and rest. Proc Natl Acad Sci U S A 2009;106(31): 13040–5.

109. Fukunaga M, Horovitz SG, van Gelderen P, et al. Large-amplitude, spatially correlated fluctuations in BOLD fMRI signals during extended rest and early sleep stages. Magn Reson Imaging 2006;24(8):979–92.

110. Vincent JL, Patel GH, Fox MD, et al. Intrinsic functional architecture in the anaesthetized monkey brain. Nature 2007;447(7140):83–6.

111. Lu H, Zuo Y, Gu H, et al. Synchronized delta oscillations correlate with the resting-state functional MRI signal. Proc Natl Acad Sci U S A 2007;104(46): 18265–9.

112. Greicius MD, Kiviniemi V, Tervonen O, et al. Persistent default-mode network connectivity during light sedation. Hum Brain Mapp 2008;29(7):839–47.

113. Larson-Prior LJ, Zempel JM, Nolan TS, et al. Cortical network functional connectivity in the descent to sleep. Proc Natl Acad Sci U S A 2009;106(11): 4489–94.

114. Beckmann CF, DeLuca M, Devlin JT, et al. Investigations into resting-state connectivity using independent component analysis. Philos Trans R Soc Lond B Biol Sci 2005;360(1457):1001–13.

115. Fox MD, Snyder AZ, Vincent JL, et al. Intrinsic fluctuations within cortical systems account for intertrial variability in human behavior. Neuron 2007;56(1): 171–84.

116. van den Heuvel MP, Hulshoff Pol HE. Exploring the brain network: a review on resting-state fMRI functional connectivity. Eur Neuropsychopharmacol 2010; 20(8):519–34.

117. Fox MD, Snyder AZ, Vincent JL, et al. The human brain is intrinsically organized into dynamic, anticorrelated functional networks. Proc Natl Acad Sci U S A 2005; 102(27):9673–8.

118. Fox MD, Zhang D, Snyder AZ, et al. The global signal and observed anticorrelated resting state brain networks. J Neurophysiol 2009;101(6):3270–83.

119. Zhang D, Snyder AZ, Fox MD, et al. Intrinsic functional relations between human cerebral cortex and thalamus. J Neurophysiol 2008;100(4):1740–8.

120. Raichle ME. A paradigm shift in functional brain imaging. J Neurosci 2009; 29(41):12729–34.

121. Raichle ME. The restless brain. Brain Connect 2011;1(1):3–12.

122. Tau GZ, Peterson BS. Normal development of brain circuits. Neuropsychopharmacology 2010;35(1):147–68.
123. Fransson P, Skiold B, Engstrom M, et al. Spontaneous brain activity in the newborn brain during natural sleep–an fMRI study in infants born at full term. Pediatr Res 2009;66(3):301–5.
124. Fransson P, Skiold B, Horsch S, et al. Resting-state networks in the infant brain. Proc Natl Acad Sci U S A 2007;104(39):15531–6.
125. Doria V, Beckmann CF, Arichi T, et al. Emergence of resting state networks in the preterm human brain. Proc Natl Acad Sci U S A 2010;107(46):20015–20.
126. Smyser CD, Snyder AZ, Neil JJ. Functional connectivity MRI in infants: exploration of the functional organization of the developing brain. Neuroimage 2011; 56(3):1437–52.
127. Tournier JD, Calamante F, Connelly A. Robust determination of the fibre orientation distribution in diffusion MRI: non-negativity constrained super-resolved spherical deconvolution. Neuroimage 2007;35(4):1459–72.
128. Van Essen DC, Ugurbil K, Auerbach E, et al. The Human Connectome Project: a data acquisition perspective. Neuroimage 2012;62(4):2222–31.
129. Van Essen DC, Ugurbil K. The future of the human connectome. Neuroimage 2012;62(2):1299–310.

Pathogenesis and Prevention of Intraventricular Hemorrhage

Praveen Ballabh, MD

KEYWORDS

- Germinal matrix hemorrhage • Intraventricular hemorrhage • Astrocytes • Pericytes
- Angiogenesis • Glucocorticoids • Premature infants • Indomethacin

KEY POINTS

- Pathogenesis of intraventricular hemorrhage (IVH) is ascribed to the intrinsic weakness of germinal matrix vasculature and to the fluctuation in the cerebral blood flow.
- The germinal matrix displays accelerated angiogenesis, which orchestrates formation of nascent vessels that lack pericytes, display immature basal lamina low in fibronectin, and has astrocyte end-feet coverage deficient in glial fibrillary acidic protein. These morphologic and molecular factors contribute to the fragility of the germinal matrix vasculature.
- The fluctuations in the cerebral blood flow is attributed to the cardiorespiratory and hemodynamic instability frequently associated with extremely premature infants, including hypotension, hypoxia, pneumothorax, patent ductus arteriosus, and others.
- Prenatal glucocorticoids have emerged as the most effective intervention to prevent IVH. Therapies designed to enhance the stability of the germinal matrix vasculature and reduce fluctuation of cerebral blood flow could lead to strategies that are more effective in preventing IVH.

INTRODUCTION

In the United States, about 12,000 premature infants develop intraventricular hemorrhage (IVH) every year. The incidence of moderate-to-severe IVH has remained almost stationary during the last 2 decades.[1,2] IVH is a major problem in premature infants, as a large number of them develop neurologic sequelae.[3] Approximately 50% to 75% of preterm survivors with IVH develop cerebral palsy, mental retardation, and/or hydrocephalus.[3,4] Approximately, a quarter of nondisabled survivors develop psychiatric disorders and problems with executive function.[5–7] According to the US Census Bureau and the NICHD Neonatal Research Network, more than 3600 new cases of

Source of Funding: NIH/NINDS grant RO1 NS071263.

Conflict of Interest: None.

Department of Pediatrics, Cell Biology and Anatomy, Regional Neonatal Center, New York Medical College, Maria Fareri Children's Hospital, Westchester Medical Center, 100 Woods Road, Valhalla, NY 10595, USA

E-mail address: Pballabh@msn.com

Clin Perinatol 41 (2014) 47–67

http://dx.doi.org/10.1016/j.clp.2013.09.007   **perinatology.theclinics.com**

mental retardation each year are children who were born premature and suffered IVH.[8,9] Hence, IVH and its resultant neurologic and psychiatric sequelae continue to be a major public health concern worldwide.

IVH typically initiates in the periventricular germinal matrix.[10] This brain region is known to developmental neurobiologists as the ganglionic eminence (**Fig. 1**A). The germinal matrix consists of neuronal and glial precursor cells (see **Fig. 1**B, C) and is most prominent on the head of caudate nucleus. The subependymal germinal matrix is highly vascular and is selectively vulnerable to hemorrhage. After 24 gestational weeks (gw), thickness of the germinal matrix decreases, and it almost disappears by 36 to 37 gw. When hemorrhage in the germinal matrix is substantial, the underlying ependyma breaks and germinal matrix hemorrhage progresses to IVH, as blood fills the lateral cerebral ventricle.

PATHOGENESIS OF IVH

Pathogenesis of IVH is multifactorial, complex, and heterogeneous. An inherent fragility of the germinal matrix vasculature sets the ground for hemorrhage, and

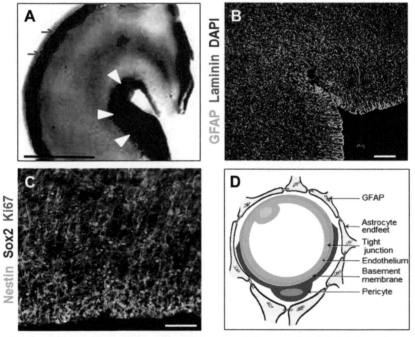

Fig. 1. Morphology of germinal matrix. (*A*) Representative cresyl violet staining of coronal section of the right-sided cerebral hemisphere of a 23-week preterm infant. Note cortical plate (*arrows*) and germinal matrix (*arrowheads*). Germinal matrix (*violet staining*) surrounds the whole ventricle, but is most conspicuous at the head of caudate nucleus. Scale bar, 0.5 cm. (*B*) Representative immunofluorescence of cryosection from germinal matrix of a 23-week premature infant labeled with DAPI (*blue*), GFAP (*green*), and laminin (*vascular marker, red*). Note germinal matrix is highly vascular (*vascular endothelium in red*) and enriched with GFAP (+) glial cells (*green*). (*C*) Coronal brain section was double labeled with nestin (*progenitor cells, green*), Sox2 (*radial glia, blue*), and Ki67 (*red, proliferation marker*). Note nestin and Sox2 positive cells are abundant in the germinal matrix. Scale bar; 100 (*B*) and 50 μm (*C*). (*D*) Schematic drawing of the blood brain barrier in cross-section showing endothelium, endothelial tight junction, basal lamina, pericyte, and astrocyte end-feet.

fluctuation in the cerebral blood flow induces the rupture of vasculature (**Box 1**). If there are associated platelet or coagulation disorders, the homeostasis mechanisms are impaired, which might accentuate the hemorrhage. Vaginal delivery, low Apgar score, severe respiratory distress syndrome, pneumothorax, hypoxia, hypercapnia, seizures, patent ductus arteriosus, infection, and others seem to increase primarily the fluctuations in the cerebral blood flow and thus represent important risk factors to the development of IVH.

What Renders the Germinal Matrix Vasculature Fragile?

Blood vessels in the brain are unique as they form a blood-brain barrier (BBB). The BBB is a complex dynamic interface between blood and the brain and consists of endothelial tight junctions, basal lamina, pericytes, and astrocyte end-feet in inside-out fashion (see **Fig. 1**D).[11,12] Logically, deficiency in any of the components of the BBB can weaken the vasculature and increase the propensity to hemorrhage. The author and his co-workers have evaluated each of these components in the human germinal matrix and have unraveled several dissimilarities in the cellular and molecular components of this germinal matrix vasculature compared to the embryonic white matter and the cortical plate (**Box 2**).

High vascular density and rapid angiogenesis in the germinal matrix

The germinal matrix exhibits rapid angiogenesis in contrast to other brain regions.[13] This rapid endothelial proliferation contributes to the high vascular density of the germinal matrix. Both the vascular density and the cross-sectional area of the vasculature are higher in the human germinal matrix compared to the cortical plate (cerebral cortex) and embryonic white matter from 17 to 35 gw.[14] In addition, the abundance of vessels and cross-sectional area of vasculature increases with advancing gestational age in the second and third trimester of pregnancy.[14] Intriguingly, vessels in the germinal matrix are circular in coronal sections, whereas blood vessels in cerebral cortex and white matter are flat and elongated. The circular shape of the vessels suggests vasculature immaturity, which is consistent with the rapid ongoing angiogenesis in the germinal matrix. The high vascularity and rapid endothelial turnover is unique to the germinal matrix and can be attributed to the high metabolic demand of this brain region, which has a preponderance of proliferating, maturing, and migrating neuronal and glial precursor cells.

Paucity of pericytes in the germinal matrix vasculature

Pericytes are perivascular cells of the capillaries, venules, and arterioles (**Fig. 2**).[15] They are enclosed in the basal lamina and wrap around the endothelial cells. They have complex and critical role to play in regulating angiogenesis, providing structural support to the vasculature, maintaining the BBB, and controlling neurovascular unit — endothelium, astrocytes, and neurons.[16–18] Pericytes are the key players in the various stages of angiogenesis, including initiation, sprout extension, migration, and maturation of blood vessels.[19] In response to angiogenic stimuli, they degrade basal lamina

---

Box 1

Pathogenesis of germinal matrix vasculature

1. Fragility of germinal matrix vasculature
2. Fluctuation in the cerebral blood flow
3. Platelet and coagulation disorder

> **Box 2**
> **Fragility of germinal matrix vasculature**
>
> 1. Paucity of pericytes
> 2. Reduced fibronectin in the basal lamina
> 3. Reduced GFAP expression in the astrocyte end-feet

and migrate out of the microvasculature, and on completion of angiogenesis, they resume their position to strengthen vessels by synthesizing extracellular matrix and inducing endothelial maturation. Pericyte recruitment is regulated primarily by 4 ligand-receptor systems; the ligands include transforming growth factor β (TGFβ), platelet-derived growth factor-B (PDGFB), angiopoietin, and sphingosine-1-phosphate.[20] Deficiency of any of these ligands in transgenic animals results in failure of pericyte recruitment and consequent dilation of the vessels with increased propensity to hemorrhage.[21]

Quantification of pericyte coverage and density in the brain of human preterm infants and fetuses has been performed in immunolabeled sections and electron micrographs. These studies have revealed that the density of perivascular cells and their periendothelial coverage in the germinal matrix are reduced compared to the white matter and cerebral cortex on both ultrastructural and histochemical evaluation.[22] Importantly, TGFβ expression is reduced in the germinal matrix microvasculature, which might be contributing to the paucity of pericytes.[22] Indeed, low TGFβ concentration promotes endothelial proliferation, and conversely, high TGFβ levels enhance capillary stabilization by facilitating pericyte recruitment. To conclude, rapid angiogenesis in the presence of low TGFβ results in abundance of angiogenic vessels deficient in pericytes, which leads to fragility of the germinal matrix microvasculature.

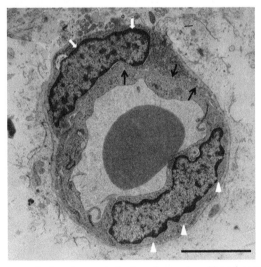

Fig. 2. Electron micrograph showing endothelium (*arrowheads*) and pericyte (*white arrows*) separated by basal laminia (*black arrows*) in the white matter of 3-day-old preterm rabbit pup (E29). Note pericyte wraps around the endothelium and outer to the basal lamina. Scale bar, 4 μm.

Deficient fibronectin in the basal lamina

Basal lamina is a key component of the BBB that surrounds pericytes and separates pericytes from astrocyte end-feet and endothelium.[12,23] Its formation and maintenance is assured by the endothelium, astrocytes, and pericytes. This contributes to the structural integrity of vasculature by virtue of its anchoring function. Basal lamina is comprised of laminin, collagen, fibronectin, heparan sulfate proteoglycan, and perlecan.[12,24,25] Knock-out experiments have revealed the necessity of these molecules in the formation of blood vessels and maintenance of the vascular stability.[26–28] Quantification of the constituents of basal lamina in human fetuses and preterm infants (postmortem) has revealed that fibronectin levels are significantly reduced in the germinal matrix vasculature compared to the cortex and white matter (**Fig. 3**A).[29] However, other components of the basement membrane, including laminin (α1, α4, and α5), α1 (IV) collagen, α5 (IV) collagen, and perlecan, are similarly expressed in the 3 brain regions. Given that polymerization of fibronectin into extracellular matrix controls stability of the vasculature and that fibronectin null mice exhibit cerebral hemorrhage, deficient fibronectin in the germinal matrix is likely to contribute to the fragility of germinal matrix vasculature.[30,31] Because TGFβ upregulates fibronectin and other components of the extracellular matrix, diminished TGFβ in the germinal matrix is consistent with low levels of fibronectin in the germinal matrix. Thus, upregulating TGFβ might elevate fibronectin levels in the basal lamina and strengthen the germinal matrix vasculature. However, TGFβ is a ubiquitously expressed growth factor; and there is no available strategy to increase the expression selectively of this molecule in the germinal matrix vasculature.

Consistent with these studies, another report has shown that there is no significant difference in the expression of Collagen I, II, and IV between the germinal matrix and other brain regions of premature human infants.[32] However, in beagle puppies, immunoreactivity of laminin and collagen V in the germinal matrix is greater at post-natal d4 compared to d1, and indomethacin treatment further increases the intensity of immunosignals for laminin and collagen V in the germinal matrix[33,34]; this suggests that deficiencies of these 2 molecules in germinal matrix vasculature of beagle puppies might contribute to the vascular weakness of this brain region. Together, the constituents of the basal lamina add to the stability of the vasculature; and a deficiency of fibronectin level in the basal lamina of the human germinal matrix might contribute to the vascular fragility of this brain region.

Reduced glial fibrillary acidic protein expression in the astrocyte end-feet

Astrocytes extend processes from the soma in all directions that cover the blood vessels. These astrocytic processes are known as end-feet, which unsheathe 99% of the BBB endothelium in adult brains.[35] The astrocytes contribute to the development of the BBB and regulate its function. Specifically, they provide structural integrity and control permeability of the BBB.[12] Moreover, they are essential for function of neurons and the neurovascular unit. Astrocyte end-feet contain intermediate filaments, which form the cytoskeleton of the astrocytes. Glial fibrillary acidic protein (GFAP) is a key component of these intermediate filaments. Studies in autopsy materials from fetuses and premature infants have shown that perivascular coverage by GFAP+ astrocyte end-feet is less in the germinal matrix compared to the cerebral cortex and the embryonic white matter (see **Fig. 3**B).[36] Because GFAP provides structural integrity and mechanical strength to the astrocyte end-feet,[37–39] fragility of the germinal matrix vasculature can also be ascribed to reduced GFAP expression in the astrocyte end-feet.

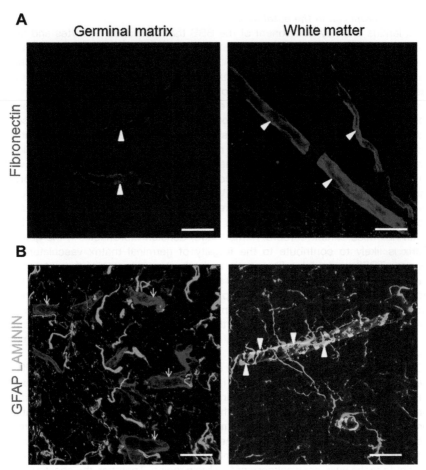

Fig. 3. Germinal matrix vasculature is deficient in fibronectin and lack GFAP+ astrocyte end-feet coverage. (*A*) Representative immunofluorescence of cryosection from germinal matrix and white matter of a 24-week premature human infant labeled with fibronectin (*red*)-specific antibody. Fibronectin is strongly expressed in the white matter, whereas it is weakly expressed in the germinal matrix (*arrowheads*). Scale bar; 20 μm. (*B*) Cryosection from germinal matrix and white matter of a 24-week premature infant was double labeled with CD34-specific (*endothelium, red*) and GFAP-specific (*astrocyte, green*) antibodies. GFAP positive astrocyte end-feet are intimately associated with the outer endothelial surface in the white matter (*arrowheads*). However, GFAP positive astrocytes are not covering endothelium in the germinal matrix (*arrows*). Scale bar, 20 μm.

Overall Mechanism of Germinal Matrix Vascular Fragility

Germinal matrix exhibits rapid angiogenesis, in contrast to the other brain regions. The accelerated endothelial proliferation of this brain region is triggered by high levels of vascular endothelial growth factor (VEGF) and angiopoeitin-2 and reduced expression of TGF-β (**Fig. 4**).[13] Because hypoxia is a key stimulant of these growth factors,[40] we have evaluated hypoxia-inducible factor-1α and have performed hypoxyprobe test. The author and his colleagues have noted that hypoxia-inducible factor-1α levels are elevated in the human germinal matrix compared to the cerebral cortex and white

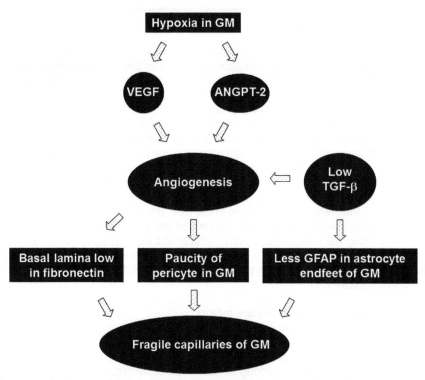

Fig. 4. Mechanisms underlying fragility of germinal matrix vasculature: hypoxic germinal matrix triggers upregulation of VEGF and angiopoieitn-2 expression. These growth factors induce angiogenesis. The angiogenic vessels of the germinal matrix exhibit paucity of pericytes and deficiency of fibronectin in immature basal lamina. Additionally, astrocyte endfeet in the germinal matrix vasculature display reduced expression of GFAP. These factors contribute to the fragility of the germinal matrix.

matter (unpublished data). In addition, hypoxyprobe [1-(2-hydroxy-3-piperidinyl)pro-pyl 2-nitroimidazole hydrochloride] test shows lower oxygen gradient in the germinal matrix compared to the adjacent white matter.[10] It seems that oxygen demand and utilization of this brain region is high as a result of its high metabolic activity. Indeed, germinal matrix harbors neuronal and glial precursor cells, which are in various phases of proliferation, migration, and maturation. Angiogenic vessels in the germinal matrix are naked endothelial tubes exhibiting paucity of pericytes and immature basal lamina low in fibronectin. In addition, GFAP is weakly expressed in the astrocyte end-feet. Together, a scarcity of pericytes, low fibronectin levels in the basement membrane, and reduced GFAP expression in the astrocyte end-feet contributes to the weakness of the germinal matrix BBB and to the vulnerability to hemorrhage. Importantly, IVH develops in the first 3 days of post-natal life, and premature infants are relatively immune to hemorrhage after this period irrespective of the gestational age. This reduced propensity to hemorrhage after 3 days in preterm infants might be because of an increase in blood and tissue oxygen concentration after birth suppressing VEGF, angiopoetin-2 levels, and the angiogenesis. A shutdown in angiogenesis shortly after birth would mature the angiogenic vessels, making them resistant to rupture despite fluctuation in the cerebral blood flow (CBF).

Disturbance in CBF

Fluctuation in the CBF

In premature infants with respiratory distress syndrome, 2 patterns of CBF velocity have been demarcated: one, stable pattern with equal peak and trough of systolic and diastolic flow velocity and other, fluctuating waveform with continuous alteration in systolic and diastolic flow velocity.[41,42] Fluctuating CBF velocity during the first day of life strongly correlates with the occurrence of IVH and more importantly, elimination of this fluctuation in the CBF by intravenous pancuronium infusion markedly reduces the incidence of IVH.[41–43] Because these studies were done in mid 1980s, it is possible that fluctuation in the CBF was related to the use of intermittent mandatory ventilation, giving rise to asynchrony between infant and ventilator breath, which can be eradicated by the use of paralytic agents. However, most of the neonatal units currently use synchronized ventilator modes, which minimizes infants "fighting" the ventilator and thus reduces fluctuations in the CBF velocity.[44] Moreover, routine use of neuromuscular blocking agents in ventilated infants is not recommended because of uncertain long-term neurologic adverse effects of these agents. Other factors that contribute to the fluctuation of CBF velocity include patent ductus arteriosus, hypercarbia, hypotension, severe respiratory distress syndrome, and rapid infusion of sodium bicarbonate (**Table 1**).[43,45–47]

Impaired autoregulation in premature infants

Cerebral autoregulation is the capability of the blood vessels in the brain to retain a constant CBF in spite of fluctuations in the blood pressure. The pressure passivity—impaired autoregulation—of CBF is associated with lower gestational age and birth weight and is commonly noted in sick, ventilated, and hemodynamically unstable premature infants. Cerebral autoregulation has been evaluated in preterm infants using several methods, including Doppler, xenon clearance, near infrared spectroscopy (NIRS), and spatially resolved spectroscopy (SRS).[48–51] Although these techniques involve continuous and repeated monitoring, the results of these studies have not been consistent. It was reported that NIRS identifies infants with impairment in cerebral autoregulation and that this is associated with high likelihood of severe IVH.[52] Subsequent investigators realized continuous monitoring of CBF over extended period, because cerebral blood pressure passivity is not an "all-or-none phenomena", but it can occur over varied time intervals.[49] In very low birth weight (VLBW) infants, continuous monitoring of cerebral perfusion by NIRS and mean arterial blood pressure has shown that CBF is pressure passive for an average of 20% of the time; and there is strong correlation between pressure passive state and hypotension with lower birth weight and gestational age.[49] Additionally, there is no association between impaired autoregulation and the occurrence of IVH.[49] Another subsequent report, in which CBF was measured by SRS, showed strong association between diminished autoregulation and subsequent mortality; however, impaired autoregulation was not associated with the development of IVH.[50] In a recent study on continuous monitoring of VLBW using NIRS, it has been shown that the correlation of regional cerebral oxygen saturation and mean blood pressure indicates pressure passivity of the CBF, and these metrics may predict the occurrence of IVH.[53] Hence, the role of impaired autoregulation in the development of IVH needs further evaluation.

Perinatal risk factors for IVH, fluctuation in the CBF, and germinal matrix fragility

Several risk factors are associated with IVH, which directly or indirectly increase either the fluctuation in the CBF or the fragility of the germinal matrix microvasculature (see **Table 1**). Hypotension is common in premature infants; however, there is conflicting

Table 1
Neonatal risk factors in the pathogenesis of IVH

Major Pathogenic Mechanism	Putative Mechanisms[a]	Risk Factors	Preventive Measures
Disturbance in CBF	Fluctuation in CBF	• Suctioning and handling	• No routine suctioning
		• Hypercarbia, hypoxia, acidosis	• Optimize ventilation
		• Asynchrony between infants and ventilator breathe	• Synchronized ventilation by the use of assist control or synchronized mandatory ventilation modes
		• Severe RDS	
		• Patent ductus arteriosis	• Indomethacin/ ibuprofen
		• Rapid infusion of NaHCO$_3$	• Slow infusion over extended period
	High cerebral venous pressure	• Pneumothorax, high ventilator pressure	• Gentle ventilation
		• Prolonged labor	• Individualized approach as appropriate
	Abnormal blood pressure	• Hypotension	• As appropriate for the infant
		• Hypertension	
		• Sepsis	
		• Dehydration	
	Pressure passive circulation	Extreme prematurity and low birth weight (<1000 g)	• As appropriate for the infant
		Clinically unstable resulting from respiratory compromise, sepsis, or other reasons	
Inherent fragility of germinal matrix vasculature	Might be worsened by an inflammatory injury to the BBB	Hypoxic ischemic insult Sepsis	Prenatal GCs stabilize the microvasculature by increasing: 1. Pericyte coverage 2. GFAP expression in astrocytes 3. Fibronectin in basal lamina
Platelet and coagulation disturbances	Hemostatic failure	Thrombocytopenia Disseminated intravascular coagulopathy	Replacement of blood products

[a] Correlation of mechanisms with the risk factors and preventive measures is based on available evidence and author's speculations.

data on the association between IVH and hypotension.[49,54–57] A correlation between hypotension and CBF seems to be complex, and hypotension may not indicate reduced or disturbed CBF.[58] An increase in central venous pressure (CVP) might contribute to the onset of IVH. Indeed, CVP is elevated in pneumothorax and in infants on mechanical ventilation using high mean airway pressure. Moreover, germinal matrix hemorrhage has been demonstrated to be mainly of venous origin in a study on autopsy materials from premature human infants.[59] Prolonged positive pressure ventilation is also known to increase BBB permeability.[60] A rapid infusion of sodium bicarbonate might contribute to the development of IVH. It is possible that a rapid infusion of a large dose of sodium bicarbonate will increase serum osmolality and arterial CO_2 resulting in vasodilation and rupture of the microvasculature in the germinal matrix. However, there is disagreement on a causative role of bicarbonate in the development of IVH.[61–63] Other risk factors for IVH include early onset sepsis, maternal chorioamnionitis, development of respiratory distress syndrome, recurrent tracheal suctioning, prolonged labor, hypoxia, hypercarbia, and others (see **Table 1**). It appears that most of these conditions contribute to the occurrence of IVH by disturbing the CBF. However, sepsis and hypoxia-ischemia might cause molecular and morphologic changes in the microvasculature, which may weaken the vessels of the germinal matrix. Coagulopathy does not seem to play a key role in pathogenesis of IVH, but can modify the risk and severity of IVH. A Cochrane systematic review showed that vitamin K administration did not affect the incidence of IVH.[64] Fresh frozen plasma administration has also been tried without success.[65] However, several studies have reported that thrombocytopenia is a risk factor for IVH.[66–68]

Genetic Factors and IVH

Mutations in the type IV procollagen gene, COL4A1, are associated with IVH in dizygotic preterm twins.[69] Because inflammatory mediators and coagulation factors might have a role in the development of IVH, polymorphisms of proinflammatory cytokines and mutations in the coagulation factors have been evaluated as candidate genes that modify the severity and risk of IVH. Mutations in factor V Leiden, prothrombin G20210A, and interleukin (IL)-1 beta have been implicated in the development of grade I and II IVH.[70–72] Polymorphisms of IL-6 and TNFα are proposed as genetic modifiers of IVH risk.[73,74] In addition, polymorphism of methylenetetrahydrofolate reductase (MTHFR) gene has been reported in infants with IVH. C677T polymorphism in MTHFR enzyme is associated with high plasma homocysteine levels, which is a known risk factor for vascular disease.[75] Together, mutations in coagulation, thrombophilia, and inflammation-related genes might contribute to the development of IVH.

PREVENTION OF IVH
Rationale of Preventive Therapies

Because IVH is primarily attributed to increased vascular fragility and disturbance in CBF, the strategies should be directed to strengthening the germinal matrix vasculature and to stabilizing the CBF. Germinal matrix has a subset of vessels that are angiogenic, immature, and lack pericytes, and they thrive because of high levels of VEGF and angiopoietin-2.[13,22] These blood vessels exhibit high fragility and propensity to bleed. It appears that the immature neovasculature are pruned within a few days of premature delivery, thus stabilizing the germinal matrix microvasculature. This is because oxygen concentration increases above intrauterine level shortly after birth, which possibly downregulates the VEGF levels in the germinal matrix. Indeed, preterm infants become relatively immune to the development of IVH after post-natal day 3. Prenatal glucocorticoids (GCs) or antenatal celecoxib also downregulate VEGF levels, which leads to apoptosis of naked endothelial cells, lacking pericyte coverage.[13,76] Hence, prenatal use of angiogenic inhibitors—GCs or celecoxib—trims the nascent vessels, but not the functional vessels protected by pericytes, thereby orchestrating a vascular network consisting of stable blood vessels.[22,76–78] Fluctuations in the CBF are related to routine procedures performed in neonatal units, such as suctioning, handling, placing intravenous lines, and common problems associated with prematurity, including respiratory distress syndrome, patent ductus arteriosus, apneic episodes, seizures, hypoxemia, hypercarbia, and others (see **Table 1**). Hence, fluctuations in the CBF can be minimized by reducing the stimulation to the infant and appropriately managing the common complications of prematurity. Overall preventive approach is listed in **Table 2**.

Prenatal Pharmacologic Treatments to Prevent IVH

Glucocorticoids
In the United States, the preterm birth rate is about 12.5%, and approximately 75% women in premature labor with gestational age of less than 34 weeks are treated with either betamethasone or dexamethasone.[79] Several studies have confirmed that prenatal GC reduces both severity and incidence of IVH.[80,81] The beneficial effect of prenatal GC is attributed to stabilization of the microvasculature of the germinal matrix and alleviation of disturbance in the CBF. Prenatal GC, as discussed earlier, suppresses angiogenesis in the germinal matrix microvasculature and thus trims the nascent and fragile vasculature, which are vulnerable to hemorrhage. Thus, GC exposure stabilizes the BBB of the germinal matrix, and infants treated with prenatal GC exhibit greater pericyte coverage, higher fibronectin levels, and more GFAP in the astrocyte end-feet of the blood vessels of the germinal matrix compared to untreated infants.[22,29,76] Moreover, it reduces the incidence and severity of respiratory distress syndrome, which might minimize fluctuation in the CBF. Post-natal betamethasone also reduces cerebral flow velocity possibly by exerting a vasoconstrictor effect on cerebral vessels in preterm infants.[82] Similarly, prenatal betamethasone has been shown to reduce CBF by increasing cerebrovascular resistance in fetal sheep model.[83]

The optimal effects of prenatal GC have been observed after a complete course of 2 doses of betamethasone or 4 doses of dexamethasone when administered within a week of delivery of the premature newborn.[84] However, benefits have also been noted with incomplete courses of GCs.[85] Comparison of the 2 GCs—betamethasone and dexamethasone—has not conclusively shown superiority of one over the other and

Table 2 Prevention of intraventricular hemorrhage	
Prenatal interventions	a. Prevent preterm delivery b. Maternal transport to regional neonatal center c. Prenatal GCs d. Agents of unproven benefit: Prenatal phenobarbitone, vitamin K, and magnesium sulfate
Care during infant delivery	Optimize obstetric care and prevent prolonged labor
Post-natal interventions	a. Delay cord clamping and optimize neonatal resuscitation b. Minimize handling and suctioning, synchronized and gentle ventilation, prompt treatment of patent ductus arteriosus, maintaining normal O_2 and CO_2, preventing apneic episodes and seizures c. Correction of coagulation and bleeding disorders d. Indomethacin: Reduces IVH, but does not enhance long-term outcome e. Agents of unproven benefit: Phenobarbitone, vitamin E, etamsylate

clinicians should choose whatever is available.[85] Betamethasone-exposed infants exhibit less severe respiratory distress syndrome, but more IVH, compared to prenatal dexamethasone–treated infants.[84,86] There has been concern that prenatal dexamethasone might increase the incidence of periventricular leukomalacia.[87] However, a subsequent study on a larger population clearly showed that there is no difference in the incidence of cystic PVL between dexamethasone- and betamethasone-exposed infants.[88] This study also noted that both GCs are equally efficacious in preventing severe IVH; however there is a trend toward better efficacy for dexamethasone compared to betamethasone.[88] Importantly, prenatal betamethasone is associated with a reduced risk for neonatal death compared with dexamethasone.[88] Together, there is no recommendation for the use of one GC over the other, despite multiple clinical trials undertaken. Another key issue related to the use of prenatal steroid is single versus repeated course. Unfortunately, there is no agreement among the experts on the advantage of single versus multiple course of GCs.[85] There are concerns that multiple course of prenatal GC might have adverse effects on brain and other organ systems.

Phenobarbital and magnesium sulfate

As etiopathogenesis of IVH was more mysterious in 80s than now, several agents without a concrete rationale were tried to prevent IVH. Phenobarbital and vitamin K are important to mention here, as these medications attracted the attention of investigators. Initial studies showed some protective effect of phenobarbital; however, subsequent clinical trials failed to confirm the protective effect of phenobarbital in preventing IVH.[89–93] Maternal treatment of vitamin K or magnesium sulfate to prevent IVH did not demonstrate any benefit either.[64,94–96]

Post-natal Pharmacologic Treatment to Prevent IVH

Indomethacin

Indomethacin, commonly used in premature neonates to close patent ductus arteriosus, has been shown to prevent IVH in several clinical trials. Indomethacin, a nonselective cyclo-oxygenase (COX) inhibitor, suppresses both COX1 and COX2 isoforms to reduce prostaglandin synthesis. It attenuates cerebral vascular hyperemic responses induced by hypoxia, hypercapnia, hypertension, and asphyxia.[97,98] It reduces alterations in the BBB permeability after cerebral ischemia and promotes maturation of basement membrane by increasing the expression of laminin and collagen V.[33,34,99] The maturation of basal lamina on indomethacin treatment can be attributed to COX2 inhibition, which suppresses angiogenesis and matures the germinal matrix vasculature.[13]

In several clinical trials, indomethacin treatment has shown short-term benefit of reducing the incidence of IVH.[100–102] Secondary analyses of a multicenter study based on gender have shown that indomethacin treatment reduces the rate of IVH in male infants, but not in female infants.[103] However, another study on a larger population of preterm infants showed just a weak differential effect of indomethacin by sex.[104] Because indomethacin reduces the occurrence of IVH, it was anticipated that this treatment would improve the neurodevelopment outcome of the infants. However, indomethacin treatment failed to reduce the rate of cerebral palsy, deafness, and blindness on long-term follow-up.[105,106] A meta-analysis of 19 clinical trials also did not show any improvement in the long-term outcome of indomethacin-treated infants.[107,108] Together, indomethacin prophylaxis has immediate benefits of reduction in symptomatic patent ductus arteriosus and severe IVH; however, this does not affect long-term neurodevelopmental outcomes. Hence, indomethacin is not recommended for routine prophylaxis against IVH. However, indomethacin is still being used in some neonatal units depending on clinical circumstances and personal preferences.

Ibuprofen is another nonselective COX inhibitor that has shown promise in closing patent ductus arteriosus. This compound does not reduce CBF, in contrast to indomethacin. More importantly, ibuprofen does not prevent IVH in premature infants.[109,110]

Other clinical trials of unproven benefit

Post-natal phenobarbital has been used in several clinical trials to prevent IVH in 1980s, based on the premise that it might reduce abrupt changes in the CBF during tracheal suctioning, handling, and motor activity.[111–115] However, phenobarbital did not reduce the incidence of IVH significantly. Another agent that drew the attention of investigators in 1980s was etamsylate. This compound reduces prostaglandin synthesis and promotes platelet adhesiveness. In addition, etamsylate induces polymerization of hyaluronic acid in the vascular basement membrane, which might promote homeostasis and minimize bleeding. However, large clinical trials showed that etamsylate neither reduced the incidence of IVH nor enhanced the neurodevelopmental outcome of premature infants.[116,117] Pathogenesis of IVH has always puzzled the investigators and thus, a role of free radicals in the etiology of IVH cannot be totally excluded. Hence, vitamin E—a potent antioxidant—has been tried to prevent IVH in preterm infants without appreciable benefits.[118,119] To address the need to minimize asynchrony between infant and ventilator breath, pancuronium has been tried in 1980s and was found to reduce fluctuation in CBF and also the incidence of IVH.[42] A relatively recent meta-analysis identified 6 clinical trials in which the use of neuromuscular blocking agent during mechanical ventilation was compared with no paralysis in newborn infants.[120] It was concluded that neuromuscular paralyses with pancuronium reduced the rate of IVH. However, owing to complications associated with neuromuscular paralysis, routine use of pancuronium in extremely premature infants has not been recommended. The role of activated recombinant factor VII (rVIIa) in promoting coagulation is promising, and it has been hypothesized that early (prophylactic) administration of rVIIa to extremely premature infants would reduce the incidence of IVH. However, IVH is not primarily a coagulation disorder, and this hypothesis does not seem to be logical.

Optimizing Care of Fetuses and Premature Newborns

Prenatal interventions

Interhospital transport of extremely premature infants is associated with increased incidence and severity of IVH. This correlation has remained constant in recent years.[121] Hence, pregnant mothers in preterm labor should be transported to a tertiary care center specializing in high-risk delivery. Prolonged labor might increase the risk of IVH and should be managed appropriately. Data on the incidence of IVH in cesarean section versus vaginal delivery are inconsistent,[122,123] and thus, infants are delivered based on the decisions made by obstetricians.

Post-natal interventions

There is no specific recommendation about neonatal resuscitation of premature infants to prevent IVH. However, restoration of normal oxygenation and ventilation immediately at birth is important as hypoxemia and hypercarbia can cause fluctuation in the CBF, which might contribute to IVH. Although preventing metabolic acidosis and accomplishing normal perfusion is important, a rapid sodium bicarbonate infusion might add to the risk of IVH. After infants have been transferred to the neonatal unit, gentle and synchronized ventilation, prompt closure of ductus arteriosus, and maintenance of normal O_2 and CO_2 levels in the arterial blood are important preventive measures. Preventing pneumothorax, apneic episodes, seizures, as well as minimizing tracheal suctioning and handling will prevent disturbances in the CBF. Reducing stimulation and gentle caretaking decreases the incidence of IVH.[124] Effect of surfactant treatment on the development of IVH is unclear. Use of high-frequency ventilators does not increase the risk of IVH,[125] and therefore, an individualized approach in selection of appropriate ventilator should be pursued.

Together, the incidence of IVH has remained unchanged over the last couple of decades, despite advances in care of newborns. Use of prenatal GCs remains the most effective strategy in the prevention of IVH.

SUMMARY

IVH is a major complication of prematurity. IVH usually initiates in the periventricular germinal matrix and progresses to IVH on the rupture of the underlying ependyma. The pathogenesis of IVH is ascribed to the intrinsic fragility of germinal matrix vasculature and to fluctuations in the CBF. The germinal matrix exhibits accelerated angiogenesis, which orchestrates formation of nascent vessels that lack pericytes, display immature basal lamina low in fibronectin, and have astrocyte end-feet coverage deficient in GFAP. These morphologic and molecular factors contribute to the fragility of the germinal matrix vasculature. Importantly, pressure passive circulation is frequent in the premature infants, and CBF fluctuates with the changes in a) internal milieu (O_2, CO_2, pH, osmolarity), b) central venous pressure, c) blood pressure and d) cardiac output secondary to inadequate ventilation, pneumothorax, severe lung disease, hemodynamic instability, sepsis, dehydration, patent ductus arteriosus, frequent suctioning, increased handling, and other factors. Recent studies have suggested roles of genes encoding coagulation factors, inflammatory cytokines, and collagen in the pathogenesis of IVH. Prenatal GCs are the most effective in preventing IVH and are the standard care. There is no long-term advantage of using post-natal indomethacin. There is a need of improved therapy to prevent IVH and its neurodevelopmental sequelae. Therapies designed to enhance the stability of the germinal matrix vasculature and reduce fluctuation of CBF might lead to more effective strategies in preventing IVH.

ACKNOWLEDGMENTS

Authors thank Drs Laura Ment and Barabara Stonstreet for the critical review of the article and Joanne Abrahams for the assistance with images.

REFERENCES

1. Fanaroff AA, Stoll BJ, Wright LL, et al. Trends in neonatal morbidity and mortality for very low birthweight infants. Am J Obstet Gynecol 2007;196(2):147.e1–8.
2. Jain NJ, Kruse LK, Demissie K, et al. Impact of mode of delivery on neonatal complications: trends between 1997 and 2005. J Matern Fetal Neonatal Med 2009;22(6):491–500.
3. Sherlock RL, Anderson PJ, Doyle LW, et al. Neurodevelopmental sequelae of intraventricular haemorrhage at 8 years of age in a regional cohort of ELBW/very preterm infants. Early Hum Dev 2005;81(11):909–16.
4. Luu TM, Ment LR, Schneider KC, et al. Lasting effects of preterm birth and neonatal brain hemorrhage at 12 years of age. Pediatrics 2009;123(3):1037–44.
5. Indredavik MS, Vik T, Evensen KA, et al. Perinatal risk and psychiatric outcome in adolescents born preterm with very low birth weight or term small for gestational age. J Dev Behav Pediatr 2010;31(4):286–94.

6. Nosarti C, Giouroukou E, Micali N, et al. Impaired executive functioning in young adults born very preterm. J Int Neuropsychol Soc 2007;13(4):571–81.

7. Whitaker AH, Feldman JF, Lorenz JM, et al. Neonatal head ultrasound abnormalities in preterm infants and adolescent psychiatric disorders. Arch Gen Psychiatry 2011;68(7):742–52.

8. Rushing S, Ment LR. Preterm birth: a cost benefit analysis. Semin Perinatol 2004;28(6):444–50.

9. McCrea HJ, Ment LR. The diagnosis, management, and postnatal prevention of intraventricular hemorrhage in the preterm neonate. Clin Perinatol 2008;35(4): 777–92, vii.

10. Ballabh P. Intraventricular hemorrhage in premature infants: mechanism of disease. Pediatr Res 2010;67(1):1–8.

11. Ballabh P, Braun A, Nedergaard M. The blood-brain barrier: an overview: structure, regulation, and clinical implications. Neurobiol Dis 2004;16(1):1–13.

12. Persidsky Y, Ramirez SH, Haorah J, et al. Blood-brain barrier: structural components and function under physiologic and pathologic conditions. J Neuroimmune Pharmacol 2006;1(3):223–36.

13. Ballabh P, Xu H, Hu F, et al. Angiogenic inhibition reduces germinal matrix hemorrhage. Nat Med 2007;13(4):477–85.

14. Ballabh P, Braun A, Nedergaard M. Anatomic analysis of blood vessels in germinal matrix, cerebral cortex, and white matter in developing infants. Pediatr Res 2004;56(1):117–24.

15. Sa-Pereira I, Brites D, Brito MA. Neurovascular unit: a focus on pericytes. Mol Neurobiol 2012;45(2):327–47.

16. Balabanov R, Dore-Duffy P. Role of the CNS microvascular pericyte in the blood-brain barrier. J Neurosci Res 1998;53(6):637–44.

17. Jain RK. Molecular regulation of vessel maturation. Nat Med 2003;9(6):685–93.

18. Armulik A, Genove G, Mae M, et al. Pericytes regulate the blood-brain barrier. Nature 2010;468(7323):557–61.

19. Hirschi KK, D'Amore PA. Control of angiogenesis by the pericyte: molecular mechanisms and significance. EXS 1997;79:419–28.

20. Gaengel K, Genove G, Armulik A, et al. Endothelial-mural cell signaling in vascular development and angiogenesis. Arterioscler Thromb Vasc Biol 2009; 29(5):630–8.

21. Lindahl P, Johansson BR, Leveen P, et al. Pericyte loss and microaneurysm formation in PDGF-B-deficient mice. Science 1997;277(5323):242–5.

22. Braun A, Xu H, Hu F, et al. Paucity of pericytes in germinal matrix vasculature of premature infants. J Neurosci 2007;27(44):12012–24.

23. Stratman AN, Davis GE. Endothelial cell-pericyte interactions stimulate basement membrane matrix assembly: influence on vascular tube remodeling, maturation, and stabilization. Microsc Microanal 2012;18(1):68–80.

24. Tilling T, Engelbertz C, Decker S, et al. Expression and adhesive properties of basement membrane proteins in cerebral capillary endothelial cell cultures. Cell Tissue Res 2002;310(1):19–29.

25. Hallmann R, Horn N, Selg M, et al. Expression and function of laminins in the embryonic and mature vasculature. Physiol Rev 2005;85(3):979–1000.

26. Forsberg E, Kjellen L. Heparan sulfate: lessons from knockout mice. J Clin Invest 2001;108(2):175–80.

27. Gould DB, Phalan FC, Breedveld GJ, et al. Mutations in Col4a1 cause perinatal cerebral hemorrhage and porencephaly. Science 2005;308(5725): 1167–71.

28. George EL, Georges-Labouesse EN, Patel-King RS, et al. Defects in mesoderm, neural tube and vascular development in mouse embryos lacking fibronectin. Development 1993;119(4):1079–91.

29. Xu H, Hu F, Sado Y, et al. Maturational changes in laminin, fibronectin, collagen IV, and perlecan in germinal matrix, cortex, and white matter and effect of beta-methasone. J Neurosci Res 2008;86(7):1482–500.

30. Mao Y, Schwarzbauer JE. Fibronectin fibrillogenesis, a cell-mediated matrix assembly process. Matrix Biol 2005;24(6):389–99.

31. Sottile J, Hocking DC, Langenbach KJ. Fibronectin polymerization stimulates cell growth by RGD-dependent and -independent mechanisms. J Cell Sci 2000;113(Pt 23):4287–99.

32. Anstrom JA, Thore CR, Moody DM, et al. Morphometric assessment of collagen accumulation in germinal matrix vessels of premature human neonates. Neuropathol Appl Neurobiol 2005;31(2):181–90.

33. Ment LR, Stewart WB, Ardito TA, et al. Beagle pup germinal matrix maturation studies. Stroke 1991;22(3):390–5.

34. Ment LR, Stewart WB, Ardito TA, et al. Indomethacin promotes germinal matrix microvessel maturation in the newborn beagle pup. Stroke 1992;23(8):1132–7.

35. Hawkins BT, Davis TP. The blood-brain barrier/neurovascular unit in health and disease. Pharmacol Rev 2005;57(2):173–85.

36. El-Khoury N, Braun A, Hu F, et al. Astrocyte end-feet in germinal matrix, cerebral cortex, and white matter in developing infants. Pediatr Res 2006;59(5):673–9.

37. Liedtke W, Edelmann W, Bieri PL, et al. GFAP is necessary for the integrity of CNS white matter architecture and long-term maintenance of myelination. Neuron 1996;17(4):607–15.

38. Trimmer PA, Reier PJ, Oh TH, et al. An ultrastructural and immunocytochemical study of astrocytic differentiation in vitro: changes in the composition and distribution of the cellular cytoskeleton. J Neuroimmunol 1982;2(3–4):235–60.

39. Ribotta MG, Menet V, Privat A. Glial scar and axonal regeneration in the CNS: lessons from GFAP and vimentin transgenic mice. Acta Neurochir Suppl 2004; 89:87–92.

40. Mu D, Jiang X, Sheldon RA, et al. Regulation of hypoxia-inducible factor 1alpha and induction of vascular endothelial growth factor in a rat neonatal stroke model. Neurobiol Dis 2003;14(3):524–34.

41. Perlman JM, McMenamin JB, Volpe JJ. Fluctuating cerebral blood-flow velocity in respiratory-distress syndrome. Relation to the development of intraventricular hemorrhage. N Engl J Med 1983;309(4):204–9.

42. Perlman JM, Goodman S, Kreusser KL, et al. Reduction in intraventricular hemorrhage by elimination of fluctuating cerebral blood-flow velocity in preterm infants with respiratory distress syndrome. N Engl J Med 1985;312(21): 1353–7.

43. Van Bel F, Van de Bor M, Stijnen T, et al. Aetiological role of cerebral blood-flow alterations in development and extension of peri-intraventricular haemorrhage. Dev Med Child Neurol 1987;29(5):601–14.

44. Rennie JM, South M, Morley CJ. Cerebral blood flow velocity variability in infants receiving assisted ventilation. Arch Dis Child 1987;62(12):1247–51.

45. Mullaart RA, Hopman JC, De Haan AF, et al. Cerebral blood flow fluctuation in low-risk preterm newborns. Early Hum Dev 1992;30(1):41–8.

46. Mullaart RA, Hopman JC, Rotteveel JJ, et al. Cerebral blood flow fluctuation in neonatal respiratory distress and periventricular haemorrhage. Early Hum Dev 1994;37(3):179–85.

47. Coughtrey H, Rennie JM, Evans DH. Variability in cerebral blood flow velocity: observations over one minute in preterm babies. Early Hum Dev 1997;47(1): 63–70.
48. du Plessis AJ. Cerebrovascular injury in premature infants: current understanding and challenges for future prevention. Clin Perinatol 2008;35(4):609–41, v.
49. Soul JS, Hammer PE, Tsuji M, et al. Fluctuating pressure-passivity is common in the cerebral circulation of sick premature infants. Pediatr Res 2007;61(4): 467–73.
50. Wong FY, Leung TS, Austin T, et al. Impaired autoregulation in preterm infants identified by using spatially resolved spectroscopy. Pediatrics 2008;121(3): e604–11.
51. Caicedo A, De Smet D, Naulaers G, et al. Cerebral tissue oxygenation and regional oxygen saturation can be used to study cerebral autoregulation in prematurely born infants. Pediatr Res 2011;69(6):548–53.
52. Tsuji M, Saul JP, du Plessis A, et al. Cerebral intravascular oxygenation correlates with mean arterial pressure in critically ill premature infants. Pediatrics 2000;106(4):625–32.
53. Alderliesten T, Lemmers PM, Smarius JJ, et al. Cerebral oxygenation, extraction, and autoregulation in very preterm infants who develop peri-intraventricular hemorrhage. J Pediatr 2013;162(4):698–704.e2.
54. Weindling AM, Wilkinson AR, Cook J, et al. Perinatal events which precede periventricular haemorrhage and leukomalacia in the newborn. Br J Obstet Gynaecol 1985;92(12):1218–23.
55. Muller AM, Morales C, Briner J, et al. Loss of CO2 reactivity of cerebral blood flow is associated with severe brain damage in mechanically ventilated very low birth weight infants. Eur J Paediatr Neurol 1997;1(5–6):157–63.
56. Watkins AM, West CR, Cooke RW. Blood pressure and cerebral haemorrhage and ischaemia in very low birthweight infants. Early Hum Dev 1989;19(2):103–10.
57. Miall-Allen VM, de Vries LS, Whitelaw AG. Mean arterial blood pressure and neonatal cerebral lesions. Arch Dis Child 1987;62(10):1068–9.
58. Lightburn MH, Gauss CH, Williams DK, et al. Cerebral blood flow velocities in extremely low birth weight infants with hypotension and infants with normal blood pressure. J Pediatr 2009;154(6):824–8.
59. Ghazi-Birry HS, Brown WR, Moody DM, et al. Human germinal matrix: venous origin of hemorrhage and vascular characteristics. AJNR Am J Neuroradiol 1997;18(2):219–29.
60. Stonestreet BS, McKnight AJ, Sadowska G, et al. Effects of duration of positive-pressure ventilation on blood-brain barrier function in premature lambs. J Appl Physiol 2000;88(5):1672–7.
61. Van de Bor M, Van Bel F, Lineman R, et al. Perinatal factors and periventricular-intraventricular hemorrhage in preterm infants. Am J Dis Child 1986;140(11): 1125–30.
62. Wigglesworth JS, Keith IH, Girling DJ, et al. Hyaline membrane disease, alkali, and intraventricular haemorrhage. Arch Dis Child 1976;51(10):755–62.
63. Dykes FD, Lazzara A, Ahmann P, et al. Intraventricular hemorrhage: a prospective evaluation of etiopathogenesis. Pediatrics 1980;66(1):42–9.
64. Crowther CA, Crosby DD, Henderson-Smart DJ. Vitamin K prior to preterm birth for preventing neonatal periventricular haemorrhage. Cochrane Database Syst Rev 2010;(1):CD000229.
65. Beverley DW, Pitts-Tucker TJ, Congdon PJ, et al. Prevention of intraventricular haemorrhage by fresh frozen plasma. Arch Dis Child 1985;60(8):710–3.

66. Van de Bor M, Briet E, Van Bel F, et al. Hemostasis and periventricular-intraventricular hemorrhage of the newborn. Am J Dis Child 1986;140(11): 1131–4.

67. Lupton BA, Hill A, Whitfield MF, et al. Reduced platelet count as a risk factor for intraventricular hemorrhage. Am J Dis Child 1988;142(11):1222–4.

68. Shirahata A, Nakamura T, Shimono M, et al. Blood coagulation findings and the efficacy of factor XIII concentrate in premature infants with intracranial hemorrhages. Thromb Res 1990;57(5):755–63.

69. Bilguvar K, DiLuna ML, Bizzarro MJ, et al. COL4A1 mutation in preterm intraventricular hemorrhage. J Pediatr 2009;155(5):743–5.

70. Debus O, Koch HG, Kurlemann G, et al. Factor V Leiden and genetic defects of thrombophilia in childhood porencephaly. Arch Dis Child Fetal Neonatal Ed 1998;78(2):F121–4.

71. Gopel W, Gortner L, Kohlmann T, et al. Low prevalence of large intraventricular haemorrhage in very low birthweight infants carrying the factor V Leiden or prothrombin G20210A mutation. Acta Paediatr 2001;90(9):1021–4.

72. Ryckman KK, Feenstra B, Shaffer JR, et al. Replication of a genome-wide association study of birth weight in preterm neonates. J Pediatr 2012;160(1): 19–24.e4.

73. Gopel W, Hartel C, Ahrens P, et al. Interleukin-6-174-genotype, sepsis and cerebral injury in very low birth weight infants. Genes Immun 2006;7(1):65–8.

74. Adcock K, Hedberg C, Loggins J, et al. The TNF-alpha -308, MCP-1 -2518 and TGF-beta1 +915 polymorphisms are not associated with the development of chronic lung disease in very low birth weight infants. Genes Immun 2003;4(6): 420–6.

75. Harteman JC, Groenendaal F, van Haastert IC, et al. Atypical timing and presentation of periventricular haemorrhagic infarction in preterm infants: the role of thrombophilia. Dev Med Child Neurol 2012;54(2):140–7.

76. Vinukonda G, Dummula K, Malik S, et al. Effect of prenatal glucocorticoids on cerebral vasculature of the developing brain. Stroke 2010;41(8):1766–73.

77. Jain RK. Normalization of tumor vasculature: an emerging concept in antiangiogenic therapy. Science 2005;307(5706):58–62.

78. Winkler F, Kozin SV, Tong RT, et al. Kinetics of vascular normalization by VEGFR2 blockade governs brain tumor response to radiation: role of oxygenation, angiopoietin-1, and matrix metalloproteinases. Cancer Cell 2004;6(6):553–63.

79. Meadow WL, Bell A, Sunstein CR. Statistics, not memories: what was the standard of care for administering antenatal steroids to women in preterm labor between 1985 and 2000? Obstet Gynecol 2003;102(2):356–62.

80. Roberts D, Dalziel S. Antenatal corticosteroids for accelerating fetal lung maturation for women at risk of preterm birth. Cochrane Database Syst Rev 2006;(3):CD004454.

81. Shankaran S, Bauer CR, Bain R, et al. Relationship between antenatal steroid administration and grades III and IV intracranial hemorrhage in low birth weight infants. The NICHD Neonatal Research Network. Am J Obstet Gynecol 1995; 173(1):305–12.

82. Cambonie G, Mesnage R, Milesi C, et al. Betamethasone impairs cerebral blood flow velocities in very premature infants with severe chronic lung disease. J Pediatr 2008;152(2):270–5.

83. Lohle M, Muller T, Wicher C, et al. Betamethasone effects on fetal sheep cerebral blood flow are not dependent on maturation of cerebrovascular system and pituitary-adrenal axis. J Physiol 2005;564(Pt 2):575–88.

84. Brownfoot FC, Crowther CA, Middleton P. Different corticosteroids and regimens for accelerating fetal lung maturation for women at risk of preterm birth. Cochrane Database Syst Rev 2008;(4):CD006764.
85. Wapner R, Jobe AH. Controversy: antenatal steroids. Clin Perinatol 2011;38(3): 529–45.
86. Feldman DM, Carbone J, Belden L, et al. Betamethasone vs dexamethasone for the prevention of morbidity in very-low-birthweight neonates. Am J Obstet Gynecol 2007;197(3):284.e1–4.
87. Baud O, Foix-L'Helias L, Kaminski M, et al. Antenatal glucocorticoid treatment and cystic periventricular leukomalacia in very premature infants. N Engl J Med 1999;341(16):1190–6.
88. Lee BH, Stoll BJ, McDonald SA, et al. Adverse neonatal outcomes associated with antenatal dexamethasone versus antenatal betamethasone. Pediatrics 2006;117(5):1503–10.
89. Shankaran S, Cepeda EE, Ilagan N, et al. Pharmacokinetic basis for antenatal dosing of phenobarbital for the prevention of neonatal intracerebral hemorrhage. Dev Pharmacol Ther 1986;9(3):171–7.
90. Shankaran S, Cepeda EE, Ilagan N, et al. Antenatal phenobarbital for the prevention of neonatal intracerebral hemorrhage. Am J Obstet Gynecol 1986; 154(1):53–7.
91. Thorp JA, Ferrette-Smith D, Gaston LA, et al. Combined antenatal vitamin K and phenobarbital therapy for preventing intracranial hemorrhage in newborns less than 34 weeks' gestation. Obstet Gynecol 1995;86(1):1–8.
92. Thorp JA, Parriott J, Ferrette-Smith D, et al. Antepartum vitamin K and phenobarbital for preventing intraventricular hemorrhage in the premature newborn: a randomized, double-blind, placebo-controlled trial. Obstet Gynecol 1994; 83(1):70–6.
93. Kaempf JW, Porreco R, Molina R, et al. Antenatal phenobarbital for the prevention of periventricular and intraventricular hemorrhage: a double-blind, randomized, placebo-controlled, multihospital trial. J Pediatr 1990;117(6): 933–8.
94. Mitani M, Matsuda Y, Shimada E, et al. Short- and long-term outcomes in babies born after antenatal magnesium treatment. J Obstet Gynaecol Res 2011;37(11): 1609–14.
95. Basu SK, Chickajajur V, Lopez V, et al. Immediate clinical outcomes in preterm neonates receiving antenatal magnesium for neuroprotection. J Perinat Med 2012;40(2):185–9.
96. Perlman JM, Risser RC, Gee JB. Pregnancy-induced hypertension and reduced intraventricular hemorrhage in preterm infants. Pediatr Neurol 1997;17(1):29–33.
97. Coyle MG, Oh W, Stonestreet BS. Effects of indomethacin on brain blood flow and cerebral metabolism in hypoxic newborn piglets. Am J Physiol 1993; 264(1 Pt 2):H141–9.
98. Coyle MG, Oh W, Petersson KH, et al. Effects of indomethacin on brain blood flow, cerebral metabolism, and sagittal sinus prostanoids after hypoxia. Am J Physiol 1995;269(4 Pt 2):H1450–9.
99. Zuckerman SL, Mirro R, Armstead WM, et al. Indomethacin reduces ischemia-induced alteration of blood-brain barrier transport in piglets. Am J Physiol 1994;266(6 Pt 2):H2198–203.
100. Schmidt B, Davis P, Moddemann D, et al. Long-term effects of indomethacin prophylaxis in extremely-low-birth-weight infants. N Engl J Med 2001;344(26): 1966–72.

101. Ment LR, Oh W, Ehrenkranz RA, et al. Low-dose indomethacin and prevention of intraventricular hemorrhage: a multicenter randomized trial. Pediatrics 1994; 93(4):543–50.
102. Fowlie PW, Davis PG. Prophylactic indomethacin for preterm infants: a systematic review and meta-analysis. Arch Dis Child Fetal Neonatal Ed 2003;88(6):F464–6.
103. Ment LR, Vohr BR, Makuch RW, et al. Prevention of intraventricular hemorrhage by indomethacin in male preterm infants. J Pediatr 2004;145(6):832–4.
104. Ohlsson A, Roberts RS, Schmidt B, et al. Male/female differences in indomethacin effects in preterm infants. J Pediatr 2005;147(6):860–2.
105. Ment LR, Vohr B, Oh W, et al. Neurodevelopmental outcome at 36 months' corrected age of preterm infants in the Multicenter Indomethacin Intraventricular Hemorrhage Prevention Trial. Pediatrics 1996;98(4 Pt 1):714–8.
106. Ment LR, Vohr B, Allan W, et al. Outcome of children in the indomethacin intraventricular hemorrhage prevention trial. Pediatrics 2000;105(3 Pt 1):485–91.
107. Fowlie PW, Davis PG. Prophylactic intravenous indomethacin for preventing mortality and morbidity in preterm infants. Cochrane Database Syst Rev 2002;(3):CD000174.
108. Fowlie PW, Davis PG, McGuire W. Prophylactic intravenous indomethacin for preventing mortality and morbidity in preterm infants. Cochrane Database Syst Rev 2010;(7):CD000174.
109. Dani C, Bertini G, Pezzati M, et al. Prophylactic ibuprofen for the prevention of intraventricular hemorrhage among preterm infants: a multicenter, randomized study. Pediatrics 2005;115(6):1529–35.
110. Van Overmeire B, Allegaert K, Casaer A, et al. Prophylactic ibuprofen in premature infants: a multicentre, randomised, double-blind, placebo-controlled trial. Lancet 2004;364(9449):1945–9.
111. Bedard MP, Shankaran S, Slovis TL, et al. Effect of prophylactic phenobarbital on intraventricular hemorrhage in high-risk infants. Pediatrics 1984;73(4):435–9.
112. Donn SM, Roloff DW, Goldstein GW. Prevention of intraventricular haemorrhage in preterm infants by phenobarbitone. A controlled trial. Lancet 1981;2(8240): 215–7.
113. Anwar M, Kadam S, Hiatt IM, et al. Phenobarbitone prophylaxis of intraventricular haemorrhage. Arch Dis Child 1986;61(2):196–7.
114. Morgan ME, Massey RF, Cooke RW. Does phenobarbitone prevent periventricular hemorrhage in very low-birth-weight babies?: a controlled trial. Pediatrics 1982;70(2):186–9.
115. Kuban KC, Leviton A, Krishnamoorthy KS, et al. Neonatal intracranial hemorrhage and phenobarbital. Pediatrics 1986;77(4):443–50.
116. Cooke RW, Morgan ME. Prophylactic ethamsylate for periventricular haemorrhage. Arch Dis Child 1984;59(1):82–3.
117. Benson JW, Drayton MR, Hayward C, et al. Multicentre trial of ethamsylate for prevention of periventricular haemorrhage in very low birthweight infants. Lancet 1986;2(8519):1297–300.
118. Fish WH, Cohen M, Franzek D, et al. Effect of intramuscular vitamin E on mortality and intracranial hemorrhage in neonates of 1000 grams or less. Pediatrics 1990;85(4):578–84.
119. Brion LP, Bell EF, Raghuveer TS. Vitamin E supplementation for prevention of morbidity and mortality in preterm infants. Cochrane Database Syst Rev 2003;(4):CD003665.
120. Cools F, Offringa M. Neuromuscular paralysis for newborn infants receiving mechanical ventilation. Cochrane Database Syst Rev 2005;(2):CD002773.

121. Mohamed MA, Aly H. Transport of premature infants is associated with increased risk for intraventricular haemorrhage. Arch Dis Child Fetal Neonatal Ed 2010;95(6):F403–7.

122. Anderson GD, Bada HS, Shaver DC, et al. The effect of cesarean section on intraventricular hemorrhage in the preterm infant. Am J Obstet Gynecol 1992; 166(4):1091–9 [discussion: 1099–101].

123. Wadhawan R, Vohr BR, Fanaroff AA, et al. Does labor influence neonatal and neurodevelopmental outcomes of extremely-low-birth-weight infants who are born by cesarean delivery? Am J Obstet Gynecol 2003;189(2):501–6.

124. Szymonowicz W, Yu VY, Walker A, et al. Reduction in periventricular haemorrhage in preterm infants. Arch Dis Child 1986;61(7):661–5.

125. Henderson-Smart DJ, Cools F, Bhuta T, et al. Elective high frequency oscillatory ventilation versus conventional ventilation for acute pulmonary dysfunction in preterm infants. Cochrane Database Syst Rev 2007;(3):CD000104.

Neuroimaging of White Matter Injury, Intraventricular and Cerebellar Hemorrhage

Manon J.N.L. Benders, MD, PhD, Karina J. Kersbergen, MD,
Linda S. de Vries, MD, PhD*

KEYWORDS

- White matter injury • IVH • PWML • Cerebellar hemorrhage • cPVL • Imaging • MRI

KEY POINTS

- Cerebral ultrasound is reliable for the detection of large hemorrhages and cystic periventricular leukomalacia. MRI is more sensitive for detection of cerebellar hemorrhages, punctate and diffuse white matter injury.
- The combination of conventional imaging with sequences such as diffusion-weighted imaging, diffusion tensor imaging, and susceptibility weighted imaging can be used as an noninvasive method of improving detection and understanding of the underlying pathophysiology.
- Further studies are needed to assess neurodevelopmental outcome in infants with noncystic white matter injury.

Neuroimaging of preterm infants has become part of routine clinical care in the neonatal intensive care unit (NICU). Cranial ultrasound (cUS) is still considered the method of first choice for a sick preterm infant in the NICU. Besides the advantage of being a bedside technique, another advantage of cUS is that the examination can be performed as often as indicated, which allows visualization of the evolution of the lesion. Without sequential cUS, it may be difficult to make a distinction between a cyst following a periventricular hemorrhagic infarction (PVHI) (**Fig. 1**) and cystic periventricular leukomalacia (c-PVL). In the past, performing sequential cUS has also helped to recognize risk factors, including hypercapnia in germinal matrix–intraventricular hemorrhage (GMH-IVH) and hypocarbia in c-PVL.[1,2]

MRI is increasingly performed in extremely preterm infants at least once during the admission period, either during the acute phase following stabilization, at discharge,

Disclosures: The authors have nothing to disclose.
Department of Neonatology, Wilhelmina Children's Hospital, University Medical Center Utrecht, KE 04.123.1, PO Box 85090, Utrecht 3508 AB, The Netherlands
* Corresponding author.
E-mail address: l.s.devries@umcutrecht.nl

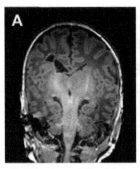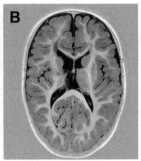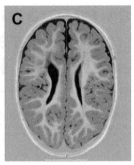

Fig. 1. MRI, T1-weighted image at term-equivalent age and at 2 years of age in a preterm born infant (gestational age 26 weeks). A single cyst is seen adjacent to but not communicating with the lateral ventricle. A PVHI is noted on sequential cUS. Asymmetry in myelination is seen (*A*). At 2 years, an interruption of the posterior limb of the internal capsule is seen as well an area of low signal intensity adjacent to the mildly dilated right ventricle (*B, C*). The child developed a mild unilateral spastic cerebral palsy.

and/or at term equivalent age (TEA). MRI may show lesions, which are not always easy to interpret and may be a cause of concern for parents.[3] Several studies have compared cUS and MRI contemporaneously. All investigators concluded that cUS is highly effective in diagnosing severe white matter lesions such as c-PVL and PVHI, but that MRI is necessary to identify smaller cerebellar hemorrhages (CBHs) and more subtle white matter injury (WMI), such as punctate white matter lesions (PWML) or diffuse extensive high signal intensity (DEHSI), which may further improve prediction of outcome.[4–7]

GMH-IVH

Even though WMI is now considered the main determinant of cerebral palsy (CP) later in infancy, a severe GMH-IVH is still a serious condition in preterm infants, which is still associated with a high mortality. cUS is reliable for the diagnosis of a severe GMH-IVH but less so for recognizing a small GMH outside the region of the caudate nucleus. To make a distinction between a GMH only and a GMH associated with a small IVH is more difficult with cUS than with MRI; however, the diagnosis can be made more reliably using the posterior fontanelle as an additional acoustic window.[8]

Whether a small GMH-IVH may have an effect on outcome is still uncertain. An adverse effect was recently suggested, showing a reduced cortical volume on TEA MRI.[9] However, the diagnosis of the GMH-IVH was made using cUS. Whether associated subtle WMI, not detected using cUS, played an additional or even a more important role needs to be established with prospective cUS and preferably serial MRI studies.[9–11] In the EPIPAGE (Etude Epidémiologique sur les Petits Ages Gestationnels) study, 6.8% and 8.1% of infants with a grade I and II GMH-IVH, respectively, developed CP. Once again, however, this was based on cUS instead of MRI data.[12] In another large cohort, no difference was found between infants without a hemorrhage and those with a grade I or II GMH-IVH.[13] In this study there were, again, a high percentage of infants who developed CP: 8% and 9% of infants without or with grade I to II GMH-IVH, respectively. This is likely to be explained by associated WMI not recognized with cUS.

According to Papile and colleagues,[14] a severe hemorrhage, grade III and IV, can be reliably diagnosed with cUS, even though associated WMI and/or cerebellar lesions may not be detected. As the outcome of a grade III hemorrhage (a large GMH-IVH with a blood clot filling the ventricle>50% and resulting in acute dilatation of the lateral ventricle) is considerably better than that of a PVHI (sometimes still called a grade IV), these two should not be taken together. A large GMH-IVH, complicated by posthemorrhagic ventricular dilation (PHVD) and a PVHI, carries an increased risk of adverse neurologic sequelae. PVHI may look like a large globular lesion communicating with the lateral ventricle, with subsequent evolution into a porencephalic cyst (PC) (**Fig. 2**). However, a PVHI may be more triangular with the apex of the lesion adjacent to, but not necessarily in communication with, the lateral ventricle. This type of PVHI does not evolve into a PC, but tends to evolve into one or more cysts, which remain separate from the lateral ventricle (see **Fig. 1**).

As the amount of blood determines the development of PHVD, the risk of developing PVHD is greater in infants with grade III than in those with a PVHI.[15] The size of the lateral ventricles can be measured with sequential cUS, which will help to determine when best to intervene. The most commonly used measures are the anterior horn width (AHW) and thalamo-occipital distance (TOD), according to Davies and colleagues,[16] as well as ventricular width, according to Levene[17] (**Fig. 3**). New reference values for the ventricular width, AHW, and TOD were recently published with an age range of 24 to 42 weeks.[18] When PHVD is severe, it may become difficult to access the periventricular white matter with cUS (see **Fig. 3**C) because there will be compression of the white matter and the white matter may no longer fit within the field of view. Because associated WMI may be missed in infants with severe PHVD, MRI will be of additional value.

CBH

Cerebellar injury is now more often reported, which may be due to the increased survival of extremely preterm infants[19,20] because the incidence of cerebellar injury increases with decreasing gestational age (GA). In addition, the use of both cUS, using the mastoid window, and particularly MRI, which has become standard clinical care in many centers worldwide in extremely preterm infants, has improved detection of more subtle punctate lesions in the cerebellum. cUS will only detect cerebellar lesions reliably when they exceed 4 mm.[21] Extremely preterm infants are at an increased risk to develop cerebellar injury because they have a vulnerable germinal matrix in the fourth ventricle and an extensive granular layer covering the cerebellar surface.[22] The cerebellum is rapidly developing (fivefold increase in volume from 24 to 40 weeks

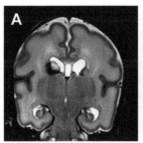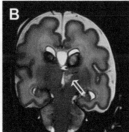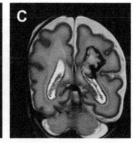

Fig. 2. MRI, T2-weighted sequence. (*A*) Preterm infant, gestational age (GA) 30 weeks, small GMH-IVH on the right. (*B, C*) Preterm infant, GA 27 weeks showing a bilateral GMH-IVH, larger on the left and associated with a PVHI on the left. Also note a lenticulostriate infarct (*open arrow*) seen as a wedge shaped lesion in the left thalamus (*B*).

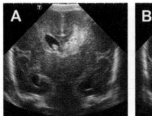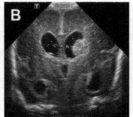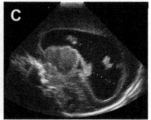

Fig. 3. Preterm infant, gestational age 25 weeks. cUS on day 3 (*A*) and day 12 (*B, C*) showing a large left-sided IVH and PVHI (*A*). PHVD developed with severe dilatation of the left occipital horn (31 mm, *C*). *Dotted lines* A and C in figure *B* are measurements of ventricular width, while B and D are measurements of the AHW. The *dotted line* in figure *C* is a measurement of the TOD.

corrected age) and, therefore, maybe especially vulnerable.[23] Injury to the cerebellum is often related to cognitive and behavioral deficits later in life.[24,25]

Information about the incidence of CBH using either cUS or MRI in cohort studies of extremely preterm infants is still limited. When using cUS with the mastoid fontanelle, the incidence varies between 3% and 9%, but it was 15% in a more recent cohort.[26] When using MRI, the incidence increases dramatically and can be as high as almost 20%, mainly due to recognition of punctate lesions (**Fig. 4**).[21]

Previous studies have shown that large CBH affect the sickest and most immature infants.[26] The pathogenesis of large and small CBHs may be different. For the large CBH, it is described that circulatory factors, such as a patent ductus arteriosus and the need for inotropic support, in the presence of impaired cerebrovascular autoregulation, exposes the immature capillary beds of the subependymal and subpial germinal matrix to fluctuations in arterial pressure. This may lead to rupture of immature vessels.[26] These circulatory risk factors were not found for small CBHs.

Primary CBH in preterm infants may originate in the external granular layer, from the germinal matrices that are present in the subependymal region around the fourth ventricle. The vulnerable capillaries, present in these structures, can easily rupture, especially with the circulatory changes in the vulnerable preterm infant.[27]

Besides the actual lesion in the cerebellar tissue, there are additional deleterious effects such as the toxicity of blood breakdown products (eg, heme and iron) in the cerebrospinal fluid because of (supratentorial) hemorrhage. This iron accumulation and free radical attack is associated with cerebellar atrophy.[24,28,29]

MRI studies are particularly valuable in the identification of cerebellar injury in premature infants. CBH is more often seen in the presence of supratentorial cerebral lesions, such as a large IVH with or without ventricular dilatation,[29] PVHI, or WMI.[30] Other investigators have noted that unexplained ventricular dilatation can be seen in the context of CBH.[31] It is described that these supratentorial lesions are related to reduced cerebellar volumes due to interruption of the cerebello-thalamo-cortical pathways. These pathways project from the cerebellum to the contralateral cerebral cortex and vice versa. Disruption of supratentorial neural systems, leading to crossed cerebello-cerebral diaschisis, might play a role in long-term neurodevelopmental impairment (**Fig. 5**).[32] Cerebellar volume of the preterm infant, assessed at TEA, is associated with cognitive developmental outcome at 2 years corrected age.[33]

WMI

Neuroimaging studies indicate that WMI in its various forms is by far the most common type of injury in preterm infants, occurring in 50% or more of very low birth weight

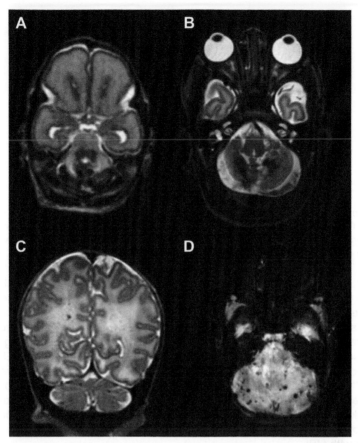

Fig. 4. Preterm infant, GA 25 weeks. MRI, T2-weighted sequence coronal view, showing large bilateral cerebellar hemorrhages on the scan performed at 30-weeks postmenstrual age (*A*). The MRI performed at TEA, axial view still clearly shows the hemorrhages as well as cerebellar atrophy, especially on the right side (*B*). Another preterm infant, GA 34 weeks, MRI, T2-weighted sequence, coronal view with a few punctate lesions (*C*). Many more punctate lesions were, however, identified in the cerebellum using susceptibility weighted imaging (*D*).

(VLBW) infants.[34] In the literature, WMI is often divided into two types: cystic and diffuse PVL.[35] The cystic type consists of focal necrosis deep in the periventricular white matter involving the loss of cellular elements. Within several weeks, this evolves generally to multiple cystic lesions, known as c-PVL, clearly visualized by cUS (**Fig. 6**). Currently, this severe lesion is less often observed (3%) in VLWB infants.[36] In noncystic WMI, it is most likely to be a more diffuse process. White matter necrosis is more often microscopic with paucity of myelinating (mature and immature) oligodendrocytes throughout the cerebral white matter, which might evolve over several weeks to astrogliosis and microgliosis. Often, this type of WMI is not reliably detected by cUS, although it may sometimes be suggested by the presence of inhomogeneous echogenicity. This form is referred to as noncystic WMI.[37]

Performing sequential cUS is very important in detecting cystic WMI because the cysts will become apparent after 2 to 4 weeks but they are often no longer seen at TEA. Instead, ventriculomegaly suggestive of white matter loss can be seen on the

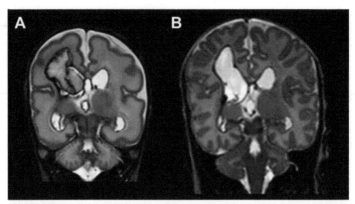

Fig. 5. Preterm infant, GA 26 weeks, T2-weighted image, coronal views at 30 and 40 weeks postmenstrual age, with a large IVH with right-sided PVHI, as seen on the early scan (*A*). The subsequent contralateral cerebello-cerebral diaschisis is clearly visible on the T2-weighted sequence at 40-weeks postmenstrual age (*A*). Also note the development of a PC (*B*).

TEA MRI. However, the role of cUS is limited in detecting noncystic WMI. MRI, a more sensitive type of imaging, shows more subtle and diffuse WMI.[38,39] Noncystic WMI is often referred to as diffuse excessive high signal intensity (DEHSI) or punctate white matter lesions (PWML). Several recent papers have shown that a very large proportion of preterm neonates show DESHI on their TEA MRI, especially when imaged on a 3 Tesla scanner. When imaged after a postmenstrual age of 50 weeks, DESHI was no longer identified. In addition, no relation with neurodevelopmental outcome is yet found.[40–42] Therefore, it is likely that DESHI is a prematurity-related developmental phenomenon, instead of WMI, even though increased apparent diffusion coefficient (ADC) values were reported by the group who coined the term DEHSI.[38] PWML is suggested by inhomogeneous echogenicity seen on cUS, but can only be reliably detected with MRI.

Apart from conventional T1-weighted and T2-weighted imaging, additional imaging techniques can further increase sensitivity and may help improve the prediction of outcome. In particular, diffusion-weighted imaging (DWI) and diffusion tensor imaging (DTI) are increasingly being used. DWI is especially useful in the acute stage for detection of cytotoxic edema, which is present for about a week after the insult and may help to predict subsequent cystic evolution.[43] DTI can identify altered microstructure in the white matter of the corticospinal tracts by evaluating fractional anisotropy (FA) values or fibertracking.[44] FA values in the white matter of the centrum semiovale were reported as significantly lower in infants with DEHSI.[45] Similar findings were found with quantitative fiber tracking, with which WMI was noted to adversely affect the volume and length of the corpus callosum (CC) and posterior limb of the internal capsule (PLIC) bundles (**Fig. 7**).[46] Thinning or atrophy of the CC suggests primary damage in the commissural tracts and reflects degeneration secondary to white-matter lesions. Thinning of the CC is commonly seen in preterm infants and is associated with a worse outcome.[47] Volumetric and microstructural abnormalities are described in the thalamus in preterm children with WMI, likely reflecting neuronal loss and axonal injury.[48,49]

PWML

PWML are small, focal patches of different signal intensity, most often seen in the periventricular white matter or intermediate white matter. Typically, they are seen as

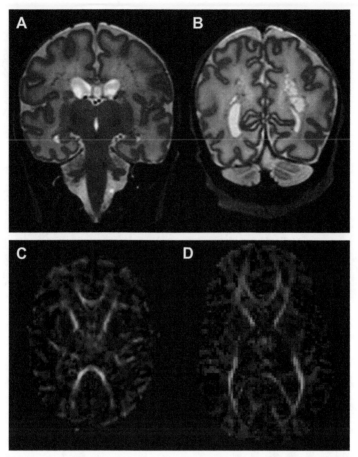

Fig. 6. Preterm infant, GA 32 +1 weeks, who developed c-PVL. MRI, T2-weighted sequence, coronal views, performed on day 24. Note both PWML and ventriculomegaly due to white matter loss (*A*) and extensive cystic lesions (*B*). Using diffusion tensor imaging, the direction encoded color (DEC) map at TEA shows an abnormal development of the posterior limb of the internal capsule (PLIC) and optic radiation (*C*). For comparison, a DEC image with normal appearance of the PLIC in a preterm infant at TEA (*D*).

hyperintense focal lesions on T1-weighted imaging and hypointense lesions on T2-weighted imaging. The reported incidence ranges from around 20% to more than 50% of premature infants.[5,7,39,40,50,51]

Several appearances are described. Lesions are arranged either linear, isolated, or in clusters, and are located in the border of the ventricle, adjacent to the ventricles, in the intermediate white matter or deeper in the centrum semiovale.[4,50,52] The number of lesions can differ greatly and severity is often judged by a cut-off. In infants imaged before term, more than three lesions or lesions greater than 2 mm, but involving less than 5% of the hemisphere, are considered moderate. When more than 5% of the hemisphere is involved, they are considered severe. For infants imaged at TEA, a cut-off of more than six lesions is most often used to define PWML as moderate-severe.[4,7,39,53]

The underlying pathophysiology of PWML in not yet completely understood and there is not much histologic material available.[4,50,54-56] Concurrent with the

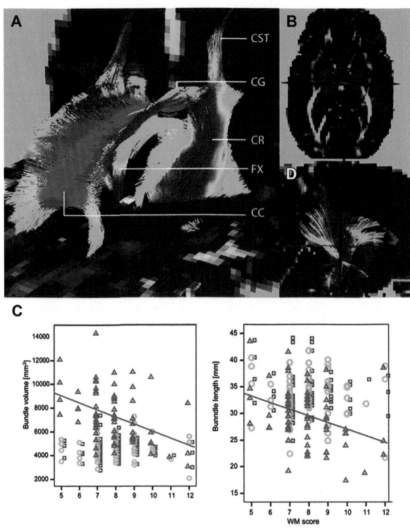

Fig. 7. Quantitative imaging of corpus callosum (CC) and PLIC bundles in relation to WMI. Graphs show the relation of volume (*C, left*) and length bundles (*C, right*) of PLIC left and right and CC with WMI score (higher score equals more severity, according to Woodward et al[66]). CG, cingulum; CR, corona radiata; CST, corticospinal tract; FX, fornix. (*Adapted from* Van Pul C, Van Kooij BJ, de Vries LS, et al. Quantitative fiber tracking in the corpus callosum and internal capsule reveals microstructural abnormalities in preterm infants at term-equivalent age. AJNR Am J Neuroradiol 2012;33:680–1; with permission.)

differences in appearance, it is reasonable to suspect several possible underlying mechanisms. Childs and colleagues[4] described pathologic states in two cases, with focal areas of gliosis corresponding with the site of the PWML on MRI in one infant, whereas the other showed focal areas of ischemic damage. Other histologic studies showed clusters of activated microglia and focal areas of hemorrhage.[50,55,56] These limited data suggest that PWML is caused by both hypoxic-ischemic and hemorrhagic processes. Apart from premature infants, PWML are also often found in infants with congenital heart disease, even before cardiac surgery is performed.[57,58] A larger pathology study in this group showed diffuse gliosis in the white matter, suggestive of hypoxia-ischemia as an underlying cause.[59]

Intrauterine inflammation is described as an important factor for development of WMI,[35,60] but the relation with PWML is not so clear. Other clinical risk factors, such as intrauterine growth retardation, hypotension, and late-onset sepsis were studied, but no clear relationship with the occurrence of PWML was shown.[56,61] Hemorrhagic PWML were more often seen in the presence of an associated GMH-IVH.[55]

Although PWML are usually identified on conventional T1- and T2-weighted imaging, using additional sequences, such as DWI or susceptibility weighted imaging (SWI), on a regular basis may provide more information about the causes of PWML. Especially in the acute stage, a decreased ADC calculated from DWI suggests an ischemic origin. Sequences with a high sensitivity for hemorrhage, such as SWI, can help distinguish between hemorrhagic and nonhemorrhagic PWML (**Fig. 8**).[55] A low DWI signal can also be caused by signal distortion due to hemorrhage. Therefore, the combination of the two sequences in particular will allow a differentiation between the different types of PWML.

Studies using DTI have shown that PWML can have a more global effect on the white matter. ADC values at TEA are lower throughout the white matter in infants with PWML compared with controls without brain damage[38] and a tract-based spatial statistics study showed a lower FA in the corticospinal tracts outside the immediate region of injury, suggesting diffuse injury to these tracts in infants with PWML.[44] Lower brain maturation scores at TEA, found in a study comparing conventional imaging of infants with PWML to those with normal appearing MRI, also suggest a more global effect of PWML on brain maturation.[62]

Although most premature infants are imaged around TEA, a growing number of units also perform earlier or serial MRI. Several studies describing early or serial imaging in premature infants found that all lesions are visible on MRI around 3 weeks after birth, and showed that only a very small percentage of infants will develop new lesions between the first and second TEA scan.[4,5,51,52,63] Some of these studies also demonstrated a decrease in the amount and intensity of the lesions at TEA compared with the early scan,[51] suggesting that an early scan might be more sensitive to demonstrate the total lesion burden, although the total amount of lesions remained stable in other cohorts.[5,7] Comparatively little is known about the evolution of PWML after the neonatal period. In one study, the investigators performed repeat MRI at 18 months

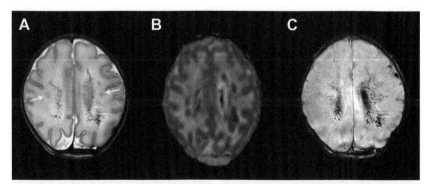

Fig. 8. At T2-weighted imaging multiple PWML, both linear and isolated (*arrows*) are visible (*A*). Preterm infant (gestation age 32 weeks, imaged at 33 weeks), showing both ischemic and hemorrhagic PWML. The ADC map shows several areas of restricted diffusion (*B*). On the SWI, the linear PWML are clearly visible, whereas the isolated ones are not (*C*).

of age and showed gliotic lesions of the same size and location as the PWML on the neonatal scan. This was especially true for those infants with more than six PWML on their first scan.[53]

Neurodevelopmental outcome in infants with PWML so far seems favorable, although outcome data beyond 2 years of age are still lacking. Lesion load and origin seem to play a role in determining outcome. Infants with supposedly hemorrhagic lesions and with fewer than six lesions of any kind at TEA are reported to perform well.[50,51,53] Lower developmental indices are reported in infants with supposedly ischemic lesions, a high lesion burden of more than six lesions at TEA, and/or associated white matter lesions.[40,41,50,52]

However, as several of these studies suggest, these outcome data are all limited to a young age. It is plausible that these lesions will cause milder cognitive impairment or learning and/or behavioral problems, often found at school age in prematurely born children. Serial cohort studies with long-term follow-up are needed to provide an answer to this hypothesis.

SUMMARY

In the VLBW infant, GMH-IVHs are still common with an incidence of 10% to 20%.[15,16] Although the incidence of severe WMI such as c-PVL in extremely preterm infants is declining, other lesions such as CBH and PWML are commonly recognized, especially with the increased use of MRI. Development of CP is explained by a severe hemorrhage (grade III and PVHI) or c-PVL seen on neonatal cUS or MRI. The size and, especially, the site of the lesion will reliably predict whether the infant is likely to develop neurologic sequelae.[64,65] For the prediction of cognitive outcome after prematurity, more advanced MRI techniques are required.[66] In recent years, a diverse spectrum of neuronal-axonal disturbances involving thalamus, basal ganglia, and cerebral cortex is commonly found in premature infants, usually in association with WMI.[7] It is now apparent that an additional and clinically important component of this neuronal-axonal constellation is the involvement of the cerebellum.[22] The relation between milder WMI such as PWML and neurodevelopmental outcome remains uncertain and this must be evaluated in serial cohort studies.

MRI enables noninvasive exploration of acute injury and postinjury alterations in structural and functional connectivity associated with preterm birth. This might be of crucial importance, not only for assessing long-term neurodevelopmental impairment but also for neuroprotective intervention trials. Advanced imaging techniques will provide data on the disturbances of neuronal-axonal constellation by studying both

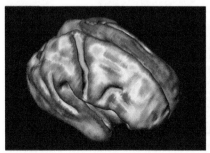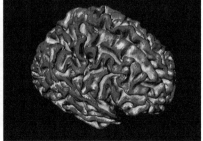

Fig. 9. Surfaces of the brain at 30 weeks (*left*) and 40 weeks (*right*) colored according to their mean curvature; blue represents areas of high curvature. (*Courtesy of* P. Moeskops, MSc, Image Sciences Institute, University Medical Center, Utrecht.)

connectivity and cortical development in relation to WMI. A relatively new technique, functional MRI connectivity, combined with advanced image analysis tools, such as voxel-based morphometry and morphology-based analysis of cortical folding (**Fig. 9**), may provide complementary data for understanding development, injury, and recovery in the developing brain.

Currently, MRI is the most sensitive noninvasive neuroimaging technique to assess brain development, anatomic integrity, microstructural connectivity, and functional performance. Therefore, it should be the method of choice to evaluate the effect of (future) neuroprotective treatments, ranging from pharmacologic drugs to stem cell therapies.

REFERENCES

1. Vela-Huerta MM, Amador-Licona M, Medina-Ovando N, et al. Factors associated with early severe intraventricular haemorrhage in very low birth weight infants. Neuropediatrics 2009;40:224–7.
2. Shankaran S, Langer JC, Kazzi SN, et al. Cumulative index of exposure to hypocarbia and hyperoxia as risk factors for periventricular leukomalacia in low birth weight infants. Pediatrics 2006;118:1654–9.
3. Pearce R, Baardsnes J. Term MRI for small preterm babies: do parents really want to know and why has nobody asked them? Acta Paediatr 2012;101:1013–5.
4. Childs AM, Cornette L, Ramenghi LA, et al. Magnetic resonance and cranial ultrasound characteristics of periventricular white matter abnormalities in newborn infants. Clin Radiol 2001;56:647–55.
5. Debillon T, N'Guyen S, Muet A, et al. Limitations of ultrasonography for diagnosing white matter damage in preterm infants. Arch Dis Child Fetal Neonatal Ed 2003;88:F275–9.
6. Maalouf EF, Duggan PJ, Counsell SJ, et al. Comparison of findings on cranial ultrasound and magnetic resonance imaging in preterm infants. Pediatrics 2001;107:719–27.
7. Miller SP, Cozzio CC, Goldstein RB, et al. Comparing the diagnosis of white matter injury in premature newborns with serial MR imaging and transfontanel ultrasonography findings. AJNR Am J Neuroradiol 2003;24:1661–9.
8. Correa F, Enriquez G, Rossello J, et al. Posterior fontanelle sonography: an acoustic window into the neonatal brain. AJNR Am J Neuroradiol 2004;25:1274–82.
9. Vasileiadis GT, Gelman N, Han VK, et al. Uncomplicated intraventricular hemorrhage is followed by reduced cortical volume at near-term age. Pediatrics 2004;114:e367–72.
10. Patra K, Wilson-Costello D, Taylor HG, et al. Grades I-II intraventricular hemorrhage in extremely low birth weight infants: effects on neurodevelopment. J Pediatr 2006;149:169–73.
11. Vavasseur C, Slevin M, Donoghue V, et al. Effect of low grade intraventricular hemorrhage on developmental outcome of preterm infants. J Pediatr 2007;151:e6–7.
12. Beaino G, Khoshnood B, Kaminski M, et al. Predictors of the risk of cognitive deficiency in very preterm infants: the EPIPAGE prospective cohort. Acta Paediatr 2011;100:370–8.
13. Payne AH, Hintz SR, Hibbs AM, et al. Neurodevelopmental outcomes of extremely low-gestational-age neonates with low-grade periventricular-intraventricular hemorrhage. JAMA Pediatr 2013;167:451–9.

14. Papile LA, Burstein J, Burstein R, et al. Incidence and evolution of subependymal and intraventricular hemorrhage: a study of infants with birth weights less than 1,500 gm. J Pediatr 1978;92:529–34.

15. Brouwer A, Groenendaal F, van Haastert IL, et al. Neurodevelopmental outcome of preterm infants with severe intraventricular hemorrhage and therapy for posthemorrhagic ventricular dilatation. J Pediatr 2008;152:648–54.

16. Davies MW, Swaminathan M, Chuang SL, et al. Reference ranges for the linear dimensions of the intracranial ventricles in preterm neonates. Arch Dis Child Fetal Neonatal Ed 2000;82:F218–23.

17. Levene MI. Measurement of the growth of the lateral ventricles in preterm infants with real-time ultrasound. Arch Dis Child 1981;56:900–4.

18. Brouwer MJ, de Vries LS, Groenendaal F, et al. New reference values for the neonatal cerebral ventricles. Radiology 2012;262:224–33.

19. Costeloe KL, Hennessy EM, Haider S, et al. Short term outcomes after extreme preterm birth in England: comparison of two birth cohorts in 1995 and 2006 (the EPICure studies). BMJ 2012;345:e7976.

20. Serenius F, Kallen K, Blennow M, et al. Neurodevelopmental outcome in extremely preterm infants at 2.5 years after active perinatal care in Sweden. JAMA 2013;309:1810–20.

21. Steggerda SJ, Leijser LM, Wiggers-de Bruine FT, et al. Cerebellar injury in preterm infants: incidence and findings on US and MR images. Radiology 2009; 252:190–9.

22. Volpe JJ. Cerebellum of the premature infant: rapidly developing, vulnerable, clinically important. J Child Neurol 2009;24:1085–104.

23. Chang CH, Chang FM, Yu CH, et al. Assessment of fetal cerebellar volume using three-dimensional ultrasound. Ultrasound Med Biol 2000;26:981–8.

24. Tam EW, Rosenbluth G, Rogers EE, et al. Cerebellar hemorrhage on magnetic resonance imaging in preterm newborns associated with abnormal neurologic outcome. J Pediatr 2011;158:245–50.

25. Limperopoulos C, Bassan H, Gauvreau K, et al. Does cerebellar injury in premature infants contribute to the high prevalence of long-term cognitive, learning, and behavioral disability in survivors? Pediatrics 2007;120:584–93.

26. Limperopoulos C, Benson CB, Bassan H, et al. Cerebellar hemorrhage in the preterm infant: ultrasonographic findings and risk factors. Pediatrics 2005; 116:717–24.

27. Volpe JJ. Neurology of the Newborn. Chapter 10: Intracranial Hemorrhage: subdural, Primary Subarachnoid, Cerebellar, Intraventricular (Term Infant), and Miscellaneous. 2008. p. 495–501.

28. Tam EW, Ferriero DM, Xu D, et al. Cerebellar development in the preterm neonate: effect of supratentorial brain injury. Pediatr Res 2009;66:102–6.

29. Tam EW, Miller SP, Studholme C, et al. Differential effects of intraventricular hemorrhage and white matter injury on preterm cerebellar growth. J Pediatr 2011; 158:366–71.

30. Argyropoulou MI, Xydis V, Drougia A, et al. MRI measurements of the pons and cerebellum in children born preterm; associations with the severity of periventricular leukomalacia and perinatal risk factors. Neuroradiology 2003;45:730–4.

31. Ecury-Goossen GM, Dudink J, Lequin M, et al. The clinical presentation of preterm cerebellar haemorrhage. Eur J Pediatr 2010;169:1249–53.

32. Tien RD, Ashdown BC. Crossed cerebellar diaschisis and crossed cerebellar atrophy: correlation of MR findings, clinical symptoms, and supratentorial diseases in 26 patients. AJR Am J Roentgenol 1992;158:1155–9.

33. Van Kooij BJ, Benders MJ, Anbeek P, et al. Cerebellar volume and proton magnetic resonance spectroscopy at term, and neurodevelopment at 2 years of age in preterm infants. Dev Med Child Neurol 2012;54:260–6.

34. Volpe JJ. The encephalopathy of prematurity—brain injury and impaired brain development inextricably intertwined. Semin Pediatr Neurol 2009;16:167–78.

35. Volpe JJ. Brain injury in premature infants: a complex amalgam of destructive and developmental disturbances. Lancet Neurol 2009;8:110–24.

36. van Haastert IC, Groenendaal F, Uiterwaal CS, et al. Decreasing incidence and severity of cerebral palsy in prematurely born children. J Pediatr 2011;159: 86–91.

37. Back SA. Perinatal white matter injury: the changing spectrum of pathology and emerging insights into pathogenetic mechanisms. Ment Retard Dev Disabil Res Rev 2006;12:129–40.

38. Counsell SJ, Allsop JM, Harrison MC, et al. Diffusion-weighted imaging of the brain in preterm infants with focal and diffuse white matter abnormality. Pediatrics 2003;112:1–7.

39. Leijser LM, de Bruine FT, Steggerda SJ, et al. Brain imaging findings in very preterm infants throughout the neonatal period: part I. Incidences and evolution of lesions, comparison between ultrasound and MRI. Early Hum Dev 2009;85: 101–9.

40. de Bruine FT, van den Berg-Huysmans AA, Leijser LM, et al. Clinical implications of MR imaging findings in the white matter in very preterm infants: a 2-year follow-up study. Radiology 2011;261:899–906.

41. Jeon TY, Kim JH, Yoo SY, et al. Neurodevelopmental outcomes in preterm infants: comparison of infants with and without diffuse excessive high signal intensity on MR images at near-term-equivalent age. Radiology 2012;263:518–26.

42. Hart A, Whitby E, Wilkinson S, et al. Neuro-developmental outcome at 18 months in premature infants with diffuse excessive high signal intensity on MR imaging of the brain. Pediatr Radiol 2011;41:1284–92.

43. Inder T, Huppi PS, Zientara GP, et al. Early detection of periventricular leukomalacia by diffusion-weighted magnetic resonance imaging techniques. J Pediatr 1999;134:631–4.

44. Bassi L, Chew A, Merchant N, et al. Diffusion tensor imaging in preterm infants with punctate white matter lesions. Pediatr Res 2011;69:561–6.

45. Skiold B, Horsch S, Hallberg B, et al. White matter changes in extremely preterm infants, a population-based diffusion tensor imaging study. Acta Paediatr 2010; 99:842–9.

46. Van Pul C, Van Kooij BJ, de Vries LS, et al. Quantitative fiber tracking in the corpus callosum and internal capsule reveals microstructural abnormalities in preterm infants at term-equivalent age. AJNR Am J Neuroradiol 2012;33: 678–84.

47. Stewart AL, Rifkin L, Amess PN, et al. Brain structure and neurocognitive and behavioural function in adolescents who were born very preterm. Lancet 1999;353:1653–7.

48. Ball G, Boardman JP, Aljabar P, et al. The influence of preterm birth on the developing thalamocortical connectome. Cortex 2013;49:1711–21.

49. Ball G, Boardman JP, Rueckert D, et al. The effect of preterm birth on thalamic and cortical development. Cereb Cortex 2012;22:1016–24.

50. Cornette LG, Tanner SF, Ramenghi LA, et al. Magnetic resonance imaging of the infant brain: anatomical characteristics and clinical significance of punctate lesions. Arch Dis Child Fetal Neonatal Ed 2002;86:F171–7.

51. Dyet LE, Kennea N, Counsell SJ, et al. Natural history of brain lesions in extremely preterm infants studied with serial magnetic resonance imaging from birth and neurodevelopmental assessment. Pediatrics 2006;118:536–48.

52. Miller SP, Ferriero DM, Leonard C, et al. Early brain injury in premature newborns detected with magnetic resonance imaging is associated with adverse early neurodevelopmental outcome. J Pediatr 2005;147:609–16.

53. Sie LT, Hart AA, van HJ, et al. Predictive value of neonatal MRI with respect to late MRI findings and clinical outcome. A study in infants with periventricular densities on neonatal ultrasound. Neuropediatrics 2005;36:78–89.

54. Felderhoff-Mueser U, Rutherford MA, Squier WV, et al. Relationship between MR imaging and histopathologic findings of the brain in extremely sick preterm infants. AJNR Am J Neuroradiol 1999;20:1349–57.

55. Niwa T, de Vries LS, Benders MJ, et al. Punctate white matter lesions in infants: new insights using susceptibility-weighted imaging. Neuroradiology 2011;53:669–79.

56. Rutherford MA, Supramaniam V, Ederies A, et al. Magnetic resonance imaging of white matter diseases of prematurity. Neuroradiology 2010;52:505–21.

57. Ortinau C, Beca J, Lambeth J, et al. Regional alterations in cerebral growth exist preoperatively in infants with congenital heart disease. J Thorac Cardiovasc Surg 2012;143:1264–70.

58. Block AJ, McQuillen PS, Chau V, et al. Clinically silent preoperative brain injuries do not worsen with surgery in neonates with congenital heart disease. J Thorac Cardiovasc Surg 2010;140:550–7.

59. Kinney HC, Panigrahy A, Newburger JW, et al. Hypoxic-ischemic brain injury in infants with congenital heart disease dying after cardiac surgery. Acta Neuropathol 2005;110:563–78.

60. Khwaja O, Volpe JJ. Pathogenesis of cerebral white matter injury of prematurity. Arch Dis Child Fetal Neonatal Ed 2008;93:F153–61.

61. Leijser LM, Steggerda SJ, de Bruine FT, et al. Brain imaging findings in very preterm infants throughout the neonatal period: part II. Relation with perinatal clinical data. Early Hum Dev 2009;85:111–5.

62. Ramenghi LA, Fumagalli M, Righini A, et al. Magnetic resonance imaging assessment of brain maturation in preterm neonates with punctate white matter lesions. Neuroradiology 2007;49:161–7.

63. Maalouf EF, Duggan PJ, Rutherford MA, et al. Magnetic resonance imaging of the brain in a cohort of extremely preterm infants. J Pediatr 1999;135:351–7.

64. Rademaker KJ, Groenendaal F, Jansen GH, et al. Unilateral haemorrhagic parenchymal lesions in the preterm infant: shape, site and prognosis. Acta Paediatr 1994;83:602–8.

65. Roze E, Harris PA, Ball G, et al. Tractography of the corticospinal tracts in infants with focal perinatal injury: comparison with normal controls and to motor development. Neuroradiology 2012;54:507–16.

66. Ment LR, Hirtz D, Huppi PS. Imaging biomarkers of outcome in the developing preterm brain. Lancet Neurol 2009;8:1042–55.

Chorioamnionitis in the Pathogenesis of Brain Injury in Preterm Infants

Vann Chau, MD[a,c,d,*], Deborah E. McFadden, MD[d,e,f],
Kenneth J. Poskitt, MDCM[d,f,g], Steven P. Miller, MDCM, MAS[a,b,c,d]

KEYWORDS

- Placental infection • White matter injury • Neurodevelopment • Cerebral palsy
- Magnetic resonance imaging • Diffusion tensor imaging
- Magnetic resonance spectroscopic imaging

KEY POINTS

- Chorioamnionitis, or placental infection, can lead to a fetal inflammatory response syndrome (FIRS) and the release of proinflammatory cytokines.
- FIRS is believed to contribute to brain injuries such as cystic periventricular leukomalacia (PVL) in the premature newborn.
- Three meta-analyses have linked chorioamnionitis to cystic PVL and cerebral palsy. Yet, the relationship between chorioamnionitis and brain injury was attenuated in newer studies. This difference may have resulted from heterogeneity of the studies (different methodologies) reviewed, or possibly as a result of improved neonatal intensive care.
- Large multicenter studies using rigorous definitions of chorioamnionitis on placental pathologies, quantitative magnetic resonance techniques, and standardized follow-up assessments would help clarify the impact of chorioamnionitis on brain health and outcomes.

Conflict of Interest: The authors declare that they have no conflict of interest. S.P. Miller is currently the Bloorview Children's Hospital Chair in Pediatric Neuroscience and was previously supported by a Tier 2 Canada Research Chair in Neonatal Neuroscience, and Michael Smith Foundation for Health Research Scholar Award.

[a] Division of Neurology, Department of Pediatrics, The Hospital for Sick Children, 555 University Avenue, Toronto, Ontario, M5G 1X8, Canada; [b] Neurosciences and Mental Health Program, Research Institute, 555 University Avenue, Toronto, Ontario, M5G 1X8, Canada; [c] University of Toronto, Department of Pediatrics, 563 Spadina Crescent, Toronto, Ontario, M5S 2J7, Canada; [d] Child & Family Research Institute, 950 28th Avenue, Vancouver, British Columbia, V5Z 4H4, Canada; [e] Department of Pathology, BC Children's & Women's Health Center, 4480 Oak Street, Vancouver, British Columbia, V6H 3V4, Canada; [f] University of British Columbia, Departments of Pediatrics, Pathology and Radiology, 2329 West Mall, Vancouver, British Columbia, V6T 1Z4, Canada; [g] Departments of Pediatrics and Radiology, BC Children's & Women's Health Center, 4480 Oak Street, Vancouver, British Columbia, V6H 3V4, Canada
* Corresponding author. Department of Pediatrics (Neurology), The Hospital for Sick Children, University of Toronto, 555 University Avenue, Room 6546, Hill Wing, Toronto, Ontario M5G 1X8, Canada.
E-mail address: vann.chau@sickkids.ca

Clin Perinatol 41 (2014) 83–103
http://dx.doi.org/10.1016/j.clp.2013.10.009
0095-5108/14/$ – see front matter © 2014 Elsevier Inc. All rights reserved.

CHORIOAMNIONITIS AND PREMATURITY

Chorioamnionitis refers to an inflammation of placental tissue, either of mixed fetal-maternal origin (choriodecidual space) or solely fetal origin (chorioamniotic membranes, amniotic fluid, and umbilical cord).[1] Most infections are believed to occur through an ascending process along the uterine cavity, although only a few bacterial culture positive cases can be documented.[2] Pathogens that are most commonly associated with chorioamnionitis are of low virulence and lead to subclinical inflammatory processes. These pathogens include *Ureaplasma urealyticum* and *Mycoplasma hominis* and are best detected with newer techniques such as polymerase chain reaction.[2] Given the associations between polymorphisms in immunoregulatory genes and chorioamnionitis, it has been suggested that both the maternal and fetal immune systems play important roles in the development of chorioamnionitis.[3,4]

In the United States, the incidence of preterm birth continues to increase despite notable progress in antenatal care, accounting for 12% to 13% of all live births.[5] Preterm birth places a considerable burden on families, and society, because it is an important risk factor for death before the first birthday[6] and for long-term neurologic and developmental disabilities.[7,8] Chorioamnionitis is now recognized as a major cause of spontaneous preterm delivery.[2] It is especially common at younger gestational ages, with an incidence that is inversely proportional to gestational age; up to 80% of infants born at 23 weeks of gestation have evidence of chorioamnionitis.[9] A recent multicenter study of preterm newborns has shown this close relationship of microbial colonization and inflammation on placental tissue with spontaneous preterm deliveries.[10,11]

CLINICAL AND HISTOLOGIC CHORIOAMNIONITIS

The definition and criteria of clinical chorioamnionitis (**Table 1**) have been inconsistent across studies. In addition to being nonspecific, signs and symptoms of chorioamnionitis are found in a few cases (usually the more serious instances) and include maternal fever and tachycardia, leukocytosis or increased C-reactive protein, uterine tenderness, and foul-smelling vaginal discharges.[12,13] When the fetus is directly exposed to inflammation of the amniotic fluid or the placental-fetal circulation, the resulting fetal response is known as fetal inflammatory response syndrome (FIRS).[14] The fetus may then show tachycardia.[12,13] Funisitis and increased cord blood interleukin 6 (IL-6) are considered to reflect the more serious end of the FIRS.[14] Other blood markers, mainly proinflammatory cytokines, are also believed to reflect FIRS: IL-1 and tumor necrosis factor α (TNF-α).[14]

Clinically defined chorioamnionitis correlates poorly with findings on histopathologic examination of the placenta.[15] Thus, placental examination is the diagnostic gold standard.[16] Normally sterile (**Fig. 1**) placental tissues that are invaded by pathogens, which can usually be detected by culture or polymerase chain reaction,[17,18] show typical histologic indicators of an acute inflammatory process (see **Table 1**). Infiltration by polymorphonuclear cells (neutrophils) is the most prominent feature (**Fig. 2**). Neutrophils can be found in different maternal tissues or spaces as well as fetal placental membranes or within the walls of blood vessels. Karyorrhexis, necrosis, debris, and degeneration of vascular smooth muscle cell are present in more severe cases.[19]

Many previous studies have reported inconsistent associations between chorioamnionitis and different postnatal outcomes (**Table 2**). Although most of these associations are discussed, this review focuses mainly on the associations of chorioamnionitis with brain injury and neurodevelopmental outcomes.

Table 1
Clinical and histopathologic criteria of chorioamnionitis

Chorioamnionitis	Fetus	Mother
Clinical Diagnosis[a]		
Symptoms/signs	Fetal tachycardia (>160 bpm)	Maternal fever (≥37.8°C) Maternal tachycardia (>120 bpm) Uterine tenderness Foul-smelling vaginal discharges
Laboratory results		Increased C-reactive protein Leukocytosis (>14,000 cells/mm³) in the absence of other source of infection
Histopathologic Examination[b]		
Stage	1. Early (ie, with chorionic vasculitis or umbilical phlebitis) 2. Intermediate (ie, with umbilical vasculitis or umbilical panvasculitis) 3. Advanced (ie, with necrotizing funisitis or concentric umbilical perivasculitis)	1. Early (ie, acute subchorionitis or chorionitis) 2. Intermediate (ie, acute chorioamnionitis) 3. Advanced (ie, necrotizing chorioamnionitis)
Grade	1. Mild to moderate (no special terminology) 2. Severe (ie, with severe fetal inflammatory response or with intense chorionic [umbilical] vasculitis)	1. Mild to moderate (no special terminology) 2. Severe (ie, severe acute chorioamnionitis or with subchorionic microabscesses)

[a] The core feature for clinical diagnosis is maternal fever. In clinical research, 2 more signs/symptoms or abnormal laboratory results are needed to make the diagnosis.[100] However, in clinical practice, the definition of clinical chorioamnionitis is commonly based on the presence of maternal fever and 1 more sign/symptom or laboratory results from the list in the table.[101]
[b] Based on and modified from Redline and colleagues' criteria.[19]

CYSTIC PERIVENTRICULAR LEUKOMALACIA, NONCYSTIC FOCAL WHITE MATTER INJURY, AND CEREBRAL PALSY

Over the last decade, the incidence of cystic periventricular leukomalacia (PVL), which refers to injury of cerebral white matter with periventricular focal necrosis in a characteristic distribution,[20] has decreased dramatically in premature newborns.[21,22] In contrast, multifocal noncystic white matter injury (WMI) is increasingly recognized as the most prevalent pattern of brain injury in this population.[21] The severity of WMI, best visualized with magnetic resonance imaging (MRI), is associated with adverse neurodevelopmental outcome at 12 to 18 months of age.[7,8,23] The magnetic resonance (MR) signal changes that characterize this form of WMI (ie, multifocal WMI) are most easily recognized in the first weeks of life (**Fig. 3**), becoming more difficult to detect near term-equivalent age.[7]

Experimental studies attribute the exquisite vulnerability of the preterm brain to WMI as resulting from specific developmentally regulated cell populations that are vulnerable to oxidative stress,[24] ischemia,[25] and inflammation.[26] More specifically, perinatal infections[27,28] as well as increased inflammatory cytokines[29–31] are recognized risk factors for WMI. The myelination failure associated with WMI results primarily from arrested maturation of the oligodendrocyte lineage at the preoligodendrocyte stage.[32]

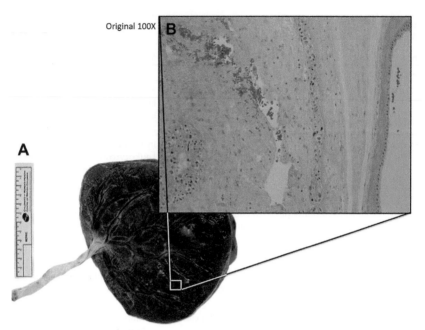

Fig. 1. Gross and microscopic (original magnification x100) images showing uninflamed placenta. Fetal membranes are translucent (*A*), and histologic examination shows no inflammatory cells (*B*).

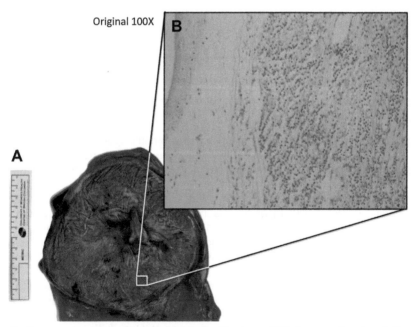

Fig. 2. Gross and microscopic (original magnification x100) images showing inflamed placenta. Fetal membranes are opaque, thickened, and show green discoloration (*A*). Histologic examination shows abundant acute inflammatory cells and debris (*B*).

The persistence of this susceptible cell population also maintains white matter vulnerability to recurrent insults.[33] Furthermore, there is now increasing recognition of gray matter injuries in preterm neonates, with abnormalities increasingly recognized in the cerebral cortex, thalamus, and cerebellum.[20,34,35]

Cerebral palsy (CP) refers to a group of permanent disorders of the development of movement and posture, causing activity limitation, that are attributed to nonprogressive disturbances that occurred during the development of fetal or infant's brain.[36] Although the brain abnormality is theoretically nonprogressive, the clinical manifestations usually evolve. In addition to motor impairment, children with CP often show musculoskeletal problems, perceptual abnormalities, and communication and behavioral disorders.[37] Severe intellectual disability, visual impairment, and epilepsy are seen respectively in 31%, 11%, and 21%.[38] CP is particularly prevalent in children born preterm, reaching 100 per 1000 in those born before 28 weeks' gestation,[39] although the incidence seems to be decreasing.[22,40] Although cystic PVL, periventricular hemorrhagic infarction, and severe intraventricular hemorrhage (IVH) are well known causes of CP in preterm born children, the role of perinatal infection and inflammation in the pathogenesis of brain injury in this population is increasingly recognized.[41]

PROPOSED MECHANISMS OF BRAIN INJURY VIA FIRS

The current model of brain injury resulting from chorioamnionitis is based on the involvement of inflammatory processes that occur at distance, via the release of proinflammatory cytokines (**Fig. 4**). Involvement of local cytokine production in intrauterine infections was first noted after the discovery of increased concentrations of proinflammatory molecules in amniotic fluid with preterm deliveries.[42,43] Other supportive evidence originates from postmortem immunohistochemical studies, which revealed a higher expression of TNF-α, IL-1, and IL-6 in brain sections of premature infants with PVL exposed to infections compared with brains with PVL but not exposed to infection.[44]

In animal studies, both locally produced and systemic cytokines caused by FIRS disrupt the tight junction structure of brain vessels, leading to increased permeability for cytotoxic proteins. TNF-α directly damages oligodendrocytes or their progenitors.[45] This insult is untimely, because it occurs during a critical period of fetal brain development with active myelination.[46] With the activation of microglia, the process of myelination is compromised via the apoptosis of the developing oligodendrocytes, which leads to WMI through 2 specific mechanisms. First, the microglial production of proinflammatory cytokines not only affects the cerebral fetal white matter oligodendrocytes[47] but also secondarily induces neuronal loss and impaired neuronal guidance.[48] In inflamed fetal brains, maturation and differentiation of immature oligodendrocytes into fully functional cells are inhibited by the presence of critically high levels of proinflammatory cytokines.[49,50] In addition, by increasing the permeability of the developing blood-brain barrier[46] and impairing the cerebral blood flow,[51] proinflammatory cytokines may affect the central nervous system. Second, microglial activation generates reactive oxygen and nitrogen species, which in turn injure the developing oligodendrocytes.[52] Together, these 2 processes result in white matter lesions and impairment of myelination.[27]

Bacteremia, complicated or not with endotoxemia, occurring in the context of perinatal infections may cause a loss of cerebral autoregulation, which in turn may contribute to fetal brain injury.[53] In animal models, an endotoxin extracted from the cell wall of gram-negative bacteria called lipopolysaccharide has been shown to affect

Table 2
Summary of study characteristics associating histologic chorioamnionitis, brain abnormalities, and abnormal neurodevelopment in preterm infants (<32 weeks' gestation or <1500 g)

Study Using Histologic Criteria to Define Chorioamnionitis[a]	Study Design	Brain Abnormalities OR (95% CI)	Neuroimaging Modality	Outcomes OR (95% CI)	Adjusting Factors
Prospective Studies					
Verma et al,[102] 1997	Prospective cohort (305/745)[b]	IVH and PVL Both ns	cUS	—	GA, BWT
DiSalvo et al,[103] 1998	Prospective cohort (515/1095)	IVH 2.5 (0.97-6.5)	cUS	—	GA, labor, route of delivery
Hansen et al,[104] 1999	Prospective cohort (N/A/1131)	IVH and PVL Both ns	cUS	—	Labor, route of delivery, ROM
Leviton et al,[61] 1999	Prospective cohort (353/1078)	PVL 10.8 (95% CI not given)	cUS	—	GA, BWT, ROM, preeclampsia
Dexter et al,[82] 2000	Prospective cohort (164/287)	IVH grade 3 and 4 RR 1.6 (1.1-2.4)	cUS	DD at 7 mo ns	Gender, BWT, GA, IVH, multiple gestation, antibiotic use, preterm labor, PROM, ROM
Bass[c] et al,[105] 2002	Prospective cohort (14/73)	PVL P<.05 (56% vs 15%)	cUS	—	—
De Felice et al,[106] 2005	Prospective cohort (67/116)	IVH 3 and 4 P<.0001 (41% vs 4.1%)	cUS	—	GA, gender
Kent et al,[99] 2005	Prospective cohort (72/220)	IVH P = .002 (57% vs 34%)	cUS	CP P = .03 (33% vs 3%)	Results for subgroup of patients not exposed to full dose of antenatal steroid
Polam et al,[107] 2005	Prospective cohort (102/177)	IVH P = .04 (30% vs 13%)	cUS	DD and CP Both ns	GA, gender, antenatal steroid, intrapartum antibiotics
Sarkar et al,[108] 2005	Prospective cohort (29/62)	IVH ns	cUS	—	13 perinatal risk factors, including GA
Andrews et al,[17] 2006	Prospective cohort (222/446)	IVH and PVL Both ns	cUS	—	GA, race, gender

Study	Design (n)	IVH/PVL	cUS and MRI	DD	Adjustments
Kaukola et al,[62] 2006	Prospective cohort (25/54)	IVH 8.2 (1.6–34)	cUS and MRI	DD 15.2 (1.3–18.1) NB: if HCA combined with placental perfusion defect	For IVH: vaginal delivery, CRIB score, lowest mean blood pressure For DD: GA, BWT
Redline et al,[109] 2007	Prospective cohort (69/129)	—	—	CP and DD Both ns	GA, gestational size, neonatal risk score, SES
Andrews et al,[110] 2008	Prospective cohort (N/A/261)	—	—	CP and DD ns	GA, ethnicity, SES
Reiman et al,[60] 2008	Prospective cohort (53/121)	Regional brain volumes ns	MRI	—	Gender, BWT
Zanardo et al,[111] 2008	Prospective cohort (68/287)	IVH ns PVL P = .01 (6% vs 0.5%)	cUS	—	—
Been et al,[15] 2009	Prospective cohort (121/301)	IVH P<.05 (25% vs 13%) PVL ns	cUS	—	GA
Chau et al,[67] 2009	Prospective cohort (31/92)	IVH, PVL, and brain development All ns	MRI, DTI, MRSI	—	GA, regions of interest, twin pairs
Suppiej et al,[112] 2009	Prospective cohort (41/104)	IVH and PVL ns	cUS	Speech delay 2.4 (1.3–4.2) Motor delay ns Hearing loss P<.05	—
Hendson et al,[113] 2011	Prospective cohort (303/628)	IVH P = .01 (20% vs 12%) PVL ns	cUS	CP and DD ns	GA, PROM, antenatal steroids, intrapartum antibiotics, mode of delivery, gender, multiple gestation

(continued on next page)

Table 2
(continued)

Study Using Histologic Criteria to Define Chorioamnionitis[a]	Study Design	Brain Abnormalities OR (95% CI)	Neuroimaging Modality	Outcomes OR (95% CI)	Adjusting Factors
Rovira et al,[114] 2011	Prospective cohort (87/177)	IVH and PVL Both ns	cUS	Moderate to severe disability 4.1 (1.1–15.1)	GA, BWT, 5-min Apgar
Case-Control Studies					
Murphy et al,[115] 1995	Case-control (59/234)	—		CP 4.2 (1.4–12.0)	GA
O'Shea et al,[116] 1998	Case-control (14/21)	—		CP ns	GA
Redline et al,[117] 2000	Nested case-control (72/119)	—		Neurologic impairment 13.2 (1.3–137.0)	Multiple placental lesion, oxygen therapy at 36 wk gestation, severe cUS abnormalities
Gray et al,[118] 2001	Case-control (75/137)	—		CP ns	Matched analysis
Grether et al,[119] 2003	Case-control (246/330)	—		CP ns	GA, preeclampsia, time between admission and delivery
Wharton et al,[120] 2004	Case-control (46/76)	PVL 2.9 (1.0–8.1)	cUS	—	GA
Vigneswaran et al,[121] 2004	Case cohort (76/204)	—		CP ns	—
Costantine et al,[122] 2007	Case-control (19/57)	—		CP 3.7 (1.2–11.9)	Gender
Schlapbach et al,[123] 2010	Case-control (33/99)	—		CP and DD ns	GA, BWT, weight at 2 y of age, BPD, mechanical ventilation

Retrospective Studies

Study	Design	Outcome	Imaging	Outcome	Adjusted factors
Salafia et al,[124] 1995	Retrospective cohort (139/406)	Early IVH 1.4 (1.1–1.8)	cUS	—	GA, steroids, volume expansion, MgSO4
Kosuge et al,[125] 2000	Retrospective cohort (44/81)	IVH and PVL Both ns	cUS	CP, MR Both ns	18 perinatal risk factors, including GA
Vergani et al,[126] 2000	Retrospective cohort (43/119)	IVH 1.8 (1.7–1.9)	cUS	—	RDS
Ogunyemi et al,[127] 2003	Retrospective cohort (76/204)	IVH 1.7 (1.2–23)	cUS	—	—
Sato et al,[68] 2011	Retrospective cohort (158/302)	IVH and PVL Both ns	MRI	—	GA
Horvath et al,[128] 2012	Retrospective cohort (43/128)	—	—	CP 4.1 (1.1–15.0)	GA, BWT
Nasef et al,[129] 2013	Retrospective cohort (95/274)	PVL ns	cUS	CP, infant mortality and ROP All ns	Mode of delivery, PROM
Soraisham et al,[130] 2013	Retrospective cohort (197/384)	IVH P = .001 (28% vs 14%) PVL P = .02 (2.5% vs 0%)	cUS	CP 2.5 (1.1–5.4) Deafness and blindness Both ns	GA, gestational hypertension, PROM >24 h

Abbreviations: 95% CI, 95% confidence interval; BWT, birth weight; CP, cerebral palsy; CRIB, clinical risk index for babies; cUS, cranial ultrasound; DD, developmental delay; DTI, diffusion tensor imaging; GA, gestational age; HCA, histologic acute chorioamnionitis; IVH, intraventricular hemorrhage; MgSO4, magnesium sulfate; MR, magnetic resonance; MRI, magnetic resonance imaging; MRSI, magnetic resonance spectroscopic imaging; N/A, number not found; ns, nonsignificant; OR, odds ratio; PROM, premature rupture of membranes; PVL, periventricular leukomalacia; RDS, respiratory distress syndrome; ROM, rupture of membranes; ROP, retinopathy of prematurity; RR, relative risk; SES, socioeconomic status.

[a] Given that the criteria for clinical chorioamnionitis are nonspecific, this table summarizes only the studies that use histologic criteria to define chorioamnionitis. This list is nonexhaustive.

[b] Refers to number chorioamnionitis/total number of patients.

[c] Placental pathology was not examined in every patient.

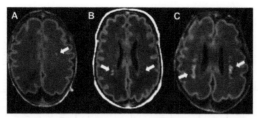

Fig. 3. WMI is seen on MRI as foci of abnormal white matter T1 hyperintensity (*arrows*) in the absence of marked T2 hypointensity, or by low-intensity T1 foci (cysts). Different scoring systems have been proposed to grade the severity of WMI. The one shown here was developed at the University of California San Francisco[7] and categorizes WMI as: (*A*) minimal ($\leq$3 lesions of <2 mm); (*B*) moderate (>3 lesions or lesions >2 mm, but involving no more than 5% of the hemisphere), or (*C*) severe (>5% of hemispheric involvement).

systemically the fetal cardiovascular function by decreasing the placental blood flow, with clear evidence of circulatory decentralization (ie, placental blood flow was nearly arrested while hyperperfusion of peripheral organs occurred).[53] The decrease in placental blood flow was accompanied by sustained hypotension, hypoxemia, and acidosis, causing dysregulation of cerebral blood flow. Experimental studies also

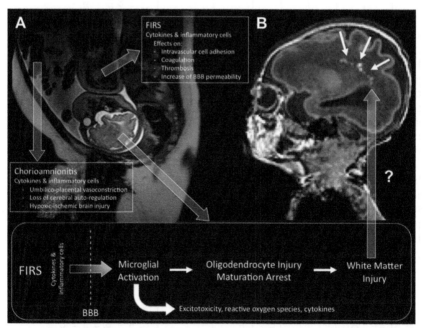

Fig. 4. Proposed mechanisms of WMI after exposure to FIRS. Rapid increase of proinflammatory cytokines follows the development of FIRS (*A*). At the placenta level, release of proinflammatory cytokines can cause umbilicoplacental vasoconstriction and lead to hypoxic-ischemic brain injury in the fetus, with loss of cerebral autoregulation.[53] In the fetus, systemic cytokines in the bloodstream readily cross the blood-brain barrier (BBB) and can damage the oligodendrocytes, either by direct cytoxicity or indirectly through the activation of microglia.[131] WMI can be seen as multifocal foci of hyperintensity (*arrows*) on this sagittal T1-weighted image (*B*). This image is an example of severe WMI.

suggest that the immature fetal brain becomes sensitized to hypoxia-ischemia during antenatal infection via bacterial endotoxins,[54] making it more vulnerable to subsequent hypoxic-ischemic injury. In addition to myelination reduction or failure, excitotoxic and inflammatory processes contributing to white matter damage are also hypothesized to lead to secondary loss of tissue in the cerebral cortex or deep gray matter.[48]

Besides the inflammatory mechanism described earlier, activated coagulation factors in premature infants with a systemic inflammatory response may also play a pathogenic role for cerebral WMI, through vessel occlusion, resulting brain ischemia, and promotion of inflammation.[55]

CHORIOAMNIONITIS AND IVH

Although several studies have proposed histologic chorioamnionitis as a risk factor for IVH (see **Table 2**), this association was not consistently observed in other studies.[56–59] The pathophysiology of IVH has not been studied as well as with WMI. Reviews and original studies seem to mix both IVH and WMI together under the generic term of brain injury. Given its more extensive documentation, this review focuses more on WMI and CP.

RELATIONSHIP BETWEEN CHORIOAMNIONITIS AND WMI

Many studies have examined the association of chorioamnionitis with cystic PVL and neurodevelopmental outcomes in children born preterm and have reached variable conclusions (see **Table 2**). The first meta-analysis, published in 2000,[56] reported that both clinical and histopathologic chorioamnionitis were significantly associated with CP. Although most individual reports failed to detect a significant association, the pooled odds ratio (OR) found chorioamnionitis to be an independent risk factor for both CP and cystic PVL (relative risk of 1.6 and 2.1, respectively).[56] These investigators highlighted that the findings from individual studies were often conflicting because of heterogeneous methodologies used to detect chorioamnionitis and brain injury and suggested the need to adjust for pregnancy-induced hypertension when examining this association. In most studies, exposure to chorioamnionitis was diagnosed clinically rather than with placental pathology.[60–64] Another systematic review performed subsequently included newer studies that failed to show a significant association between clinical and histologic chorioamnionitis with cystic PVL or CP.[57] In this analysis, only 2 studies reported a significant association.[65,66] However, in the random-effect meta-analysis, the overall association between chorioamnionitis and cystic PVL or CP was statistically significant.[57] The most recent meta-analysis published in 2010 updated this question with new studies of interest that used novel techniques, such as polymerase chain reaction of amniotic fluid samples to detect microbial infections.[58] The findings of this new meta-analysis were in line with the 2 previous reports,[56,57] linking chorioamnionitis and CP.[58] The investigators found significant associations to CP, with pooled OR of 2.42 (95% confidence interval [CI] 1.52–3.84; $P<.001$) for clinical chorioamnionitis and of 1.83 (95% CI 1.17–2.89; $P = .009$) for histologic chorioamnionitis. The investigators concluded that the risk of CP is increased by 140% and 80% for neonates exposed respectively to clinical and histologic chorioamnionitis.[58] The investigators also noted in their review that the studies failing to show an association tended to be of small sample size, were limited to 1 large tertiary hospital, and included only preterm infants delivered between 24 and 27 weeks' gestation. In contrast, the studies that showed statistical significance used larger cohorts from well-validated population registries.[58]

Although these results are consistent with chorioamnionitis playing a role in the genesis of brain injury and CP, there are nonetheless significant differences and methodological limitations across the studies that limit the ability to draw definitive conclusions regarding causality. Contrasting the methodologies across the studies, there are several possible confounding factors, which may explain, at least in part, the inconsistent findings. As highlighted by Ylijoki and colleagues,[59] some cohort studies addressing this issue may not have the power to identify gestational age as a confounder or risk modifier. Besides, reported associations between chorioamnionitis and adverse outcome in preterm infants largely depend on the criteria used to define chorioamnionitis. Investigators used different criteria of clinical chorioamnionitis, which are subjective and nonspecific.[17] The definitions of histologic chorioamnionitis were generally more rigorous, but only a few studies used placental pathology to describe both placental maternal and fetal inflammatory responses.

Variability is also recognized in regards to overall study design (eg, cohort vs case-control), the gestational ages included in the cohorts, and in the outcome measures, including definitions of brain injury. Most of the first studies to address this question used cranial ultrasonography to report brain injury. Given the poor sensitivity and specificity of this test to detect noncystic multifocal WMI and the decrease of the prevalence of cystic PVL in extremely premature infants with contemporary intensive care,[21] the results should be interpreted in this context. The most recent prospective MRI-based studies of this issue failed to show an association between histologic chorioamnionitis and brain development, brain injury, or brain growth.[60,67,68]

Although most studies adjusted the association between chorioamnionitis and CP for gestational age at birth, few took into account other postnatal risk factors that are known to be associated with adverse neurodevelopmental outcome. Postnatal infections,[28,69,70] necrotizing enterocolitis,[70–72] and hypotension are examples of conditions that may be related to chorioamnionitis and may themselves lead to adverse neurodevelopmental outcome.[73,74] In a recent prospective cohort of premature newborns,[67] postnatal infection and hypotension requiring intervention were more significant risk factors for early WMI than histologic chorioamnionitis. In that cohort, histologic chorioamnionitis was linked to an increased risk of arterial hypotension with the need for inotropic support in early life.[75] Because systemic inflammation impairs cerebrovascular autoregulation[76] and potentiates hypoxic-ischemic insults,[77,78] chorioamnionitis might still contribute to the susceptibility of white matter insult without being a direct cause.

CHORIOAMNIONITIS: A RISK FACTOR FOR MULTIPLE COMPLICATIONS IN THE PRETERM INFANT

In addition to hypotension, chorioamnionitis has been associated with several postnatal morbidities. Although earlier studies focused mainly on the respiratory and neurologic outcomes, evidence is increasing that the effects of chorioamnionitis on health and disease may extend beyond the neonatal period and involve multiple organs.[79]

A few cohort studies have shown that histologic chorioamnionitis may be associated with an increased incidence of either culture-proven or clinically suspected sepsis in very preterm infants.[17,80,81] However, this association was not linked to increased neonatal mortality,[17,81,82] unless there is histologic evidence of fetal involvement, in which case the risk of mortality seemed higher.[83]

Like cystic PVL and CP, neonatal respiratory outcome has been associated inconsistently with chorioamnionitis. The heterogeneity in this finding may relate to inconsistent definitions of bronchopulmonary dysplasia (BPD) and inclusion criteria (such as gestational age or birth weight).[84] The first report outlined that exposure to intrauterine inflammation may decrease the risk of respiratory distress syndrome (RDS) in premature infants and increase the risk of BPD.[85] These observations correlate with the findings of increased neutrophils and higher expression of proinflammatory cytokines in lung tissues of stillborn fetuses exposed to chorioamnionitis.[86] The association between FIRS as represented by umbilical cord vasculitis/funisitis with BPD was seen in certain studies,[87] but not in others.[88,89] In at least 1 study, FIRS was protective for BPD.[90] It has been suggested that histologic chorioamnionitis causes increased cortisol secretion and accelerated lung maturation through adrenal stimulation.[91] In an animal model, pulmonary maturation induced by fetal inflammation was associated with a significantly disturbed structural development of the lung, although the specific role of cortisol was not confirmed.[92] In a recent cohort of preterm newborns, prenatal exposure to inflammation has been shown to deteriorate the response to exogenous surfactant associated with a longer need for mechanical ventilation.[93] Histologic chorioamnionitis seems to potentiate the effects of mechanical ventilation for the development of BPD,[94] with a susceptibility of the lung for further postnatal injury.[84]

A recent meta-analysis of 33 relevant studies found that clinical chorioamnionitis was significantly associated with necrotizing enterocolitis (OR 1.24; 95% CI 1.01–1.52; P = .04).[95] With histologic chorioamnionitis, the association is statistically significant only when there is fetal involvement (OR 3.29; 95% CI 1.87–5.78; P<.001).[95] These findings are relevant to the relationship of chorioamnionitis and brain injury, because necrotizing enterocolitis is a strong risk factor for WMI and abnormal neurodevelopment.[70–72]

In other studies, histologic chorioamnionitis is also believed to be linked to fetal growth restriction, especially at earlier gestational ages.[82,96] This poor postnatal growth could be caused by vasospasm and altered blood flow in the context of inflammation and cytokine release. Poor postnatal growth is now recognized as a risk for abnormal maturation of the cerebral cortex.[34] Other organs, such as the eyes, heart, thyroid, liver, adrenal glands, and skin could also be affected by chorioamnionitis.[97]

PERSPECTIVE AND FUTURE DIRECTIONS

Current evidence links chorioamnionitis with brain injury and CP, although the findings are heterogeneous. It is possible that the inconsistency in these findings across studies may relate to differences in study methodology but may also relate to advances in neonatal care over the last decade. Some investigators have made the observation that most studies reporting a positive association between chorioamnionitis and outcome were published before the wide use of antenatal steroids in clinical practice. Ylijoki and colleagues[59] noted that from the 11 articles that they reviewed and in which 80% or more of the study infants received antenatal steroids, only one found histologic chorioamnionitis to be associated with poorer psychomotor development at 18 months corrected age. More specifically, they noted that 10 of these 11 studies (91%) either did not show significant association between chorioamnionitis and outcomes, or reported their findings only from univariate analyses.[59] These findings are consistent with other studies, which showed that antenatal exposure to steroids is associated with higher Apgar scores, lower incidence of RDS, IVH, PVL, and patent ductus arteriosus, and fewer neonatal deaths.[98] In a more recent cohort,[99] histologic chorioamnionitis was associated with severe IVH and CP in infants whose did not receive 2 doses of antenatal corticosteroids, as opposed to when a full set of corticosteroids was administered. Thus, the context of chorioamnionitis is emerging as a key moderator of the relationship with adverse brain health (see **Table 2**).

Advanced quantitative brain imaging measures now provide an opportunity to examine the relationship of chorioamnionitis with altered brain maturation in contemporary cohorts with consideration of current neonatal intensive care therapies. The role of chorioamnionitis may be further clarified with the use of rigorous histologic criteria of chorioamnionitis in large multicenter studies and with quantitative MR techniques (such as diffusion tensor imaging, MR spectroscopy, deformation morphometry) and standardized assessment of motor and cognitive outcomes.

REFERENCES

1. Hagberg H, Wennerholm UB, Savman K. Sequelae of chorioamnionitis. Curr Opin Infect Dis 2002;15(3):301–6.
2. Goldenberg RL, Hauth JC, Andrews WW. Intrauterine infection and preterm delivery. N Engl J Med 2000;342(20):1500–7.
3. Annells MF, Hart PH, Mullighan CG, et al. Polymorphisms in immunoregulatory genes and the risk of histologic chorioamnionitis in Caucasoid women: a case control study. BMC Pregnancy Childbirth 2005;5(1):4.
4. Holst D, Garnier Y. Preterm birth and inflammation–the role of genetic polymorphisms. Eur J Obstet Gynecol Reprod Biol 2008;141(1):3–9.
5. Goldenberg RL, Culhane JF, Iams JD, et al. Epidemiology and causes of preterm birth. Lancet 2008;371(9606):75–84.
6. Muglia LJ, Katz M. The enigma of spontaneous preterm birth. N Engl J Med 2010;362(6):529–35.
7. Miller SP, Ferriero DM, Leonard C, et al. Early brain injury in premature newborns detected with magnetic resonance imaging is associated with adverse early neurodevelopmental outcome. J Pediatr 2005;147(5):609–16.
8. Woodward LJ, Anderson PJ, Austin NC, et al. Neonatal MRI to predict neurodevelopmental outcomes in preterm infants. N Engl J Med 2006;355(7): 685–94.
9. Onderdonk AB, Hecht JL, McElrath TF, et al. Colonization of second-trimester placenta parenchyma. Am J Obstet Gynecol 2008;199(1):52.e1–10.
10. McElrath TF, Hecht JL, Dammann O, et al. Pregnancy disorders that lead to delivery before the 28th week of gestation: an epidemiologic approach to classification. Am J Epidemiol 2008;168(9):980–9.
11. Onderdonk AB, Delaney ML, DuBois AM, et al. Detection of bacteria in placental tissues obtained from extremely low gestational age neonates. Am J Obstet Gynecol 2008;198(1):110.e1–7.
12. van Hoeven KH, Anyaegbunam A, Hochster H, et al. Clinical significance of increasing histologic severity of acute inflammation in the fetal membranes and umbilical cord. Pediatr Pathol Lab Med 1996;16(5):731–44.
13. Dammann O, Allred EN, Leviton A, et al. Fetal vasculitis in preterm newborns: interrelationships, modifiers, and antecedents. Placenta 2004;25(10):788–96.
14. Gotsch F, Romero R, Kusanovic JP, et al. The fetal inflammatory response syndrome. Clin Obstet Gynecol 2007;50(3):652–83.
15. Been JV, Rours IG, Kornelisse RF, et al. Histologic chorioamnionitis, fetal involvement, and antenatal steroids: effects on neonatal outcome in preterm infants. Am J Obstet Gynecol 2009;201(6):587.e1–8.
16. Faye-Petersen OM. The placenta in preterm birth. J Clin Pathol 2008;61(12): 1261–75.

17. Andrews WW, Goldenberg RL, Faye-Petersen O, et al. The Alabama Preterm Birth study: polymorphonuclear and mononuclear cell placental infiltrations, other markers of inflammation, and outcomes in 23- to 32-week preterm newborn infants. Am J Obstet Gynecol 2006;195(3):803–8.

18. Leviton A, Allred EN, Kuban KC, et al. Microbiologic and histologic characteristics of the extremely preterm infant's placenta predict white matter damage and later cerebral palsy. the ELGAN study. Pediatr Res 2010;67(1):95–101.

19. Redline RW, Faye-Petersen O, Heller D, et al. Amniotic infection syndrome: nosology and reproducibility of placental reaction patterns. Pediatr Dev Pathol 2003;6(5):435–48.

20. Volpe JJ. Brain injury in premature infants: a complex amalgam of destructive and developmental disturbances. Lancet Neurol 2009;8(1):110–24.

21. Hamrick SE, Miller SP, Leonard C, et al. Trends in severe brain injury and neurodevelopmental outcome in premature newborn infants: the role of cystic periventricular leukomalacia. J Pediatr 2004;145(5):593–9.

22. van Haastert IC, Groenendaal F, Uiterwaal CS, et al. Decreasing incidence and severity of cerebral palsy in prematurely born children. J Pediatr 2011;159(1): 86–91.e1.

23. Chau V, Synnes A, Grunau RE, et al. Abnormal brain maturation in preterm neonates associated with adverse developmental outcomes. Neurology 2013. in press.

24. Back SA. Perinatal white matter injury: the changing spectrum of pathology and emerging insights into pathogenetic mechanisms. Ment Retard Dev Disabil Res Rev 2006;12(2):129–40.

25. Back SA, Han BH, Luo NL, et al. Selective vulnerability of late oligodendrocyte progenitors to hypoxia-ischemia. J Neurosci 2002;22(2):455–63.

26. Degos V, Favrais G, Kaindl AM, et al. Inflammation processes in perinatal brain damage. J Neural Transm 2010;117(8):1009–17.

27. Dammann O, Kuban KC, Leviton A. Perinatal infection, fetal inflammatory response, white matter damage, and cognitive limitations in children born preterm. Ment Retard Dev Disabil Res Rev 2002;8(1):46–50.

28. Chau V, Brant R, Poskitt KJ, et al. Postnatal infection is associated with widespread abnormalities of brain development in premature newborns. Pediatr Res 2012;71(3):274–9.

29. Dammann O, Leviton A. Maternal intrauterine infection, cytokines, and brain damage in the preterm newborn. Pediatr Res 1997;42(1):1–8.

30. Yoon BH, Jun JK, Romero R, et al. Amniotic fluid inflammatory cytokines (interleukin-6, interleukin-1beta, and tumor necrosis factor-alpha), neonatal brain white matter lesions, and cerebral palsy. Am J Obstet Gynecol 1997;177(1):19–26.

31. Yoon BH, Romero R, Kim CJ, et al. High expression of tumor necrosis factor-alpha and interleukin-6 in periventricular leukomalacia. Am J Obstet Gynecol 1997;177(2):406–11.

32. Buser JR, Maire J, Riddle A, et al. Arrested preoligodendrocyte maturation contributes to myelination failure in premature infants. Ann Neurol 2012;71(1): 93–109.

33. Segovia KN, McClure M, Moravec M, et al. Arrested oligodendrocyte lineage maturation in chronic perinatal white matter injury. Ann Neurol 2008;63(4): 520–30.

34. Vinall J, Grunau RE, Brant R, et al. Slower postnatal growth is associated with delayed cerebral cortical maturation in preterm newborns. Sci Transl Med 2013;5(168):168ra8.

35. Tam EW, Miller SP, Studholme C, et al. Differential effects of intraventricular hemorrhage and white matter injury on preterm cerebellar growth. J Pediatr 2011; 158(3):366–71.

36. Rosenbaum P, Paneth N, Leviton A, et al. A report: the definition and classification of cerebral palsy April 2006. Dev Med Child Neurol Suppl 2007;109: 8–14.

37. Cooley WC. Providing a primary care medical home for children and youth with cerebral palsy. Pediatrics 2004;114(4):1106–13.

38. Surveillance of Cerebral Palsy in Europe. Surveillance of cerebral palsy in Europe: a collaboration of cerebral palsy surveys and registers. Surveillance of Cerebral Palsy in Europe (SCPE). Dev Med Child Neurol 2000;42(12):816–24.

39. Paneth N, Hong T, Korzeniewski S. The descriptive epidemiology of cerebral palsy. Clin Perinatol 2006;33(2):251–67.

40. Synnes AR, Anson S, Arkesteijn A, et al. School entry age outcomes for infants with birth weight </= 800 grams. J Pediatr 2010;157(6):989–94.e1.

41. O'Shea TM. Cerebral palsy in very preterm infants: new epidemiological insights. Ment Retard Dev Disabil Res Rev 2002;8(3):135–45.

42. Hillier SL, Witkin SS, Krohn MA, et al. The relationship of amniotic fluid cytokines and preterm delivery, amniotic fluid infection, histologic chorioamnionitis, and chorioamnion infection. Obstet Gynecol 1993;81(6):941–8.

43. Figueroa R, Garry D, Elimian A, et al. Evaluation of amniotic fluid cytokines in preterm labor and intact membranes. J Matern Fetal Neonatal Med 2005; 18(4):241–7.

44. Kadhim H, Tabarki B, Verellen G, et al. Inflammatory cytokines in the pathogenesis of periventricular leukomalacia. Neurology 2001;56(10):1278–84.

45. Back SA, Rivkees SA. Emerging concepts in periventricular white matter injury. Semin Perinatol 2004;28(6):405–14.

46. Stolp HB, Dziegielewska KM, Ek CJ, et al. Breakdown of the blood-brain barrier to proteins in white matter of the developing brain following systemic inflammation. Cell Tissue Res 2005;320(3):369–78.

47. Gavilanes AW, Strackx E, Kramer BW, et al. Chorioamnionitis induced by intra-amniotic lipopolysaccharide resulted in an interval-dependent increase in central nervous system injury in the fetal sheep. Am J Obstet Gynecol 2009;200(4): 437.e1–8.

48. Leviton A, Gressens P. Neuronal damage accompanies perinatal white-matter damage. Trends Neurosci 2007;30(9):473–8.

49. Feldhaus B, Dietzel ID, Heumann R, et al. Effects of interferon-gamma and tumor necrosis factor-alpha on survival and differentiation of oligodendrocyte progenitors. J Soc Gynecol Investig 2004;11(2):89–96.

50. Haider S, Knofler M. Human tumour necrosis factor: physiological and pathological roles in placenta and endometrium. Placenta 2009;30(2):111–23.

51. Feng SY, Phillips DJ, Stockx EM, et al. Endotoxin has acute and chronic effects on the cerebral circulation of fetal sheep. Am J Physiol Regul Integr Comp Physiol 2009;296(3):R640–50.

52. Khwaja O, Volpe JJ. Pathogenesis of cerebral white matter injury of prematurity. Arch Dis Child Fetal Neonatal Ed 2008;93(2):F153–61.

53. Garnier Y, Coumans AB, Jensen A, et al. Infection-related perinatal brain injury: the pathogenic role of impaired fetal cardiovascular control. J Soc Gynecol Investig 2003;10(8):450–9.

54. Eklind S, Mallard C, Leverin AL, et al. Bacterial endotoxin sensitizes the immature brain to hypoxic-ischaemic injury. Eur J Neurosci 2001;13(6):1101–6.

55. Leviton A, Dammann O. Coagulation, inflammation, and the risk of neonatal white matter damage. Pediatr Res 2004;55(4):541–5.
56. Wu YW, Colford JM Jr. Chorioamnionitis as a risk factor for cerebral palsy: a meta-analysis. JAMA 2000;284(11):1417–24.
57. Wu YW. Systematic review of chorioamnionitis and cerebral palsy. Ment Retard Dev Disabil Res Rev 2002;8(1):25–9.
58. Shatrov JG, Birch SC, Lam LT, et al. Chorioamnionitis and cerebral palsy: a meta-analysis. Obstet Gynecol 2010;116(2 Pt 1):387–92.
59. Ylijoki M, Ekholm E, Haataja L, et al. Is chorioamnionitis harmful for the brain of preterm infants? A clinical overview. Acta Obstet Gynecol Scand 2012;91(4): 403–19.
60. Reiman M, Kujari H, Maunu J, et al. Does placental inflammation relate to brain lesions and volume in preterm infants? J Pediatr 2008;152(5):642–7.
61. Leviton A, Paneth N, Reuss ML, et al. Maternal infection, fetal inflammatory response, and brain damage in very low birth weight infants. Developmental Epidemiology Network Investigators. Pediatr Res 1999;46(5):566–75.
62. Kaukola T, Herva R, Perhomaa M, et al. Population cohort associating chorioam-nionitis, cord inflammatory cytokines and neurologic outcome in very preterm, extremely low birth weight infants. Pediatr Res 2006;59(3):478–83.
63. Rocha G, Proenca E, Quintas C, et al. Chorioamnionitis and brain damage in the preterm newborn. J Matern Fetal Neonatal Med 2007;20(10):745–9.
64. Murata Y, Itakura A, Matsuzawa K, et al. Possible antenatal and perinatal related factors in development of cystic periventricular leukomalacia. Brain Dev 2005; 27(1):17–21.
65. Jacobsson B, Hagberg G, Hagberg B, et al. Cerebral palsy in preterm infants: a population-based case-control study of antenatal and intrapartal risk factors. Acta Paediatr 2002;91(8):946–51.
66. Yoon BH, Romero R, Park JS, et al. Fetal exposure to an intra-amniotic inflamma-tion and the development of cerebral palsy at the age of three years. Am J Ob-stet Gynecol 2000;182(3):675–81.
67. Chau V, Poskitt KJ, McFadden DE, et al. Effect of chorioamnionitis on brain development and injury in premature newborns. Ann Neurol 2009;66(2): 155–64.
68. Sato M, Nishimaki S, Yokota S, et al. Severity of chorioamnionitis and neonatal outcome. J Obstet Gynaecol Res 2011;37(10):1313–9.
69. Stoll BJ, Hansen NI, Adams-Chapman I, et al. Neurodevelopmental and growth impairment among extremely low-birth-weight infants with neonatal infection. JAMA 2004;292(19):2357–65.
70. Shah DK, Doyle LW, Anderson PJ, et al. Adverse neurodevelopment in preterm infants with postnatal sepsis or necrotizing enterocolitis is mediated by white matter abnormalities on magnetic resonance imaging at term. J Pediatr 2008; 153(2):170–5.
71. Martin CR, Dammann O, Allred EN, et al. Neurodevelopment of extremely pre-term infants who had necrotizing enterocolitis with or without late bacteremia. J Pediatr 2010;157(5):751–6.e1.
72. Schulzke SM, Deshpande GC, Patole SK. Neurodevelopmental outcomes of very low-birth-weight infants with necrotizing enterocolitis: a systematic review of observational studies. Arch Pediatr Adolesc Med 2007;161(6):583–90.
73. Kobayashi S, Fujimoto S, Koyama N, et al. Late-onset circulatory dysfunction of premature infants and late-onset periventricular leukomalacia. Pediatr Int 2008; 50(2):225–31.

74. Batton B, Zhu X, Fanaroff J, et al. Blood pressure, anti-hypotensive therapy, and neurodevelopment in extremely preterm infants. J Pediatr 2009;154(3):351–7, 357.e1.

75. Lee SY, Ng DK, Fung GP, et al. Chorioamnionitis with or without funisitis increases the risk of hypotension in very low birthweight infants on the first postnatal day but not later. Arch Dis Child Fetal Neonatal Ed 2006;91(5):F346–8.

76. Yanowitz TD, Potter DM, Bowen A, et al. Variability in cerebral oxygen delivery is reduced in premature neonates exposed to chorioamnionitis. Pediatr Res 2006; 59(2):299–304.

77. Larouche A, Roy M, Kadhim H, et al. Neuronal injuries induced by perinatal hypoxic-ischemic insults are potentiated by prenatal exposure to lipopolysaccharide: animal model for perinatally acquired encephalopathy. Dev Neurosci 2005;27(2–4):134–42.

78. Wang X, Hagberg H, Nie C, et al. Dual role of intrauterine immune challenge on neonatal and adult brain vulnerability to hypoxia-ischemia. J Neuropathol Exp Neurol 2007;66(6):552–61.

79. Been JV, Kramer BW, Zimmermann LJ. In utero and early-life conditions and adult health and disease. N Engl J Med 2008;359(14):1523–4 [author reply: 1524].

80. Baud O, Emilie D, Pelletier E, et al. Amniotic fluid concentrations of interleukin-1beta, interleukin-6 and TNF-alpha in chorioamnionitis before 32 weeks of gestation: histological associations and neonatal outcome. Br J Obstet Gynaecol 1999;106(1):72–7.

81. Dempsey E, Chen MF, Kokottis T, et al. Outcome of neonates less than 30 weeks gestation with histologic chorioamnionitis. Am J Perinatol 2005;22(3):155–9.

82. Dexter SC, Pinar H, Malee MP, et al. Outcome of very low birth weight infants with histopathologic chorioamnionitis. Obstet Gynecol 2000;96(2):172–7.

83. Lau J, Magee F, Qiu Z, et al. Chorioamnionitis with a fetal inflammatory response is associated with higher neonatal mortality, morbidity, and resource use than chorioamnionitis displaying a maternal inflammatory response only. Am J Obstet Gynecol 2005;193(3 Pt 1):708–13.

84. Been JV, Zimmermann LJ. Histological chorioamnionitis and respiratory outcome in preterm infants. Arch Dis Child Fetal Neonatal Ed 2009;94(3): F218–25.

85. Speer CP. Inflammation and bronchopulmonary dysplasia: a continuing story. Semin Fetal Neonatal Med 2006;11(5):354–62.

86. May M, Marx A, Seidenspinner S, et al. Apoptosis and proliferation in lungs of human fetuses exposed to chorioamnionitis. Histopathology 2004;45(3):283–90.

87. Matsuda T, Nakajima T, Hattori S, et al. Necrotizing funisitis: clinical significance and association with chronic lung disease in premature infants. Am J Obstet Gynecol 1997;177(6):1402–7.

88. Kent A, Dahlstrom JE. Chorioamnionitis/funisitis and the development of bronchopulmonary dysplasia. J Paediatr Child Health 2004;40(7):356–9.

89. Richardson BS, Wakim E, daSilva O, et al. Preterm histologic chorioamnionitis: impact on cord gas and pH values and neonatal outcome. Am J Obstet Gynecol 2006;195(5):1357–65.

90. Lahra MM, Beeby PJ, Jeffery HE. Intrauterine inflammation, neonatal sepsis, and chronic lung disease: a 13-year hospital cohort study. Pediatrics 2009; 123(5):1314–9.

91. Watterberg KL, Scott SM, Naeye RL. Chorioamnionitis, cortisol, and acute lung disease in very low birth weight infants. Pediatrics 1997;99(2):E6.

92. Kramer BW, Ladenburger A, Kunzmann S, et al. Intravenous lipopolysaccharide-induced pulmonary maturation and structural changes in fetal sheep. Am J Obstet Gynecol 2009;200(2):195.e1–10.

93. Been JV, Rours IG, Kornelisse RF, et al. Chorioamnionitis alters the response to surfactant in preterm infants. J Pediatr 2010;156(1):10–5.e1.

94. Van Marter LJ, Dammann O, Allred EN, et al. Chorioamnionitis, mechanical ventilation, and postnatal sepsis as modulators of chronic lung disease in preterm infants. J Pediatr 2002;140(2):171–6.

95. Been JV, Lievense S, Zimmermann LJ, et al. Chorioamnionitis as a risk factor for necrotizing enterocolitis: a systematic review and meta-analysis. J Pediatr 2013; 162(2):236–42.e2.

96. Soraisham AS, Singhal N, McMillan DD, et al. A multicenter study on the clinical outcome of chorioamnionitis in preterm infants. Am J Obstet Gynecol 2009; 200(4):372.e1–6.

97. Gantert M, Been JV, Gavilanes AW, et al. Chorioamnionitis: a multiorgan disease of the fetus? J Perinatol 2010;30(Suppl):S21–30.

98. Elimian A, Verma U, Beneck D, et al. Histologic chorioamnionitis, antenatal steroids, and perinatal outcomes. Obstet Gynecol 2000;96(3):333–6.

99. Kent A, Lomas F, Hurrion E, et al. Antenatal steroids may reduce adverse neurological outcome following chorioamnionitis: neurodevelopmental outcome and chorioamnionitis in premature infants. J Paediatr Child Health 2005;41(4): 186–90.

100. Gibbs RS, Blanco JD, St Clair PJ, et al. Quantitative bacteriology of amniotic fluid from women with clinical intraamniotic infection at term. J Infect Dis 1982;145(1):1–8.

101. Greenberg MB, Anderson BL, Schulkin J, et al. A first look at chorioamnionitis management practice variation among US obstetricians. Infect Dis Obstet Gynecol 2012;2012:628362.

102. Verma U, Tejani N, Klein S, et al. Obstetric antecedents of intraventricular hemorrhage and periventricular leukomalacia in the low-birth-weight neonate. Am J Obstet Gynecol 1997;176(2):275–81.

103. DiSalvo D. The correlation between placental pathology and intraventricular hemorrhage in the preterm infant. The Developmental Epidemiology Network Investigators. Pediatr Res 1998;43(1):15–9 [published Erratum appears in Pediatr Res 1998;43(5):570].

104. Hansen A, Leviton A. Labor and delivery characteristics and risks of cranial ultrasonographic abnormalities among very-low-birth-weight infants. The Developmental Epidemiology Network Investigators. Am J Obstet Gynecol 1999; 181(4):997–1006.

105. Bass WT, Schultz SJ, Burke BL, et al. Indices of hemodynamic and respiratory functions in premature infants at risk for the development of cerebral white matter injury. J Perinatol 2002;22(1):64–71.

106. De Felice C, Toti P, Parrini S, et al. Histologic chorioamnionitis and severity of illness in very low birth weight newborns. Pediatr Crit Care Med 2005;6(3): 298–302.

107. Polam S, Koons A, Anwar M, et al. Effect of chorioamnionitis on neurodevelopmental outcome in preterm infants. Arch Pediatr Adolesc Med 2005;159(11): 1032–5.

108. Sarkar S, Kaplan C, Wiswell TE, et al. Histological chorioamnionitis and the risk of early intraventricular hemorrhage in infants born < or =28 weeks gestation. J Perinatol 2005;25(12):749–52.

109. Redline RW, Minich N, Taylor HG, et al. Placental lesions as predictors of cerebral palsy and abnormal neurocognitive function at school age in extremely low birth weight infants (<1 kg). Pediatr Dev Pathol 2007;10(4):282–92.
110. Andrews WW, Cliver SP, Biasini F, et al. Early preterm birth: association between in utero exposure to acute inflammation and severe neurodevelopmental disability at 6 years of age. Am J Obstet Gynecol 2008;198(4):466.e1–11.
111. Zanardo V, Vedovato S, Suppiej A, et al. Histological inflammatory responses in the placenta and early neonatal brain injury. Pediatr Dev Pathol 2008;11(5):350–4.
112. Suppiej A, Franzoi M, Vedovato S, et al. Neurodevelopmental outcome in preterm histological chorioamnionitis. Early Hum Dev 2009;85(3):187–9.
113. Hendson L, Russell L, Robertson CM, et al. Neonatal and neurodevelopmental outcomes of very low birth weight infants with histologic chorioamnionitis. J Pediatr 2011;158(3):397–402.
114. Rovira N, Alarcon A, Iriondo M, et al. Impact of histological chorioamnionitis, funisitis and clinical chorioamnionitis on neurodevelopmental outcome of preterm infants. Early Hum Dev 2011;87(4):253–7.
115. Murphy DJ, Sellers S, MacKenzie IZ, et al. Case-control study of antenatal and intrapartum risk factors for cerebral palsy in very preterm singleton babies. Lancet 1995;346(8988):1449–54.
116. O'Shea TM, Klinepeter KL, Meis PJ, et al. Intrauterine infection and the risk of cerebral palsy in very low-birthweight infants. Paediatr Perinat Epidemiol 1998;12(1):72–83.
117. Redline RW, Wilson-Costello D, Borawski E, et al. The relationship between placental and other perinatal risk factors for neurologic impairment in very low birth weight children. Pediatr Res 2000;47(6):721–6.
118. Gray PH, Jones P, O'Callaghan MJ. Maternal antecedents for cerebral palsy in extremely preterm babies: a case-control study. Dev Med Child Neurol 2001;43(9):580–5.
119. Grether JK, Nelson KB, Walsh E, et al. Intrauterine exposure to infection and risk of cerebral palsy in very preterm infants. Arch Pediatr Adolesc Med 2003;157(1):26–32.
120. Wharton KN, Pinar H, Stonestreet BS, et al. Severe umbilical cord inflammation—a predictor of periventricular leukomalacia in very low birth weight infants. Early Hum Dev 2004;77(1–2):77–87.
121. Vigneswaran R, Aitchison SJ, McDonald HM, et al. Cerebral palsy and placental infection: a case-cohort study. BMC Pregnancy Childbirth 2004;4(1):1.
122. Costantine MM, How HY, Coppage K, et al. Does peripartum infection increase the incidence of cerebral palsy in extremely low birthweight infants? Am J Obstet Gynecol 2007;196(5):e6–8.
123. Schlapbach LJ, Ersch J, Adams M, et al. Impact of chorioamnionitis and preeclampsia on neurodevelopmental outcome in preterm infants below 32 weeks gestational age. Acta Paediatr 2010;99(10):1504–9.
124. Salafia CM, Minior VK, Rosenkrantz TS, et al. Maternal, placental, and neonatal associations with early germinal matrix/intraventricular hemorrhage in infants born before 32 weeks' gestation. Am J Perinatol 1995;12(6):429–36.
125. Kosuge S, Ohkuchi A, Minakami H, et al. Influence of chorioamnionitis on survival and morbidity in singletons live-born at <32 weeks of gestation. Acta Obstet Gynecol Scand 2000;79(10):861–5.
126. Vergani P, Patane L, Doria P, et al. Risk factors for neonatal intraventricular haemorrhage in spontaneous prematurity at 32 weeks gestation or less. Placenta 2000;21(4):402–7.

127. Ogunyemi D, Murillo M, Jackson U, et al. The relationship between placental histopathology findings and perinatal outcome in preterm infants. J Matern Fetal Neonatal Med 2003;13(2):102–9.

128. Horvath B, Grasselly M, Bodecs T, et al. Histological chorioamnionitis is associated with cerebral palsy in preterm neonates. Eur J Obstet Gynecol Reprod Biol 2012;163(2):160–4.

129. Nasef N, Shabaan AE, Schurr P, et al. Effect of clinical and histological chorioamnionitis on the outcome of preterm infants. Am J Perinatol 2013;30(1): 59–68.

130. Soraisham AS, Trevenen C, Wood S, et al. Histological chorioamnionitis and neurodevelopmental outcome in preterm infants. J Perinatol 2013;33(1):70–5.

131. Kuypers E, Ophelders D, Jellema RK, et al. White matter injury following fetal inflammatory response syndrome induced by chorioamnionitis and fetal sepsis: lessons from experimental ovine models. Early Hum Dev 2012;88(12):931–6.

Fault and Blame, Insults to the Perinatal Brain may be Remote from Time of Birth

Sidhartha Tan, MD

KEYWORDS

- Antenatal • Birth • Brain • Fetus • Newborn • Anoxia • Cerebral palsy

KEY POINTS

- The pathophysiology of perinatal brain injury is different from traumatic brain injury.
- It is impossible to make the distinction between single and repeated insults with certainty at the time of birth.
- There is excessive focus on events at birth when the predominance of insults causing cerebral palsy is in the antenatal period with birth-related events being a small percentage.
- The timing of the onset of the causative insult and the duration of the brain injury are often unknown.
- Better fetal biomarkers of diagnosing injury are needed in the long journey to successful prevention of bad outcomes.
- Neurodevelopmental deficits are a culmination of antenatal, natal, and postnatal events.

INTRODUCTION

The most significant problem impeding scientific progress in perinatal brain injury is the lack of knowledge of the onset, nature, and timing of the insult in the antenatal and natal period. The pathophysiological streams that cause perinatal brain injury, the plastic response, repair processes restoring to control levels, and the windows of opportunity for treatment are discussed elsewhere in this issue. This article discusses the issues around timing of insults as related to neurodevelopmental deficits, including cerebral palsy (CP).

SCIENTIFIC VERSUS LEGAL PERSPECTIVE

To the clinician, finding the timing of insults is important, not only for choosing the best future therapy but because of the legal perspective of fault and blame. Sixty percent of

NIH, NS063141, NS043285, NS051402 for support of research.

NorthShore University Health System, University Chicago Pritzker School of Medicine, 2650 Ridge Avenue, Evanston, IL 60201, USA

E-mail address: sidtan@uchicago.edu

http://dx.doi.org/10.1016/j.clp.2013.10.006
0095-5108/14/$ – see front matter © 2014 Elsevier Inc. All rights reserved.
perinatology.theclinics.com

malpractice insurance premiums paid by US obstetricians cover lawsuits for alleged birth-related CP.[1] It is instructive to understand the 2 different perspectives, one of scientific endeavor and the other of legal case building, for the latter perspective has profoundly influenced the clinical narrative. There are common themes in most legal prosecutions that deal with the etiology of CP,[2] the principal points of which are summarized in **Table 1**.

LEGAL ANALOGY

Untoward birth events in the legal perspective are considered analogous to auto collisions,[2] which immediately brings to mind the pathogenesis of traumatic brain injury. Traumatic brain injury results in a different pathophysiology than that of the global insult found in perinatal brain injury. In the perinatal period, the vulnerable cell populations differ with age. White matter injury occurs from 24 weeks to near term gestation, as late oligodendroglial progenitors are vulnerable to injury in early prematurity.[3] Neuronal injury occurs from near-term gestation to 10 weeks postnatal age with hypoxia–ischemia (H-I) with deep gray nuclei and perirolandic cortex most likely to be affected at term.

The notion of a single definable insult is borrowed from the analogy of auto collisions. Interestingly, the understanding of the pathogenesis of perinatal brain injury has come from animal models in developmental neurobiology, which mostly employ a single definable insult, such as the Vannucci model[4] and the rabbit model of CP.[5]

SINGLE DEFINABLE INSULT?

Clinical scenarios that partially or completely fit a single definable insult at the time of birth are maternal collapse, uterine rupture, cord prolapse, and sometimes placental abruption (often labeled sentinel events). In a study of similar birth sentinel events, a 12-month follow-up showed an incidence of 20% death, 41% CP, 15% developmental delay, and 24% normal,[6] the latter 2 numbers indicating the need to further understand the antecedents, plasticity, and repair responses to well-defined single insults. Even uterine rupture is associated with an incidence of only 2% to 3% death and 6% to 23% hypoxic–ischemic encephalopathy (HIE).[7,8] Blame on such sentinel events often involves a certainty of causation in the legal perspective, which is not borne out by scientific evidence. Asphyxial events, including uterine rupture, amniotic embolism, tight nuchal cord, cord prolapse, placental abruption, severe intrapartum hemorrhage, maternal cardiac arrest, and severe shoulder dystocia are associated with only 8.5% of CP patients in western Australia.[9]

Some of the clinical scenarios suggesting repeated insults are placental insufficiency conditions, preeclampsia, inflammation, seizures, and severe apnea. Repeated H-I insults may show more oxidative injury, as in rabbit H-I,[10] but not necessarily more acidemia or similar bradycardia. A pre-existing hypoxic event can worsen electrical patterns in fetal sheep after repeated umbilical cord occlusions.[11]

In all clinical scenarios, it becomes impossible to make the distinction with certainty between single and repeated insults at the time of birth; thus, there is dire need for better biomarkers.

EMPHASIS ON THE BIRTH PERIOD

The process of birth brings the expecting mother to the prolonged attention of the medical establishment. The ease of diagnostic access of the newborn baby is much more than that of the fetus, especially in diagnosing brain injury, making it convenient to study birth events and assign proportional blame.

A diagnosis of an untoward event (eg, fetal distress, nonreassuring pattern) would lead to an emergent delivery; a timely diagnosis by round-the-clock vigilance of a mother in labor is the bedrock of the legal perspective, with the argument being that further brain injury can be avoided.[2] Performing an emergent delivery is based on the reasoning that removing the fetus from an adverse maternal–placental environment would lessen the duration of H-I. The reasoning of less H-I causing less or no injury is supported by animal studies. For motor deficits, antenatal H-I at 70% gestation of 30 minutes in rabbits results in no postnatal hypertonia, with increasing incidence of hypertonia (and perinatal deaths) with 35, 37, and 40 min of H-I.[12] These studies also bring attention to the fact that a threshold of injury is needed to trigger motor deficits, and there is a certain amount of leeway in the duration of H-I before irreversible changes occur.

DURATION OF PRENATAL INSULT VERSUS INJURY

Unfortunately, motor deficits are not just caused by a certain duration of H-I. The author and colleagues have recently found that rabbit fetuses at 79% gestation have more chances of developing motor deficits if they develop an additional reperfusion–reoxygenation injury just after the cessation of H-I, even comparing outcomes in the same litter.[13] Some fetuses do not undergo reperfusion–reoxygenation injury, and these are less likely to develop later motor deficits. Thus, in a population of normal fetuses, the differences in the susceptibility to injury determine later motor deficits, which are not dependent solely on the duration of H-I. This suggestion is supported by human studies. Despite having shared genetic, demographic, and environmental risk factors, 18% to 31% of twin pairs have discordant neurodevelopmental outcomes.[14] Ethnicity also determines final CP incidence, with Asians found to have less CP than non-Hispanic whites in California.[15]

MAGNETIC RESONANCE IMAGING BIOMARKERS OF FETAL BRAIN INJURY

Because of the technological limitations of direct fetal brain sampling, most of the present biomarkers of fetal brain health depend upon blood, metabolism, or gross movement of the fetus. The biomarker for the future is noninvasive neuroimaging. In rabbit fetuses, the MRI biomarker of apparent diffusion coefficient (ADC) can differentiate between fetuses destined to have postnatal hypertonia.[13,16,17] If one tracks the ADC before, during and after H-I, the ADC response in fetal rabbits falls into 4 categories. First, some fetuses have a small drop in their ADC. These fetuses are apparently normal on neurobehavior examination after birth (**Fig. 1**, no injury). Second, ADC drops below a certain nadir threshold during H-I. Most of these fetuses will develop motor deficits after birth (see **Fig. 1**, H-I injury). Third, ADC continues to drop after end of H-I. Most of these fetuses will also develop motor deficits after birth (see **Fig. 1**, RepReOx). Finally, ADC drop is even lower during H-I (below a second threshold) and does not recover after end of H-I. These fetuses will either die or develop motor deficits. More importantly, a combination of magnetic resonance imaging (MRI) criteria, using a nadir threshold and RepReOx, can predict which fetuses will develop hypertonia after birth with sensitivity of 0.94, specificity 0.79, positive predictive value 0.93, negative predictive value 0.83. These studies have implications for people, as the presence of a significant ADC drop could be used to identify fetuses with potential brain injury and also provide an estimate of timing of insult.

Table 1
Scientific perspective versus legal perspective

Legal Perspective	Scientific Evidence	Scientific Perspective
Analogy of auto collisions (single definable insult)	1. There are clinical scenarios that partially fit this analogy, such as maternal collapse, uterine rupture, umbilical cord prolapse, placental abruption 2. Most animal models use a single definable insult	1. Analogy does not take into account multiple insults, which could be synergistic, additive, or subtractive in nature 2. Analogy does not take into account chronic insults or those with acute on chronic exacerbation 3. Not all such clinical scenarios result in disabling brain injury[6]
"If the obstetrician is not with the patient, meaningfully focusing and acting on relevant patient information during labor, the obstetrician's absence will adversely impact patient safety"[2]	1. Removing the fetus from a hostile environment improves the chances to survive without injury 2. Decreasing the duration of H-I to the brain can result in less brain injury	1. In most clinical cases, the timing of the onset and duration of the insult are unknown 2. There is presently no reliable biomarker of fetal brain injury 3. Information is based principally on EFM, with all its faults[25] 4. The only intervention option available for the obstetrician at the bedside is an emergent cesarean section or operative vaginal delivery; this intervention cannot compensate in most circumstances for past events
American College of Obstetricians and Gynecologists (ACOG) position is somewhat biased and restrictive	1. No single metabolic or heart rate biomarker is reliable in diagnosing fetal brain injury; even composite biomarkers presently are unreliable 2. There are forms of CP and intellectual disability that are not mentioned in the ACOG statement	1. Fulfillment of criteria has shown to correlate with specific form of CP[40] 2. Cases of permanent brain injury without fulfilling ACOG criteria[41] suggest that the pathophysiological streams of a systemic injury causing brain injury or a specific localized brain injury triggered by a systemic event has not been clearly distinguished

Focus on EFM in deciding more rapid delivery for avoiding potential disabling injury	1. Bradycardia accompanies global H-I quite reliably but only in the acute period	1. Timing of onset of insult cannot be determined by EFM during labor alone; EFM at best reflects only the present state and not the past state
		2. Heart rate patterns do not reflect brain injury; bradycardia both before and after delivery does not necessarily result in disabling brain injury and recovers quickly
		3. Asystole can occur without disabling brain injury
		4. EFM increases chances of cesarean section
		5. Umbilical cord acidemia theoretically is better suited for timing of insults to events around birth, although association with brain injury has not been borne out by studies[42,43]

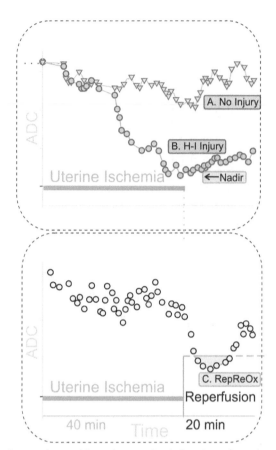

Fig. 1. 79% gestation mothers subjected to uterine ischemia and monitored in the magnet. Representative ADC values across time that show either (A) no injury later on, or (B) H-I injury, which below a certain threshold of ADC is more likely to develop motor deficits postnatally. (C) Evidence of injury in the reperfusion–reoxygenation period (RepReOx). Shaded portion can show extent of brain injury. Fetuses manifesting this pattern are more likely to develop motor deficits postnatally.

As a research tool, MRI criteria were used to investigate fetuses that are more susceptible to critical fetal brain injury. In a study examining different cell fates, the author and colleagues found higher expression in dead brain cells of neuronal nitric oxide synthase, an enzyme that is involved in production of reactive species, in premature fetuses destined to have hypertonia postnatally compared with litter mates that would be normal. This single protein change in a rabbit litter suggests that in a situation of equal injury, epigenetic changes involving different enzymes may make a particular fetus vulnerable compared with another fetus that may escape injury (**Fig. 2**). Not all fetal brains are normal or at the same vulnerability at the time of delivery.

ROUND-THE-CLOCK OBSTETRIC VIGILANCE

Just as the proverbial man searching for his lost item under a street lamp, there is an overemphasis on more vigilance around the time of delivery. A mother who comes into

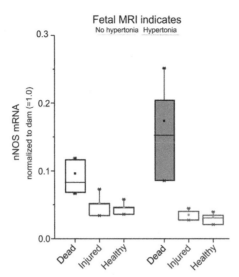

Fig. 2. 79% gestation fetuses subjected to H-I for 40 minutes while monitored by magnetic resonance imaging. Fetal brain extirpated 20 minutes after H-I and live cells sorted. Whole brain neuronal nitric oxide synthase (nNOS) gene expression increased in dead cells in E25 fetuses diagnosed by fetal magnetic resonance imaging as destined to be hypertonic ($P<.05$). In injured and healthy cells, there is no difference.

the delivery room is immediately subjected to electronic fetal monitoring (EFM) and the occasional fetal ultrasound. There are 4 points of attention to the present clinical practice.

First, it would help the clinician to have a better biomarker of fetal brain injury. The present scientific evidence points to the predominance of insults causing CP occurring in the antenatal period, with less than 10% attributed to asphyxia at birth.[18] The paucity of diagnostic modalities providing information about the fetal brain before delivery has led to an assumption that all brains are normal or at the same vulnerability at the time of delivery. Biomarkers are not available to predict which fetuses are more vulnerable, but fetal neuroimaging using noninvasive MRI is a promising biomarker that can show the response of the fetal brain to a particular insult; it is feasible in people.[19]

Second, the timing of the onset and the duration of the brain injury are often unknown in the antenatal and natal period. Thus, finding a single cause for CP becomes impossible. Without knowing timing and duration, it is often harder to provide timely intervention and future therapies. Note that the only therapy for term HIE, postnatal hypothermia, has been shown to be only useful if instituted within 6 hours of the insult.[20] The assumption that the time of delivery represents the onset of recovery from H-I is not applicable to all cases of HIE, especially when the insults are remote from the time of birth. This partly explains why hypothermia offers just an 11% reduction in risk of death or disability, from 58% to 47%.[21]

Third, the legal perspective has an excessive emphasis on heart rate.[22–24] EFM findings are supposed to trigger emergent delivery to avoid later brain injury.[25] Unfortunately, EFM is a measure of heart rate and not brain function. The institution of EFM has not reduced the incidence of CP.[25] A non-reassuring heart rate pattern is not a good diagnostic indicator of umbilical acidemia at term birth, with a sensitivity of 0.81, specificity of 0.43, positive predictive value of 0.47 and negative predictive value of 0.79.[26] Only 2.4% of the low-risk term pregnancies with severe EFM abnormalities (recurrent late or recurrent prolonged decelerations) were associated with CP.[27] In less than 1500 g infants, abnormal EFM pattern was associated with only 10.9% of children with any impairment, while 89.1% had no neurologic impairment at 2 years of age.[28] EFM has resulted in higher percentage of cesarean sections, exchanging problems from a theoretical hostile maternal–placental environment to that of a premature delivery, with risks of postnatal respiratory distress[29] and persistent pulmonary hypertension.[30]

Heart rate abnormalities can culminate in asystole. Even asystole is not a harbinger of disabling brain injury. An Apgar of 0 at 1 minute is not a good marker of later brain injury.[31] Asystole can occur at variable periods after an antenatal insult. In the author's rabbit model, it was found that a sizable number of deaths occurred at variable periods after the H-I insult, even days later.[32] This indicates the lack of relationship between asystole and timing of insult. The other implication is that successful resuscitation of the cardiovascular system assumed to be concurrent with that of the brain may not occur because of the different cell biology in different systems.

Finally, institution of a proper medical system with good communication does result in fewer cesarean sections and less litigation,[33,34] but it is unknown whether improvements in efficiency of obstetric care result in better neurodevelopmental outcomes. Poor communication is believed to contribute to a portion of stillbirths and infant deaths.[35] Again, the question arises whether one is looking in the right places if the emphasis on events around birth is also undertaken in the scientific world. With better fetal biomarkers, one could reach the target of successful prevention of bad outcomes.

ANTENATAL EVENTS

Antepartum causes were found to be the predominant cause of HIE in a study in western Australia.[36] The antepartum risk factors can be grouped under anatomic categories in the maternal-placental-fetal unit. Although HIE is just a subset of the cases of CP, it is instructive to examine the anatomic factors for the commonalities in etiology.

The maternal factors can be divided into those causing impaired oxygenation (eg, maternal asthma, pulmonary embolism and pneumonia) and those causing inadequate perfusion of maternal placenta (eg, maternal cardiorespiratory arrest, hypotension, chronic vascular disease and preeclampsia). Other factors that impact CP are lack of prenatal care, education status, and ethnicity (which may also have a postnatal component).[37]

The placental factors can be divided into potential acute factors (placental abruption, cord prolapse, uterine rupture, tight nuchal cord, true knot) and subacute factors (inflammation and vascular disorders causing placental insufficiency). Placental infarction occurs in 5% of CP cases, 2.5 times more often than controls.[38] In a series of 158 medicolegal CP cases, sentinel intrapartum events were present in only 11% of cases, but placental vascular lesions were predominant.[39]

The fetal factors include those causing impaired perfusion and oxygenation (fetomaternal hemorrhage and thrombosis).

An example of the confluence of both maternal and placental factors in affecting the fetus, and of subacute injury, is intrauterine growth retardation (IUGR). Among the antepartum risk factors in the western Australian study, IUGR showed the strongest association with HIE, with the odds ratio of 38.2, 95% confidence interval (CI) 9.4 to 154.8, of getting HIE.[36] Most babies with HIE do not meet the criteria of IUGR, but a greater proportion of HIE infants were below the tenth percentile of growth potential.[40]

Implicit in the etiology of CP are the interactions of anatomic factors with timing and duration of insults and with specific pathogenetic streams of injury (H-I, infection, inflammation, metabolic, toxic, genetic, or epigenetic) (**Fig. 3**).

If 2 children with the same insult were able to be tracked completely, these interactions would determine the final clinical phenotype of the children, and most often the outcomes would be dissimilar.[14] Conversely, if 2 children with the same phenotype were able to be tracked, differences in timing and duration of insult would likely occur.

ASYSTOLE AND DEATH

Little is known about the discordance between successful cardiovascular and brain resuscitation. All animal models are calibrated to a certain amount of injury. After cardiovascular collapse, little is known about what separates successful resuscitation with good outcome from bad outcome. The most severe animals that do not respond to 3 minutes of resuscitation are excluded in the well-known piglet model of cardiac arrest.[41] In the author's rabbit model of CP, it was found that some of the stillborn newborn kits had postural changes,[12] indicating that a percentage of deaths that could potentially have been prevented would have resulted in motor deficits in survivors.

The assumption that successful resuscitation of the cardiovascular system would also resuscitate the perinatal brain is not necessarily correct. There is a relative difficulty in getting a calibrated neurodevelopmental deficit in umbilical cord occlusion models where death occurs earlier than in placental insufficiency models.

UMBILICAL CORD ACIDEMIA

EFM variables are not considered as good as umbilical cord acidemia for timing of birth insults.[42] Neonatal seizures, other neurologic morbidities, and death are significantly more common in neonates with a pH less than or equal to 7.0, but most acidemic neonates do not have any major morbidity.[42] Both EFM variables and umbilical cord acidemia suffer from the drawback that insults remote from the time of delivery may have recovered to the normal state.

H-I IS NOT THE ONLY ETIOLOGIC FACTOR FOR CP

H-I alone can cause both bradycardia and umbilical cord acidemia, but the correlation of EFM tracings with umbilical acidemia depends upon the presence of intrauterine

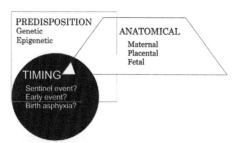

Fig. 3. Threshold of injury causing CP phenotype depends upon the interaction of timing, predisposition, anatomic and etiologic factors.

vascular pathology such as preeclampsia, abruptio placentae, and vascular pathology.[26] The presence of inflammation results in increased chances of disabling brain injury, such as chorioamnionitis[43] and vaginal infections.[44] An independent risk factor is maternal fever, often a harbinger of inflammation.[45,46] It is suspected that both the vasculopathies in placenta and inflammation can cause synergistic injury when combined with H-I.

INTERMEDIATE END POINTS OFTEN USED

There is a difference between outcomes that are intermediate in the newborn period and when the diagnosis of CP is made with conviction at 18 to 24 months. The legal perspective makes little distinction between intermediate end points such as HIE, neonatal encephalopathy, or seizures, and end points after 2 years such as CP or intellectual disability. What is lost is that only a proportion of these intermediate end points will turn out to have long-term motor and cognitive deficits. It is astounding to see during a legal argument, the etiologic leap made from the 3-hour period at birth to long-term motor and cognitive deficits, forgetting the prior 7000 hours of pregnancy[47] or the problems of the postnatal period.

POSTNATAL EVENTS THAT CONTRIBUTE

In premature infants, the presence of necrotizing enterocolitis and bacteremia double the chances of having diparetic CP and intellectual and motor deficits at 2 years, with surgical patients facing an additional quadrupling of risk.[48] Neonatal seizures also increase the chances of CP and other neurodevelopmental deficits both in term[49] and preterm infants.[50] Conversely, 37% of asphyxic newborns with seizures had normal outcome,[51] suggesting that even with a multitude of contributing factors, there is a threshold of injury that needs to be crossed before disabling injury can manifest itself.

SUMMARY

A single cause of CP is impossible to find with the present clinical biomarkers, much less pinpoint it to events at birth. A set of contributing factors may exist in an individual case, but the point at which the threshold for disabling injury is crossed is hard to determine. It is important for the scientific, clinical, and legal communities to consider all the factors that go into the direct causation of a case of CP before assigning blame. Fetal neuroimaging shows the most promise as a biomarker for timing and severity of fetal insults.

ACKNOWLEDGMENTS

Drs Emmett Hirsch and Matthew Derrick for editing the article.

REFERENCES

1. Hankins GD, MacLennan AH, Speer ME, et al. Obstetric litigation is asphyxiating our maternity services. Obstet Gynecol 2006;107:1382–5.
2. Conason RL, Pegalis SE. Neurologic birth injury. Protecting the legal rights of the child. J Leg Med 2010;31:249–86.
3. Back SA, Luo NL, Borenstein NS, et al. Late oligodendrocyte progenitors coincide with the developmental window of vulnerability for human perinatal white matter injury. J Neurosci 2001;21:1302–12.

4. Vannucci RC, Connor JR, Mauger DT, et al. Rat model of perinatal hypoxic–ischemic brain damage [review]. J Neurosci Res 1999;55:158–63.

5. Tan S, Drobyshevsky A, Jilling T, et al. Model of cerebral palsy in the perinatal rabbit. J Child Neurol 2005;20:972–9.

6. Okereafor A, Allsop J, Counsell SJ, et al. Patterns of brain injury in neonates exposed to perinatal sentinel events. Pediatrics 2008;121:906–14.

7. Barger MK, Nannini A, Weiss J, et al. Severe maternal and perinatal outcomes from uterine rupture among women at term with a trial of labor. J Perinatol 2012; 32:837–43.

8. Landon MB, Hauth JC, Leveno KJ, et al. Maternal and perinatal outcomes associated with a trial of labor after prior cesarean delivery. N Engl J Med 2004;351: 2581–9.

9. McIntyre S, Blair E, Badawi N, et al. Antecedents of cerebral palsy and perinatal death in term and late preterm singletons. Obstet Gynecol 2013;122:869–77.

10. Tan S, Zhou F, Nielsen VG, et al. Increased injury following intermittent fetal hypoxia–reoxygenation is associated with increased free radical production in fetal rabbit brain. J Neuropathol Exp Neurol 1999;58:972–81.

11. Pulgar VM, Zhang J, Massmann GA, et al. Mild chronic hypoxia modifies the fetal sheep neural and cardiovascular responses to repeated umbilical cord occlusion. Brain Res 2007;1176:18–26.

12. Derrick M, Luo NL, Bregman JC, et al. Preterm fetal hypoxia-ischemia causes hypertonia and motor deficits in the neonatal rabbit: a model for human cerebral palsy? J Neurosci 2004;24:24–34.

13. Drobyshevsky A, Luo K, Derrick M, et al. Motor deficits are triggered by reperfusion–reoxygenation injury as diagnosed by MRI and by a mechanism involving oxidants. J Neurosci 2012;32:5500–9.

14. Steingass KJ, Taylor HG, Wilson-Costello D, et al. Discordance in neonatal risk factors and early childhood outcomes of very low birth weight (<1.5 kg) twins. J Perinatol 2013;33:388–93.

15. Lang TC, Fuentes-Afflick E, Gilbert WM, et al. Cerebral palsy among Asian ethnic subgroups. Pediatrics 2012;129:e992–8.

16. Drobyshevsky A, Derrick M, Prasad PV, et al. Fetal brain magnetic resonance imaging response acutely to hypoxia–ischemia predicts postnatal outcome. Ann Neurol 2007;61:307–14.

17. Drobyshevsky A, Derrick M, Luo K, et al. Near-term fetal hypoxia–ischemia in rabbits: MRI can predict muscle tone abnormalities and deep brain injury. Stroke 2012;43:2757–63.

18. Jacobsson B, Hagberg G. Antenatal risk factors for cerebral palsy. Best Pract Res Clin Obstet Gynaecol 2004;18:425–36.

19. Guimiot F, Garel C, Fallet-Bianco C, et al. Contribution of diffusion-weighted imaging in the evaluation of diffuse white matter ischemic lesions in fetuses: correlations with fetopathologic findings. AJNR Am J Neuroradiol 2008;29:110–5.

20. Gunn AJ, Battin M, Gluckman PD, et al. Therapeutic hypothermia: from lab to NICU. J Perinat Med 2005;33:340–6.

21. Edwards AD, Brocklehurst P, Gunn AJ, et al. Neurological outcomes at 18 months of age after moderate hypothermia for perinatal hypoxic ischaemic encephalopathy: synthesis and meta-analysis of trial data. BMJ 2010;340:c363.

22. Five doctors & four nurses sued after delivery. Case on point: Livingston v. Montgomery, 0302.730 (2/27/2009)-TX. Nurs Law Regan Rep 2009;49:2.

23. OB/GYN nurse botched care—palsy resulted. Case on point: Reilly v. Ninia, 2011–01451 NYAPP2 (2/22/2011)-NY. Nurs Law Regan Rep 2011;52:4.

24. Suit alleging RNs & MDs responsible for brain injury to newborn dismissed. Case on point: C.A. v. Bentolila, A-1261–11T1 NJSUP (8/9/2012)-NJ. Nurs Law Regan Rep 2012;53:4.
25. Alfirevic Z, Devane D, Gyte GM. Continuous cardiotocography (CTG) as a form of electronic fetal monitoring (EFM) for fetal assessment during labour. Cochrane Database Syst Rev 2013;(5):CD006066.
26. Locatelli A, Incerti M, Ghidini A, et al. Factors associated with umbilical artery acidemia in term infants with low Apgar scores at 5 min. Eur J Obstet Gynecol Reprod Biol 2008;139:146–50.
27. Sameshima H, Ikenoue T, Ikeda T, et al. Unselected low-risk pregnancies and the effect of continuous intrapartum fetal heart rate monitoring on umbilical blood gases and cerebral palsy. Am J Obstet Gynecol 2004;190:118–23.
28. Nisenblat V, Alon E, Barak S, et al. Fetal heart rate patterns and neurodevelopmental outcome in very low birth weight infants. Acta Obstet Gynecol Scand 2006;85:792–6.
29. Martelius L, Janer C, Suvari L, et al. Delayed lung liquid absorption after cesarean section at term. Neonatology 2013;104:133–6.
30. Winovitch KC, Padilla L, Ghamsary M, et al. Persistent pulmonary hypertension of the newborn following elective cesarean delivery at term. J Matern Fetal Neonatal Med 2011;24:1398–402.
31. Nelson KB, Ellenberg JH. Apgar scores as predictors of chronic neurologic disability. Pediatrics 1981;68:36–44.
32. Derrick M, Englof I, Drobyshevsky A, et al. Intrauterine fetal demise can be remote from the inciting insult in an animal model of hypoxia–ischemia. Pediatr Res 2012;72(2):154–60.
33. Clark SL, Meyers JA, Frye DK, et al. Patient safety in obstetrics—the Hospital Corporation of America experience. Am J Obstet Gynecol 2011;204:283–7.
34. Clark SL, Belfort MA, Byrum SL, et al. Improved outcomes, fewer cesarean deliveries, and reduced litigation: results of a new paradigm in patient safety. Am J Obstet Gynecol 2008;199:105–7.
35. Rowe RE, Garcia J, Macfarlane AJ, et al. Does poor communication contribute to stillbirths and infant deaths? A review. J Public Health•Med 2001;23:23–34.
36. Badawi N, Kurinczuk JJ, Keogh JM, et al. Antepartum risk factors for newborn encephalopathy: the western Australian case–control study. BMJ 1998;317:1549–53.
37. Wu YW, Xing G, Fuentes-Afflick E, et al. Racial, ethnic, and socioeconomic disparities in the prevalence of cerebral palsy. Pediatrics 2011;127:e674–81.
38. Blair E, de GJ, Nelson KB. Placental infarction identified by macroscopic examination and risk of cerebral palsy in infants at 35 weeks of gestational age and over. Am J Obstet Gynecol 2011;205(2):124.e1–7.
39. Redline RW. Cerebral palsy in term infants: a clinicopathologic analysis of 158 medicolegal case reviews. Pediatr Dev Pathol 2008;11:456–64.
40. Bukowski R, Burgett AD, Gei A, et al. Impairment of fetal growth potential and neonatal encephalopathy. Am J Obstet Gynecol 2003;188:1011–5.
41. Yang ZJ, Torbey M, Li X, et al. Dopamine receptor modulation of hypoxic-ischemic neuronal injury in striatum of newborn piglets. J Cereb Blood Flow Metab 2007;27:1339–51.
42. Goldaber KG, Gilstrap LC III, Leveno KJ, et al. Pathologic fetal acidemia. Obstet Gynecol 1991;78:1103–7.
43. Wu YW, Escobar GJ, Grether JK, et al. Chorioamnionitis and cerebral palsy in term and near-term infants. JAMA 2003;290:2677–84.

44. Streja E, Miller JE, Bech BH, et al. Congenital cerebral palsy and prenatal exposure to self-reported maternal infections, fever, or smoking. Am J Obstet Gynecol 2013;209(4):332.e1–10.
45. Impey LW, Greenwood CE, Black RS, et al. The relationship between intrapartum maternal fever and neonatal acidosis as risk factors for neonatal encephalopathy. Am J Obstet Gynecol 2008;198:49.e1–6.
46. Blume HK, Li CI, Loch CM, et al. Intrapartum fever and chorioamnionitis as risks for encephalopathy in term newborns: a case-control study. Dev Med Child Neurol 2008;50:19–24.
47. Phelan JP, Martin GI, Korst LM. Birth asphyxia and cerebral palsy. Clin Perinatol 2005;32:61–76.
48. Martin CR, Dammann O, Allred EN, et al. Neurodevelopment of extremely preterm infants who had necrotizing enterocolitis with or without late bacteremia. J Pediatr 2010;157:751–6.
49. Garfinkle J, Shevell MI. Cerebral palsy, developmental delay, and epilepsy after neonatal seizures. Pediatr Neurol 2011;44:88–96.
50. Davis AS, Hintz SR, Van Meurs KP, et al. Seizures in extremely low birth weight infants are associated with adverse outcome. J Pediatr 2010;157:720–5.
51. Garfinkle J, Shevell MI. Predictors of outcome in term infants with neonatal seizures subsequent to intrapartum asphyxia. J Child Neurol 2011;26:453–9.

Pharmacologic Neuroprotective Strategies in Neonatal Brain Injury

Sandra E. Juul, MD, PhD[a],*, Donna M. Ferriero, MD, MS[b]

KEYWORDS

- Brain injury • Hypoxic-ischemic encephalopathy • Prematurity • Preconditioning

KEY POINTS

- There are many ways to achieve neuroprotection: preconditioning, salvaging, repair.
- Hypothermia is now standard of care for term hypoxic-ischemic encephalopathy so studies to investigate additional therapies will be added to that treatment.
- Strategies that target multiple mechanisms and consider age-appropriate mechanisms will be most beneficial.

MECHANISMS OF BRAIN INJURY: PRETERM VERSUS TERM

The two most common causes of neonatal brain injury in the United States are extreme prematurity and hypoxic-ischemic encephalopathy (HIE). In the United States, 1 in 8 babies is born before term (37–40 weeks), and 1.44% of babies (56,000 per year) are born with a birth weight of 1250 g or less.[1] These small, preterm babies are at high risk of death or neurodevelopmental impairment: approximately 20% die before hospital discharge, and 40% of survivors develop long-term intellectual or physical impairment, including cerebral palsy (CP).[2–4] Care of preterm infants accounts for more than half of pediatric health care dollars spent.

The brain rapidly increases in size, shape, and complexity during the second and third trimesters.[5] Neurodevelopmental compromise can result from an interruption of normal development or from damage to existing tissues. Brain development during this period is vulnerable to hypoxia-ischemia (HI), oxidant stress, inflammation, excitotoxicity, and poor nutrition. These exposures can result in structural, biochemical,

Disclosure Statement: Neither author has anything to disclose.
[a] Department of Pediatrics, University of Washington, 1959 Northeast Pacific Street, Box 356320, Seattle, WA 98195, USA; [b] Neonatal Brain Disorders Laboratory, University of California, San Francisco, 675 Nelson Rising Lane, Room 494, Box 0663, San Francisco, CA 94143, USA
* Corresponding author.
E-mail address: sjuul@uw.edu

and cell-specific injury.[6] Preoligodendrocytes, which emerge and mature between 24 and 32 weeks of development, are particularly susceptible to injury, and damage to these cells can result in white matter injury.[7] Although intracranial hemorrhage, periventricular leukomalacia, inflammatory conditions, and male gender are known risk factors for poor outcomes, little is known about how to improve these outcomes.

HIE is estimated to contribute significantly to 23% of the 4 million neonatal deaths that occur annually.[8] In the United States, HIE occurs in 1.5 to 2 live births per 1000, with a higher incidence in premature infants.[9] Untreated, the sequelae of moderate to severe HIE includes a 60% to 65% risk of mental retardation, CP, hydrocephalus, seizures, or death. Perinatal inflammation is increasingly recognized as an important contributor to neonatal HIE and poor neurodevelopmental outcomes[10]: the presence of maternal fever alone increases the risk for CP, and chorioamnionitis further increases the risks for brain injury in both preterm and term infants.[11,12] Timing of infection/inflammation relative to hypoxia is critical: it can be sensitizing (increase brain injury) if it occurs acutely or after 72 hours, but may be protective if it occurs 24 hours before hypoxia.[13] This differential response is not fully understood, but may depend on activation of fetal/neonatal Toll-like receptors in the brain.[14,15] Understanding the complex mechanisms of brain injury is essential to devising protective strategies.

THE INJURY CASCADE

Although the cellular targets of HI are different depending on age and severity of insult, the basic cascade of injury occurs in a uniform way regardless of age and continues for a prolonged period of time. Cell death occurs in 2 main phases: primary death from hypoxia and energy depletion, followed by reperfusion and increased free radical (FR) formation, excitotoxicity, and nitric oxide production with secondary energy failure and delayed death (**Fig. 1**). A tertiary phase was recently proposed, in which factors can worsen outcome, predispose a newborn to further injury, or prevent repair or regeneration after an initial insult to the brain.[16] Such mechanisms include persistent inflammation and epigenetic changes, which cause a blockade of oligodendrocyte maturation, impaired neurogenesis, impaired axonal growth, or altered synaptogenesis.

The injury process begins with energy failure creating excitotoxicity, which is caused by excessive glutamatergic activation that leads to progression of HI brain injury. Glutamate plays a key role in development, affecting progenitor cell proliferation, differentiation, migration, and survival. Glutamate accumulates in the brain after

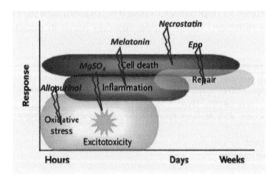

Fig. 1. The injury cascade as it occurs over time. Potential therapeutics are inserted during the course of the cascade. See text for details on these agents. Epo, erythropoietin.

HI[17] from a variety of causes, including vesicular release from axons and reversal of glutamate transporters. Glutamatergic receptors include N-methyl-D-aspartate (NMDA), alpha-3-amino-hydroxy-5-methyl-4-isoxazole propionic acid (AMPA), and kainate. Developmental differences in glutamate receptor expression contribute to the vulnerability of the immature brain (reviewed in Ref.[18]). NMDA receptor activation, although important for synaptic plasticity and synaptogenesis, can increase intracellular calcium, proapoptotic pathways via caspase-3 activation, FR formation, and lipid peroxidation, resulting in profound and widespread injury to the developing brain.

Oxidative stress is an important component of early injury, along with excitotoxicity, to the neonatal brain resulting from the excess formation of FRs (reactive oxygen species and reactive nitrogen species) under pathologic conditions. These FRs include superoxide anion (O_2^-), hydroxyl radical (OH), singlet oxygen ($^1O_2$), and hydrogen peroxide (H_2O_2). FRs target lipids, protein, and DNA, causing damage to these cellular components and initiating a cascade that results in cell death.[19]

These deleterious biological events trigger inflammatory processes that initially are harmful and later may be beneficial to the repair processes that occur after injury. The inflammatory response and cytokine production that accompany infection may play a large role in cell damage and loss. Local microglia are activated early and produce proinflammatory cytokines such as tumor necrosis factor (TNF)-alpha, interleukin (IL)-1β, and IL-6, as well as glutamate, FRs, and nitric oxide (NO), and are the main immunocompetent cells in the immature brain. Depending on the stimulus, molecular context, and timing, these cells acquire various phenotypes, which are critical to the outcome of the injury.[20]

Cell death occurs throughout the cascade, moving from a purely necrotic type to apoptosis with a continuum of phenotypes emerging in the developing brain (the apoptosis-necrosis continuum). Throughout this process, mechanistic interactions between cell death and hybrid forms of cell death occur, such as programmed or regulated necrosis or necroptosis.[21] The mechanisms behind programmed necrosis in neonatal brain injury are still being investigated but are regulated by the inflammatory processes, especially the TNF receptor superfamily, which is activated early in injury. There are many pharmacologic agents that can affect these injury phases (**Table 1**). This article highlights some of the important future therapeutics.

Table 1
Best pharmacologic candidates for impact on injury phases

Best Candidates	
Antenatal	**Postnatal**
BH4	Melatonin
Melatonin	Epo
nNOS inhibitors	NAC
Xenon	Xenon
Allopurinol	Allopurinol
Vitamin C and E	Vitamin C and E
Resveratrol	Resveratrol
NAC	Memantine
—	Topiramate

Abbreviations: BH4, tetrahydrobiopterin; NAC, N-acetyl-L-cysteine; nNOS, neuronal nitric oxide synthase.

TARGETING THE INJURY RESPONSE
Antiexcitotoxic Agents

The earliest pharmacologic strategies to protect the newborn brain were designed to block the initial phases of injury, excitotoxicity, and oxidative stress. Many of these agents failed because it is impossible to block normal developmental processes, like glutamatergic signaling, without harming the brain. Therefore, therapies designed to block the NMDA receptor resulted in increased, rather than decreased, cell death.[22] However, some agents, like magnesium sulfate, used to stop preterm labor, seemed to have beneficial effects even though they blocked the NMDA receptor. Recent clinical trials have supported the use of antenatal magnesium.[23] In 16 hospitals in Australia and New Zealand, 1062 women with fetuses younger than 30 weeks' gestation were given a loading infusion of 16 mmol followed by 8 mmol $MgSO_4$ for up to 24 hours. Substantial gross motor dysfunction (3.4% vs 6.6%; relative risk (RR), 0.51; 95% confidence interval [CI], 0.29–0.91) and combined death or substantial gross motor dysfunction were significantly reduced in the $MgSO_4$ group, although there were no significant differences in mortality or CP in survivors. In the United States, antenatal $MgSO_4$ did not reduce the risk of the composite outcome of CP or death, much like the Australian study, but was seen to reduce moderate to severe CP without increasing the risk of death.[23] However, the number needed to treat was high at 56 (95% CI, 34–164).

Another potential antiexcitotoxic agent is xenon, a noble gas used as an anesthetic agent. It has action against the NMDA receptor and has been shown to be an effective agent against hypoxic-ischemic insult both to cortical neurons in vitro and in several in vivo models.[24] Xenon lacks the dopamine-releasing properties that are present in other NMDA antagonists and does not cause increased apoptotic cell death as seen with other NMDA antagonists. Perhaps the most promising aspect of xenon pharmacology is that it increases the translational efficiency of hypoxia inducible factor-1 (HIF-1) through a mammalian target of rapamycin (mTOR) pathway[25] that has resulted in its potential application in HIE for both postinjury treatment and as a preconditioner. The prolonged increase in expression of HIF-1a by xenon causes upregulation of cytoprotective proteins such as erythropoietin (Epo), vascular endothelial growth factor (VEGF), and glucose transporter 1 protein.[25] When given with sevoflurane during labor to rats, it preconditions the fetal brain against a subsequent HI insult.[26] When given to neonatal rats in combination with hypothermia, it improves both functional and structural outcomes, even when hypothermia is delayed, and the effect is sustained through adulthood.[27]

Antioxidants

Therapies designed to reduce oxidative stress have proved to be efficacious both in the preterm and term injury states. Allopurinol was originally shown to be neuroprotective in postnatal day 7 rats after HI[28] but in humans was not seen to improve short-term or long-term outcomes in a small trial after birth asphyxia.[29] It was postulated that the drug needed to be given before reperfusion injury set in, so trials are now underway to evaluate efficacy when given to mothers who have fetuses suspected of intrauterine hypoxia. In a randomized, double-blind, placebo-controlled multicenter study that is now in progress, intravenous allopurinol is being given antenatally with the primary outcome being serum brain damage markers (S100b) and oxidative stress markers (isoprostanes and so forth) in umbilical cord blood; secondary outcome measures are neonatal mortality, serious composite neonatal morbidity, and long-term neurologic outcome.[30] There is now a randomized, placebo-controlled, double-blinded parallel group comparison study of hypothermia and allopurinol ongoing (the European ALBINO Trial). Allopurinol is being given twice: 30 minutes after birth and then 12 hours later, in addition to hypothermia in moderate to severe HIE. Outcomes will be assessed at 2 years of life.

There are many antioxidants that have been investigated in both preterm and term HI injury. Scavengers such as melatonin and vitamin E have shown promise. Lipid peroxidation inhibitors such as the lazaroids, gingko biloba, and caffeic acid, and FR reducers such as ebselen and Epo, have produced some amelioration of injury. Nitric oxide synthase inhibitors such as aminoguanidine, L-omega-nitro-arginine-methyl-ester (L-NAME), 7 nitroindazole, and newer derivatives are still being investigated.[31,32]

The most promising of these agents seems to be melatonin, which shows efficacy in both preterm and term injury. Melatonin has many targets along the injury cascade, including oxidative stress, inflammation, apoptosis, mitochondrial failure, as well as nuclear effects. The benefit is in the lack of significant side effects in children and term neonates. A recent observational study showed that melatonin levels are deficient in preterm and term newborn infants, and it is now being trialed daily for 7 days after premature birth to identify whether it will reduce the risk of prematurity-associated brain injury (MINT; ISRCTN15119574). Another investigation is underway in premature and full-term babies to identify optimal treatment doses (MELIP, NCT01340417; and MIND, NCT01340417), and there is a study to determine the effects of maternal supplementation on outcome in term infants (PREMELIP; identification number pending). An Australian study evaluating melatonin to prevent brain injury in unborn growth-restricted babies is ongoing in which mothers receive melatonin during pregnancy and oxidative stress is monitored in maternal serum, placenta, and umbilical cord blood. A composite neonatal outcome will be evaluated (NCT01695070).

Dietary manipulations may also prove promising in neuroprotection. Pomegranate juice is rich in polyphenols that can protect the neonatal mouse brain against an HI insult when given to mothers in their drinking water.[33] Even when given after the insult to neonatal animals, there is substantial protection in hippocampus, cortex, and striatum.[34] Omega-3 polyunsaturated fatty acid supplementation can reduce brain damage and improve long-term neurologic outcomes even 5 weeks after an HI insult to rodents. The effect is best appreciated in microglia, where nuclear factor kappa B activation and release of inflammatory mediators are inhibited, thus providing an antiinflammatory effect as well.[35]

Antiinflammatory Agents

As mentioned earlier, melatonin has multiple targets in the injury cascade and is a perfect candidate for manipulating inflammation. In several animal models, small and large, preterm and term, it has shown efficacy against excitotoxic lesions as well as HI. A recent study in rodents revealed that melatonin preserved white matter and learning disabilities after ibotenate lesions to the postnatal day 5 brain and was equally efficacious against IL-1β injections.[36] In a fetal sheep model at E90, cord occlusion produced substantial white matter injury that was blocked with melatonin.[37] In term brain models of HI, melatonin markedly decreased microglial activation and preserved myelination.[38] The most promising study to date in piglets revealed that melatonin, in combination with hypothermia, provided substantial improvement compared with hypothermia in preserving brain function measured by amplitude-integrated electroencephalogram, and reduced cell death in the thalamus, the region most affected by the asphyxia insult.[39] There is now a collaborative study between Hopital Robert Debre and St Thomas Hospital (Kings College London) as a proof of concept in neuroprotection study. It will be a double-blinded randomized trial of premature newborns of less than 28 weeks' gestational age. Babies will be randomized to placebo, low-dose melatonin, or high-dose melatonin, and outcome will be assessed by magnetic resonance imaging and neurodevelopmental outcome at 24 months (MINT Trial, ISRCTN15119574).

GROWTH FACTORS AS NEUROPROTECTANTS

Many growth factors have essential roles during fetal and postnatal brain development. Although the effects of some, such as brain-derived neurotrophic factor (BDNF), are largely restricted to the brain, others such as Epo, VEGF, granulocyte colony–stimulating factor (GCSF), and insulinlike growth factor 1 (IGF-1) have important somatic effects in addition to their roles in neurodevelopment. All of the factors listed earlier have been evaluated as neuroprotectant therapies for adult and neonatal brain injury. At this time, Epo is the best studied for this purpose, and is the closest to clinical use. The pleiotropic nature of these growth factors makes it essential to test meticulously for safety before clinical use, particularly because very high doses are often required for neuroprotection, given that these large molecules do not readily cross the blood-brain barrier.

Epo

Epo and its receptor (EpoR) are expressed in the developing central nervous system (CNS), and are required for normal brain development.[40] Acute exposure to hypoxia upregulates the expression of EpoR on oligodendrocytes and neurons, without a commensurate increase in Epo expression.[41] The presence of unbound cell surface EpoR drives cells of neuronal and oligodendrocyte lineage to apoptosis, whereas ligand-bound EpoR activates survival signaling pathways. With Epo binding, EpoR dimerizes to activate antiapoptotic pathways via phosphorylation of JAK2, phosphorylation, and activation of mitogen-activated protein kinase (MAPK), extracellular related kinase (ERK1/2), as well as the phosphatidylinositaol 3-kinase (PI3K/Akt) pathway and signal transducer and transcriptional activator 5 (STAT5), which are critical in cell survival.[42] Epo also stimulates production of BDNF. Epo signaling inhibits early mechanisms of brain injury by its antiinflammatory,[43,44] antiexcitotoxic,[45] antioxidant,[46,47] and antiapoptotic effects on neurons and oligodendrocytes. Repair of brain injury is also enhanced in the presence of Epo because of its positive effects on neurogenesis and angiogenesis, which are essential for plasticity and remodeling.[48,49] Epo effects are dose dependent, with multiple doses being more effective than single doses.[50,51] Epo reduces neuronal loss and learning impairment following brain injury,[52] and, even when initiated as late as 48 to 72 hours after injury, there is evidence of improved behavioral outcomes, enhanced neurogenesis, increased axonal sprouting, and reduced white matter injury in animal models of brain injury.[53,54]

Epo is now under investigation for both term and preterm brain injury. The antiinflammatory, antiexcitotoxic, and antioxidant effects are relevant to brain injury in both age groups. The specific effects of Epo in preoligodendrocytes may be most relevant to the white matter injury that characterizes preterm brain injury. Treatment approaches to acute brain injury in term infants (HIE) and preterm infants (intraventricular hemorrhage [IVH]) should differ from preventative strategies in preterm infants. In the former, a shorter duration of high-dose Epo is most appropriate, whereas for the latter, a more prolonged treatment strategy that continues during the period of oligodendrocyte vulnerability is most likely to succeed. In addition to the specific cellular effects on neurons and oligodendrocytes, this more prolonged treatment also decreases the availability and potential toxicity of free iron, caused by the erythropoietic effects of Epo, by increasing iron utilization.

Translation to Clinical Trials

Epo does not cross the placenta, so prenatal treatment is not an option. It is approved by the US Food and Drug Administration and has a robust safety profile in neonates, with more than 3000 neonates randomized to placebo-controlled trials testing its erythropoietic effects.[55] Doses required for neuroprotection are higher than those used for prevention and treatment of anemia, because only a small fraction of circulating Epo crosses the blood brain barrier. In animal models of neonatal brain injury, Epo doses of 1000 to 5000 U/kg result in sustained neuroprotection, improving both short-term and long-term structure and function.[56] Phase I/II trials have been done to establish safety and translational pharmacokinetics of Epo in preterm[57,58] and term neonates.[59] These studies suggest that 1000 U/kg/dose provides an area under the curve (AUC) most similar to a neuroprotective dose of 5000 U/kg in rodents (**Table 2**). The optimal dose and duration of treatment is likely to differ for treatment of HIE compared with preventing or treating brain injury in preterm infants, and is not yet known. Note that the pharmacokinetics in preterm and term asphyxiated infants are different, with a longer half-life noted at higher doses in infants with HIE. Phase II and III studies are now underway for neuroprotection of both extreme prematurity and HIE in term infants (**Box 1**). In the United States, a multicenter randomized controlled trial of preterm Epo neuroprotection is beginning (PENUT trial, NCT01378273). This study will use 1000 U/kg for 6 doses followed by 400 U/kg 3 times a week until 33 weeks of gestation. A Swiss trial has used 3000 U/kg for 3 doses in the first weeks of life. Enrollment is complete for this trial, with follow-up underway. The BRITE study, comparing Darbepoetin, Epo, and placebo, is showing improved outcomes in preterm neonates receiving either Darbepoetin or Epo. Erythropoietic agents (Epo and darbepoetin) are also being studied in combination with hypothermia for the treatment of HIE in term infants. Pilot studies have shown safety and early signs of benefit, and larger studies are planned or ongoing in the United States, France (NCT01732146), and China.

BDNF

BDNF is an important growth factor during fetal brain formation, particularly in the hippocampus, cerebral cortex, basal forebrain, and cerebellum. It is also active in adult neurogenesis. BDNF binds primarily to receptor tyrosine kinase B and activates MAPK and Ca^{2+}-calmodulin kinase II (CAMKII), which regulate cAMP-responsive

Table 2
Epo pharmacokinetics

	Epo Dose (U/kg)	AUC	C_{max}	$T_{1/2}$
P7 Rodents SC	5000	117,677	6224	8.4
P7 Rodents IP	5000	140,331	10,015	6.7
Preterm infants <1000 g	500	31,412 ± 2780	8078 ± 538	5.4 ± 0.6
	1000	81,498 ± 7067	14,017 ± 1293	7.1 ± 0.7
	2500	317,881 ± 22,941	46,467 ± 2987	8.7 ± 1.4
Term HIE infants	500	50,306 ± 67,426	7046 ± 814	7.2 ± 1.9
	1000	131,054 ± 17,083	13,780 ± 2674	15.0 ± 4.5
	2500	328,002 ± 61,945	33,316 ± 7377	18.7 ± 4.7

Abbreviations: AUC, area under the curve; C_{max}, maximum plasma concentration of the drug; IP, intraperitoneal; P7, postnatal day 7; SC, subcutaneously; $T_{1/2}$, half life.

Box 1
Clinical trials of neuroprotective agents

Phase 1 and 2 trials

Xenon and cooling therapy in babies at high risk of brain injury following poor condition at birth: randomized pilot study. Bristol, United Kingdom

Phase 2 and 3 trials

Safety and efficacy of topiramate in neonates with HIE treated with hypothermia (NeoNATI), Florence, Italy. NCT01241019

Neonatal Epo and therapeutic hypothermia; short-term outcome study (NEAT O Study). University of California, San Francisco, multicenter, Thrasher funded

Darbepoetin administration in newborns undergoing cooling for encephalopathy (DANCE Study) Utah, multicenter, Thrasher funded. NCT01471015

Phase 3 trials

A multicenter randomized controlled trial of therapeutic hypothermia plus magnesium sulfate ($MgSO_4$) versus therapeutic hypothermia plus placebo in the management of term and near-term babies with HIE. Turkey. NCT01646619

Optimizing cooling strategies at less than 6 hours of age for neonatal HIE. A National Institute of Child Health and Human Development (NICHD)–funded project. NCT01192776

Phase III study of efficacy of high-dose Epo to prevent HIE sequelae in term newborns. Paris, France. NCT01732146

Evaluation of systemic hypothermia initiated after 6 hours of age in infants of greater than or equal to 36 weeks' gestation with HIE: a bayesian evaluation. An NICHD-funded project. NCT00614744

Preterm Epo Neuroprotection (PENUT) Trial. A multicenter, randomized, placebo-controlled phase III 940–subject trial of Epo for the neuroprotection of extremely low gestational age neonates. An NINDS-funded project. NCT01378273

Melatonin as a Novel Neuroprotectant in Preterm Infants Trial (MINT). UK trial funded by Medical Research Council. ISRCTN15119574

---

element binding (CREB) and synapsin transcription. Neuroprotection from glutamate toxicity is mediated through PI3K and the Ras/MAPK signaling pathways, and involves an increase in B-cell lymphoma 2 (bcl-2) proteins.[60] Both exercise and caffeine increase BDNF secretion, thereby increasing recognition memory and neurogenesis.

VEGF

VEGF is a growth factor that is stimulated by HIF-1 and stimulates vasculogenesis and angiogenesis, essential processes needed for brain development and brain repair. In addition, VEGF has specific neurotrophic and neuroprotective effects in adult and neonatal models of hypoxic-ischemic brain injury.[61] These effects also involve activation of Akt and extracellular receptor kinase (ERKs). Tight regulation of this factor is needed because both overexpression and underexpression can contribute to disease.

GCSF

GCSF is a hematopoietic glycoprotein that stimulates the clonal maturation of neutrophil progenitors and increases many functional activities of mature neutrophils. In addition to these hematopoietic effects, GCSF and its receptor are expressed on neuronal cells in a variety of brain regions.[62] GCSF has shown neuroprotection in several models of brain injury, and is well tolerated at high doses. GCSF has been reported to have antiapoptotic, antiinflammatory, antiexcitotoxic, and neurotrophic properties with demonstrated improved long-term outcomes.[63] It is currently being evaluated in a phase II clinical trial for adult ischemic stroke (NCT00132470).[64]

IGF-1

IGF-1 has an important role in normal brain development, promoting neuronal growth, cellular proliferation, and differentiation in vitro, when injected directly into brain, or when given intranasally.[65] It has also been found to have neuroprotective effects, improving long-term function after hypoxic-ischemic brain injury. However, its clinical application to neurologic disorders is limited by its large molecular size, poor central uptake, and mitogenic potential.

Drug Delivery

When considering drugs for neuroprotection, drug delivery is an important consideration. For example, if a drug crosses the placenta and can be tolerated by the mother, prenatal treatment is an option, such as with xenon and melatonin. The ability to give the drug intravenously is important, given that many critically ill neonates cannot take oral medications. Some medications, such as melatonin, are presently only available as oral formulations. Inhalational agents such as xenon have the problem that, if a significant oxygen requirement exists, the ability to deliver neuroprotective concentrations (30%–50%) may be limited.

Box 2
Gaps in knowledge

1. Cytokine response
   - Innate immunity differs in newborns compared with adults
     - Th1 preponderance in newborns
     - Th2 in adults
   - When does it change?
   - How is this affected by prematurity?
   - How does this affect brain injury/repair?
2. Microglial response
   - Three activation states of CNS microglia
     - M1: classic activation (tissue defense, proinflammatory)
     - M2: alternative activation (repair, antiinflammatory, fibrosis, matrix reconstruction)
     - M3: acquired deactivation (immunosuppression, phagocytosis of apoptotic cells)
   - How are these states regulated?
   - Can this response be harnessed for healing?
   - Does it differ for preterm versus term infants?
3. Preconditioning
   - Hypoxia
   - Inflammation
     - What are the molecular mechanisms?
     - Can these mechanisms be harnessed to improve outcomes?

Small neuroactive peptides may have a therapeutic advantage compared with larger molecules such as Epo or GCSF, which are larger glycoproteins that do not cross the blood-brain barrier well. Modified neuropeptides and mimetic peptides have been designed to overcome these barriers, and are in various stages of testing.

Another novel approach is to use alternative delivery methods, targeting the inflammatory system. Polyamidoamine dendrimers have been shown to localize in activated microglia and astrocytes in the brains of newborn rabbits with CP, but not healthy controls.[66] This nanotechnology approach has been used with excellent results to deliver dendrimer-bound N-acetyl-L-cysteine (NAC) to the target inflammatory cells to suppress neuroinflammation, using much lower concentrations than are needed with systemic dosing.

Combination Therapies

As more information is gained about mechanisms of brain injury and neuroprotection, combination therapies may be applied. As mentioned earlier, some preclinical combination studies are already underway, for example, hypothermia plus xenon, and hypothermia plus Epo for the treatment of term HIE.

Gaps in Knowledge

There remain gaps in knowledge (**Box 2**). All of these must be considered in the context of the developing neonate, because immune function, cell populations, and specific vulnerabilities and response to injury change over time. As clinicians become more knowledgeable in these areas, new approaches to neuroprotection may become apparent.

REFERENCES

1. Hamilton BE, Hoyert DL, Martin JA, et al. Annual summary of vital statistics: 2010-2011. Pediatrics 2013;131:548–58.
2. O'Shea TM, Allred EN, Dammann O, et al. The ELGAN study of the brain and related disorders in extremely low gestational age newborns. Early Hum Dev 2009;85:719–25.
3. Stoll BJ, Hansen NI, Bell EF, et al. Neonatal outcomes of extremely preterm infants from the NICHD Neonatal Research Network. Pediatrics 2010;126:443–56.
4. Gargus RA, Vohr BR, Tyson JE, et al. Unimpaired outcomes for extremely low birth weight infants at 18 to 22 months. Pediatrics 2009;124:112–21.
5. Lodygensky GA, Vasung L, Sizonenko SV, et al. Neuroimaging of cortical development and brain connectivity in human newborns and animal models. J Anat 2010;217:418–28.
6. Volpe JJ. Brain injury in premature infants: a complex amalgam of destructive and developmental disturbances. Lancet Neurol 2009;8:110–24.
7. Back SA, Riddle A, McClure MM. Maturation-dependent vulnerability of perinatal white matter in premature birth. Stroke 2007;38:724–30.
8. Black RE, Cousens S, Johnson HL, et al. Global, regional, and national causes of child mortality in 2008: a systematic analysis. Lancet 2010;375:1969–87.
9. Kurinczuk JJ, White-Koning M, Badawi N. Epidemiology of neonatal encephalopathy and hypoxic-ischaemic encephalopathy. Early Hum Dev 2010;86: 329–38.
10. van Vliet EO, de Kieviet JF, Oosterlaan J, et al. Perinatal infections and neurodevelopmental outcome in very preterm and very low-birth-weight infants: a meta-analysis. JAMA Pediatr 2013;167:662–8.

11. Badawi N, Kurinczuk JJ, Keogh JM, et al. Intrapartum risk factors for newborn encephalopathy: the Western Australian case-control study. BMJ 1998;317:1554–8.

12. Wu YW, Croen LA, Shah SJ, et al. Cerebral palsy in a term population: risk factors and neuroimaging findings. Pediatrics 2006;118:690–7.

13. Eklind S, Mallard C, Arvidsson P, et al. Lipopolysaccharide induces both a primary and a secondary phase of sensitization in the developing rat brain. Pediatr Res 2005;58:112–6.

14. Vontell R, Supramaniam V, Thornton C, et al. Toll-like receptor 3 expression in glia and neurons alters in response to white matter injury in preterm infants. Dev Neurosci 2013;35(2–3):130–9.

15. Stridh L, Ek CJ, Wang X, et al. Regulation of toll-like receptors in the choroid plexus in the immature brain after systemic inflammatory stimuli. Transl Stroke Res 2013;4:220–7.

16. Fleiss B, Gressens P. Tertiary mechanisms of brain damage: a new hope for treatment of cerebral palsy? Lancet Neurol 2012;11:556–66.

17. Gucuyener K, Atalay Y, Aral YZ, et al. Excitatory amino acids and taurine levels in cerebrospinal fluid of hypoxic ischemic encephalopathy in newborn. Clin Neurol Neurosurg 1999;101:171–4.

18. Jensen FE. Developmental factors regulating susceptibility to perinatal brain injury and seizures. Curr Opin Pediatr 2006;18:628–33.

19. Buonocore G, Perrone S, Bracci R. Free radicals and brain damage in the newborn. Biol Neonate 2001;79:180–6.

20. Hagberg H, Gressens P, Mallard C. Inflammation during fetal and neonatal life: implications for neurologic and neuropsychiatric disease in children and adults. Ann Neurol 2012;71:444–57.

21. Chavez-Valdez R, Martin LJ, Northington FJ. Programmed necrosis: a prominent mechanism of cell death following neonatal brain injury. Neurol Res Int 2012; 2012:257563.

22. Ikonomidou C, Turski L. Why did NMDA receptor antagonists fail clinical trials for stroke and traumatic brain injury? Lancet Neurol 2002;1:383–6.

23. Costantine MM, Drever N. Antenatal exposure to magnesium sulfate and neuroprotection in preterm infants. Obstet Gynecol Clin North Am 2011;38:351–66, xi.

24. Wilhelm W, Hammadeh ME, White PF, et al. General anesthesia versus monitored anesthesia care with remifentanil for assisted reproductive technologies: effect on pregnancy rate. J Clin Anesth 2002;14:1–5.

25. Ma D, Lim T, Xu J, et al. Xenon preconditioning protects against renal ischemic-reperfusion injury via HIF-1alpha activation. J Am Soc Nephrol 2009;20:713–20.

26. Yang T, Zhuang L, Rei Fidalgo AM, et al. Xenon and sevoflurane provide analgesia during labor and fetal brain protection in a perinatal rat model of hypoxia-ischemia. PLoS One 2012;7:e37020.

27. Thoresen M, Hobbs CE, Wood T, et al. Cooling combined with immediate or delayed xenon inhalation provides equivalent long-term neuroprotection after neonatal hypoxia-ischemia. J Cereb Blood Flow Metab 2009;29:707–14.

28. Palmer C, Towfighi J, Roberts RL, et al. Allopurinol administered after inducing hypoxia-ischemia reduces brain injury in 7-day-old rats. Pediatr Res 1993;33: 405–11.

29. Benders MJ, Bos AF, Rademaker CM, et al. Early postnatal allopurinol does not improve short term outcome after severe birth asphyxia. Arch Dis Child Fetal Neonatal Ed 2006;91:F163–5.

30. Kaandorp JJ, Benders MJ, Rademaker CM, et al. Antenatal allopurinol for reduction of birth asphyxia induced brain damage (ALLO-Trial); a randomized

double blind placebo controlled multicenter study. BMC Pregnancy Childbirth 2010;10:8.

31. Buonocore G, Groenendaal F. Anti-oxidant strategies. Semin Fetal Neonatal Med 2007;12:287–95.

32. Yu L, Derrick M, Ji H, et al. Neuronal nitric oxide synthase inhibition prevents cerebral palsy following hypoxia-ischemia in fetal rabbits: comparison between JI-8 and 7-nitroindazole. Dev Neurosci 2011;33:312–9.

33. Loren DJ, Seeram NP, Schulman RN, et al. Maternal dietary supplementation with pomegranate juice is neuroprotective in an animal model of neonatal hypoxic-ischemic brain injury. Pediatr Res 2005;57:858–64.

34. West T, Atzeva M, Holtzman DM. Pomegranate polyphenols and resveratrol protect the neonatal brain against hypoxic-ischemic injury. Dev Neurosci 2007;29: 363–72.

35. Zhang W, Hu X, Yang W, et al. Omega-3 polyunsaturated fatty acid supplementation confers long-term neuroprotection against neonatal hypoxic-ischemic brain injury through anti-inflammatory actions. Stroke 2010;41:2341–7.

36. Ramanantsoa N, Fleiss B, Bouslama M, et al. Bench to cribside: the path for developing a neuroprotectant. Translational Stroke Research 2013;4:258–77.

37. Welin AK, Svedin P, Lapatto R, et al. Melatonin reduces inflammation and cell death in white matter in the mid-gestation fetal sheep following umbilical cord occlusion. Pediatr Res 2007;61:153–8.

38. Villapol S, Fau S, Renolleau S, et al. Melatonin promotes myelination by decreasing white matter inflammation after neonatal stroke. Pediatr Res 2011;69:51–5.

39. Robertson NJ, Faulkner S, Fleiss B, et al. Melatonin augments hypothermic neuroprotection in a perinatal asphyxia model. Brain 2013;136:90–105.

40. Yu X, Shacka JJ, Eells JB, et al. Erythropoietin receptor signalling is required for normal brain development. Development 2002;129:505–16.

41. Mazur M, Miller RH, Robinson S. Postnatal erythropoietin treatment mitigates neural cell loss after systemic prenatal hypoxic-ischemic injury. J Neurosurg Pediatr 2010;6:206–21.

42. Digicaylioglu M, Lipton SA. Erythropoietin-mediated neuroprotection involves cross-talk between Jak2 and NF-kappaB signalling cascades. Nature 2001; 412:641–7.

43. Sun Y, Calvert JW, Zhang JH. Neonatal hypoxia/ischemia is associated with decreased inflammatory mediators after erythropoietin administration. Stroke 2005;36:1672–8.

44. Juul SE, Beyer RP, Bammler TK, et al. Microarray analysis of high-dose recombinant erythropoietin treatment of unilateral brain injury in neonatal mouse hippocampus. Pediatr Res 2009;65:485–92.

45. Zacharias R, Schmidt M, Kny J, et al. Dose-dependent effects of erythropoietin in propofol anesthetized neonatal rats. Brain Res 2010;1343:14–9.

46. Kumral A, Tugyan K, Gonenc S, et al. Protective effects of erythropoietin against ethanol-induced apoptotic neurodegeneration and oxidative stress in the developing C57BL/6 mouse brain. Brain Res Dev Brain Res 2005;160:146–56.

47. Chattopadhyay A, Choudhury TD, Bandyopadhyay D, et al. Protective effect of erythropoietin on the oxidative damage of erythrocyte membrane by hydroxyl radical. Biochem Pharmacol 2000;59:419–25.

48. Iwai M, Cao G, Yin W, et al. Erythropoietin promotes neuronal replacement through revascularization and neurogenesis after neonatal hypoxia/ischemia in rats. Stroke 2007;38:2795–803.

49. Osredkar D, Sall JW, Bickler PE, et al. Erythropoietin promotes hippocampal neurogenesis in in vitro models of neonatal stroke. Neurobiol Dis 2010;38: 259–65.
50. Kellert BA, McPherson RJ, Juul SE. A comparison of high-dose recombinant erythropoietin treatment regimens in brain-injured neonatal rats. Pediatr Res 2007;61:451–5.
51. Gonzalez FF, Abel R, Almli CR, et al. Erythropoietin sustains cognitive function and brain volume after neonatal stroke. Dev Neurosci 2009;31:403–11.
52. Demers EJ, McPherson RJ, Juul SE. Erythropoietin protects dopaminergic neurons and improves neurobehavioral outcomes in juvenile rats after neonatal hypoxia-ischemia. Pediatr Res 2005;58:297–301.
53. Iwai M, Stetler RA, Xing J, et al. Enhanced oligodendrogenesis and recovery of neurological function by erythropoietin after neonatal hypoxic/ischemic brain injury. Stroke 2010;41:1032–7.
54. Reitmeir R, Kilic E, Kilic U, et al. Post-acute delivery of erythropoietin induces stroke recovery by promoting perilesional tissue remodelling and contralesional pyramidal tract plasticity. Brain 2011;134:84–99.
55. Juul S. Erythropoietin in anemia of prematurity. J Matern Fetal Neonatal Med 2012;25:80–4.
56. van der Kooij MA, Groenendaal F, Kavelaars A, et al. Neuroprotective properties and mechanisms of erythropoietin in in vitro and in vivo experimental models for hypoxia/ischemia. Brain Res Rev 2008;59:22–33.
57. Juul SE, McPherson RJ, Bauer LA, et al. A phase I/II trial of high-dose erythropoietin in extremely low birth weight infants: pharmacokinetics and safety. Pediatrics 2008;122:383–91.
58. Fauchere JC, Dame C, Vonthein R, et al. An approach to using recombinant erythropoietin for neuroprotection in very preterm infants. Pediatrics 2008;122: 375–82.
59. Wu YW, Bauer LA, Ballard RA, et al. Erythropoietin for neuroprotection in neonatal encephalopathy: safety and pharmacokinetics. Pediatrics 2012;130: 683–91.
60. Almeida RD, Manadas BJ, Melo CV, et al. Neuroprotection by BDNF against glutamate-induced apoptotic cell death is mediated by ERK and PI3-kinase pathways. Cell Death Differ 2005;12:1329–43.
61. Feng Y, Rhodes PG, Bhatt AJ. Neuroprotective effects of vascular endothelial growth factor following hypoxic ischemic brain injury in neonatal rats. Pediatr Res 2008;64:370–4.
62. Xiao BG, Lu CZ, Link H. Cell biology and clinical promise of G-CSF: immunomodulation and neuroprotection. J Cell Mol Med 2007;11:1272–90.
63. Fathali N, Lekic T, Zhang JH, et al. Long-term evaluation of granulocyte-colony stimulating factor on hypoxic-ischemic brain damage in infant rats. Intensive Care Med 2010;36:1602–8.
64. Schabitz WR, Laage R, Vogt G, et al. AXIS: a trial of intravenous granulocyte colony-stimulating factor in acute ischemic stroke. Stroke 2010;41:2545–51.
65. Popken GJ, Hodge RD, Ye P, et al. In vivo effects of insulin-like growth factor-I (IGF-I) on prenatal and early postnatal development of the central nervous system. Eur J Neurosci 2004;19:2056–68.
66. Kannan S, Dai H, Navath RS, et al. Dendrimer-based postnatal therapy for neuroinflammation and cerebral palsy in a rabbit model. Sci Transl Med 2012;4: 130ra46.

Stem Cell Therapy for Neonatal Brain Injury

Bobbi Fleiss, PhD[a,b,c,d], Pascale V. Guillot, PhD[e],
Luigi Titomanlio, MD, PhD[a,b,c], Olivier Baud, MD, PhD[a,b,c],
Henrik Hagberg, MD, PhD[d,f,g], Pierre Gressens, MD, PhD[a,b,c,d],*

KEYWORDS

- Stem cell therapy • Neuroprotection • Mesenchymal stem cells
- Amniotic stem cells • Placental stem cells • Neural stem cells
- Embryonic stem cells • Cord blood

KEY POINTS

- Preclinical studies support efficacy of stem cells in models of perinatal brain injury.
- Mechanisms underpinning these neurotherapeutic effects are not fully understood.
- Systemic comparative analysis of effects of known cells across models is required.
- Randomized clinical trials are ongoing.

INTRODUCTION

To understand how to harness the potential of stem cells as therapeutic agents requires the considered formulation and interpretation of data from studies in animal models of injury and disease. Animal models, despite their limitations, represent

Authors have no conflict of interest to disclose.

The research of the authors is supported by the Inserm (OB, LT, and PG), Paris Diderot University (OB and PG), the PremUP Foundation (OB and PG), the Seventh Framework Program of the European Union (grant agreement No. HEALTH-F2-2009-241778/Neurobid, PG), the Indo-French Center for the Promotion of Advanced Research (CEFIPRA project No. 4903-H, PG), the Leducq Foundation (HH and PG), the de Spoelberch Foundation (PG), the Grace de Monaco Foundation (PG), Medical Research Council (Sweden, 2012-2642, HH), ALF-LUA (ALFGBG2863, HH), Wellcome Trust Program Grant (WT094823MA, HH and PG), SPARKS Foundation (PVG), and the Assistance Publique-Hôpitaux de Paris ("contrat hospitalier de recherche translationnelle," PG).

[a] Inserm U676, Paris, 75019, France; [b] University Paris Diderot, Sorbonne Paris Cité, UMRS 676, Paris, 75019, France; [c] PremUP, Paris, 75019, France; [d] Department of Perinatal Imaging and Health, Department of Division of Imaging Sciences and Biomedical Engineering, King's College London, King's Health Partners, St. Thomas' Hospital, London, SE1 7EH, UK; [e] UCL Institute for Women's Health, University College London, London, WC1E 6HX, UK; [f] Department of Clinical Sciences, Sahlgrenska Academy/East Hospital, 416 85 Gothenburg, Sweden; [g] Department of Physiology and Neuroscience, Perinatal Center, Sahlgrenska Academy, Gothenburg University, 40530, Gothenburg, Sweden

* Corresponding author. Inserm U676, Robert Debré Hospital, 48 Boulevard Serurier, Paris 75019, France.

E-mail address: pierre.gressens@inserm.fr

well-defined biologic systems with levels of complexity and responsiveness compara-ble in many ways to those of human infants. To model neonatal brain injury, re-searchers have developed two complementary approaches: (1) a reductionist approach, involving inducing specific cellular and/or molecular mechanisms known to be involved in injury; or (2) recapitulating the supposed causal event.

Although the causes and outcomes of brain injury in preterm and term neonates are far from identical, they share some common cellular and molecular mechanisms. These include the processes of excitotoxicity and neuroinflammation, incorporating microglial activation, proinflammatory cytokine and chemokine production, and toll-like receptor (TLR) activation through the production of injured neural tissues of damage-associated molecular patterns (DAMPs, or alarmins). The importance of these pathways is the generally accepted rationale for using excitotoxic agents (eg, agonists of N-methyl-d-aspartate [NMDA] or a-amino-3-hydroxy-5-methyl-4-isoxazolepropionic acid [AMPA]-kainate glutamate receptors), proinflammatory cytokines, or TLR agonists to mimic mechanistic aspects of these human brain disorders in animal models.[1–4]

In neonatal brain injury, although there is no definitive consensus about the cause of brain damage, the two predominating hypotheses are a hypoxic-ischemic (HI) origin and a systemic inflammatory origin, linked to pathologies such as chorioamnionitis.[4] Accordingly, to model neonatal brain injury in a causal manner, various animal models have been developed based on (1) acute HI insults (eg, transient umbilical cord [UC] occlusion during late gestation[5]), (2) in utero asphyxiation during delivery,[6] (3) carotid artery ligation combined with transient hypoxia in the early neonatal period,[7] (4) chronic hypoxic insults (eg, protracted hypoxia during either the fetal or early postnatal period[8,9]), or (5) systemic acute or subacute inflammatory insults (ie, administration of the TLR agonists[10] or the cytokine IL-1-beta during either the late fetal or early post-natal periods[11]). See later discussion.[3,12] In addition, investigating groups have devel-oped combined models in which systemic inflammation sensitizes the developing brain to a second HI or excitotoxic insult.[13,14]

Stem cell therapies have been envisaged as having enormous potential to repair and regenerate across many fields of medicine. Although much quality research tria-ling stem cells in neonatal brain damage has been performed in various laboratories across the world, the data are still confusing and sometimes conflicting. This is likely because each research group uses different animal models, different types of stem cells, and different experimental endpoints or assessments.

This article briefly describes the major types of stem cells, reviews the animal data relating to the use of stem cells to protect and repair the neonatal brain, and mentions any safety concerns, before describing the on-going pilot clinical trials with stem cell therapy in human neonates. The article concludes with what the authors believe are the necessary questions that need answering to move this research forward and determine an optimized design for clinical trials in human neonates with brain injury.

MAJOR TYPES OF STEM CELLS

Characteristics that give stem cells therapeutic value include the capacity for some (but not all) lineages to differentiate under permissive conditions and their antiinflam-matory and immune-modulatory functions. Stem cells can be obtained from many different tissues and at all stages of life (**Table 1**).

Embryonic Stem Cells

Embryonic stem cells (ESCs) are derived from the inner mass of blastocysts and can self-renew indefinitely because they are able to maintain an identical phenotype

Table 1
Major types of stem cells and their key features

Stem Cell Source	Advantages	Disadvantages
Embryonic stem cells	Pluripotent Possibility to derive neural stem cells and other neurogenic lineages Can be used for prenatal, neonatal, and postnatal applications Self-renewing Highly expandable	Ethical restriction Not accessible for autologous use Tumorigenic
Induced pluripotent stem cells	Pluripotent Possibility to derive neural stem cells and other neurogenic lineages Can be used autologously Can be used for prenatal, neonatal and postnatal applications Self-renewing Highly expandable	Produced via ectopic expression of genetic material Epigenetic instability Epigenetic memory Poor efficiency Tumorigenic
Neural stem cells	Precursor to all neurogenic lineages	Not directly accessible in humans
Chemically-induced induced pluripotent stem cells from amniotic fluid stem cells	Pluripotent Possibility to derive neural stem cells and other neurogenic lineages Safe High efficiency Can be used autologously Can be used for prenatal, neonatal and postnatal applications Self-renewing Highly expandable	Tumorigenic
Fetal mesenchymal stem cells	Antiinflammatory and immunomodulatory Can be used autologously Can be used for prenatal, neonatal and postnatal applications Highly expandable	Multipotent Cannot undergo differentiation into ectodermic lineages Do not self-renew
Adult mesenchymal stem cells	Antiinflammatory and immunomodulatory Can be used autologously Can be used for postnatal applications	Multipotent, with lower differentiation potency compared with fetal mesenchymal stem cells Cannot undergo differentiation into ectodermic lineages Cannot be used for prenatal and neonatal applications Do not self-renew Slow growth kinetics and early senescence

(continued on next page)

Table 1 (continued)		
Stem Cell Source	**Advantages**	**Disadvantages**
Cord blood stem cells	Antiinflammatory and immunomodulatory Can be used autologously Can be used for neonatal applications	Multipotent Cannot undergo differentiation into ectodermic lineages Cannot be used for prenatal applications Do not self-renew Slow growth kinetics and early senescence
Amniotic fluid stem cells	Can be chemically reverted to pluripotency Can express early markers of neurogenic and oligodendrocyte differentiation in vitro Can be used autologously Can be used for prenatal, neonatal and postnatal applications Highly expandable	Multipotent Cannot undergo differentiation into ectodermic lineages Do not self-renew Isolated during prenatal diagnostic
Fetal placenta stem cells (from first trimester or term chorionic membrane)	Nontumorigenic Can form embryoid bodies Can produce neurons in vitro Can be used autologously Can be used for prenatal, neonatal and postnatal applications Highly expandable	Multipotent Do not self-renew

following cell division. ESCs are pluripotent, able to give rise to cell types from each of the three germ layers: ectoderm, endoderm, and mesoderm. ESCs can, therefore, differentiate into neural cells and represent an almost unlimited supply of cells for transplantation. However, they can form teratomas after transplantation[15,16] and their use induces considerable ethical concerns.

Induced Pluripotent Stem Cells

Induced pluripotent stem cells (iPSCs) are terminally differentiated somatic cells reverted to pluripotency. This process was first performed using integrating viruses to deliver the reprogramming factors Oct4, Sox2, c-Myc, and Klf4b; or Oct4, Sox2, Nanog, and Lin28.[17] Reprogramming techniques have been further refined by using nonintegrative viruses, mRNAs, and minicircle plasmids to decrease the risk of mutagenicity associated with the insertion of exogenous genetic material into the genome.[18] Recent findings suggest that endogenous expression of key pluripotency factors may favor the reprogramming process of certain cells. For example, neural stem cells (NSCs) endogenously expressing Sox2 and c-Myc could be reprogrammed via ectopic expression of Oct4 alone.[19] In addition, germline cells and epiblast stem cells, which endogenously express Oct4, could be reprogrammed to pluripotency without ectopic expression of transcription factors, solely by supplementation with small molecules.[20,21] Mouse somatic stem cells have also been reprogrammed, albeit with low efficiency, using a cocktail of chemicals.[22] A major step toward transcription factor-free chemical derivation of patient-specific pluripotent cell types was made within the author's (PVG) laboratory, by converting human c-Kit+ first and second trimester amniotic fluid stem cells (AFSCs) to functional pluripotency without ectopic expression of pluripotency factors.[23–25] These chemically reprogrammed cells are of great interest because they are not genetically modified and the hope is that risks of potential persisting proliferative activity following injection are reduced. An advantage of iPSCs is to allow autologous grafts, although the safety of these cells after transplantation remains to be fully established.

NSCs

NSCs can be derived from the embryonic or fetal brain, but are also present in the subventricular zone and dentate gyrus of the adult brain.[26,27] NSCs can be cultured and expanded in vitro as neurospheres that contain true NSCs, committed progenitors, and differentiated progeny. NSCs can differentiate into neurons of different subtypes, oligodendrocytes, and astrocytes,[28–32] but have the same potential for teratoma formation as ESCs. Reducing the ethical burden of using these cells, NSC can also be derived from chemically induced iPSC.[23]

Mesenchymal Stem Cells

Mesenchymal stem cells (MSCs) can be isolated from fetal and adult tissues throughout development (ie, first trimester fetal blood, liver and bone marrow [BM], adult BM, cord blood, and UC stroma).[33] MSCs can differentiate into all kinds of mesodermal tissues (eg, bone, cartilage, fat); however, fetal cells demonstrate a greater potential for plasticity compared with their adult counterparts. It has been suggested that MSCs can differentiate into functional neurons, although this remains highly controversial, especially after transplantation.[28,34] The immunogenicity of MSCs is extremely low because they lack expression of major histocompatibility complex class-II antigens, making them attractive therapeutic candidates. Moreover, MSCs have immunosuppressive and antiinflammatory properties.[35,36]

UC Stem Cells

UC blood (UCB) contains many types of stem cells, including MSCs,[37] endothelial progenitor cells,[38] and UCB-mononuclear cells (UCB-MNCs). The latter have shown to differentiate in vitro into virtually all types of mature cells,[39–43] including neural cells.[44–46] The advantages of UCB-MNCs include easy acquisition of cord blood at birth, limited ethical issues, and low immunogenicity.[47] UC Wharton jelly is also a source of MSCs (UC-MSCs) that exhibit greater proliferative potential compared with BM-derived MSCs (BM-MSCs).[33,48]

AFSCs

Amniotic fluid contains a subset of c-Kit+ cells that possess an intermediate phenotype between embryonic and mesenchymal stem cells, expressing features of both.[25,49] For example, AFSCs coexpress the pluripotency marker Oct4 variant 1 and the MSC cell surface marker CD73. AFSCs can be found in the amniotic fluid throughout gestation and can be readily isolated during prenatal diagnostics, holding promise for cell-based therapies and tissue engineering. AFSCs are fast growing, nontumorigenic, and are broadly multipotent, being able to differentiate into the standard tri-mesodermal lineages of bone, fat, and cartilage, as well as into renal, neurogenic, hematopoietic, cardiac, and skeletal myogenic lineages.[25]

Placental Stem Cells

Fetal placental chorionic stem cells (CSCs) can be isolated from the fetal membranes during first trimester prenatal diagnostic testing (chorionic villi sampling) or at birth. Interestingly, comparison of first-trimester versus term-derived c-Kit+ CSCs showed that early CSCs found during the first trimester are smaller in size, grow faster, show higher levels of expression of pluripotency markers, can form embryoid bodies containing lineages from the three germ layers, and have the capacity to differentiate into neural-like cells in vitro.[50]

STEM CELL THERAPY IN ANIMAL MODELS OF NEONATAL BRAIN DAMAGE
Data from Trials of NSCs

In a model of excitotoxic lesion to the immature brain (P5 mouse), injection of murine NSCs into the contralateral hemisphere at 4 or 72 hours significantly reduced brain damage and improved long-term behavior.[51] Human NSCs derived from ESCs, that were injected into the striatum 3 days after excitotoxic lesion in the same model were shown to migrate to the site of lesion, express neuronal and glial markers, and partially restore striatal neuronal number.[52] The neuroprotective capacity of murine NSCs derived from ESCs (by retinoic acid-induced differentiation) injected into the striatum after right carotid artery ligation to induce acute ischemia in P12 mice has also been tested. Illustrating the importance of timing of treatment, intrastriatal injection 2 days after ischemia reduced brain damage, whereas no effect was observed when NSCs were injected 7 days after the insult.[53] However, in this study, 30% of the animals treated with NSCs developed brain tumors. In a model of neonatal HI brain injury, human NSCs derived from ESCs injected into the forebrain 1 day after the insult induced long-term improved behavior.[54]

Data from Trials of MSCs

Numerous studies, especially those from the Utrecht group, have shown that BM-MSCs were highly neuroprotective for the developing brain.[55–58] Treatment of neonatal mice with MSCs 3 and 10 days after transient unilateral right carotid artery occlusion and exposure to low oxygen concentrations on P9 produced a 60% decrease in neuronal loss. Furthermore, there was a 46% improvement in sensorimotor function, as observed in the cylinder-rearing test, and remodeling of the corticospinal tract correlated with sensorimotor improvements. Interestingly, intranasal administration of MSCs proved to be nearly as protective as intracranial administration in these studies.[55]

In addition, a few studies have analyzed the protective effects of human UC-MSCs in the developing brain. In a rodent model of neonatal HI brain injury, intracerebral injection of human UC-MSCs reduced brain damage and improved long-term functional outcome.[59,60]

Data from Trials of UCB-MNCs

It was recently shown that human UCB-MNCs were unable to reduce neonatal excitotoxic brain injury,[61] in contrast with protection previously observed with NSCs in this model.[51] Furthermore, intraperitoneal injection of high doses of UCB-MNCs was associated with a systemic inflammatory response causing a moderate exacerbation of brain damage. Similarly, intravenous injection of human UCB-MNCs in a severe model of neonatal HI showed no improvement in functional outcome or lesion volume.[62] On the other hand, three studies have demonstrated protective effects of intraperitoneal administration of human UCB-MNCs in a rodent model of neonatal

HI brain injury based on (1) a reduction in the occurrence of spastic paresis,[63] (2) improvement in sensorimotor performance and striatal neuron survival,[64] and (3) indirect reduction of secondary cell death and facilitation of postischemic plasticity through attenuation of reactive gliosis.[65]

COMBINING HYPOTHERMIA AND STEM CELLS

The provision of therapeutic hypothermia in clinics has been an important step forward to reducing the burden of mortality in infants diagnosed with hypoxic-ischemia encephalopathy based on Apgar score, pH, and lactate levels.[66] However, to date there are no in vivo studies assessing the usefulness of combined stem cell-hypothermia treatment of neonatal brain injury. Hypothermia alters the time course of pathophysiologic events initiated by brain injury, such as energy failure and inflammation,[67] and it dramatically alters the metabolism of drugs given as adjunct therapies to treat these processes.[68,69] As such, strategic combinations of stem cell therapy with hypothermia must consider, for example, that the inflammatory signals mediating homing of stem cells to areas of need may be impaired during the application of hypothermia. In addition, the health and therapeutic capacity of stem cells may themselves be altered by hypothermia, requiring adaptations to application regimes. These considerations may be overcome via application of stem cells following cessation of hypothermia but, regardless, the combination must be considered a new therapy and tested with the same rigor.

CLINICAL DATA AND ONGOING CLINICAL TRIALS

A pilot safety study of autologous cord blood infusion was performed in 184 infants with acquired neurologic disorders.[70] This retrospective study supported the short-term safety of intravenous autologous cord blood infusion. Several randomized controlled trials (RCTs) using stem cells to treat subjects with cerebral palsy, stroke, or neonatal HI encephalopathy have been initiated and/or are shortly set to report findings (**Table 2**). There is a substantial heterogeneity in the type of cells, the route of administration, and the timing for intervention in these trials. In most trials, cells are administered from weeks to years after the brain insult, although there is no preclinical data demonstrating the efficacy of cell therapy with such a prolonged interval in the pediatric population. Three RCTS have been completed, but to the authors' knowledge, results from only one have been communicated so far. Preliminary data provided regarding outcomes from the Korean clinical trial using a combination of rehabilitation, erythropoietin, and allogeneic intravenous stem cell therapy in infants between 2 and 5 years of age with cerebral palsy have shown significant improvements in gross motor function and quality during the study period.[71] No formal analysis has yet been made to confirm that this improvement is greater then expected over time for untreated infants, but it seems that the combination therapy is more effective than rehabilitation alone, or rehabilitation and erythropoietin combined, in improving outcome measures. At Duke University, an open label study using autologous blood–derived stem cells is also set to report findings at the end of 2013. However, because of the study design, the ability to interpret the findings will be severely compromised.

ISSUES TO BE ADDRESSED

Animal data clearly supports the hypothesis that stem cells are of great benefit for protecting the neonatal brain from acquired injuries such as HI brain injury. In the authors'

Table 2
Ongoing randomized clinical trials using stem cell therapy to treat neonatal brain injury

Title	Trial Duration	Intervention	Age at Inclusion	Status	Sponsor and Trial Identifier
UCB in the treatment of stroke in children	September 2012–December 2015	Autologous human cord blood–derived stem cell injection Single intravenous injection with 2-y follow-up	6 wk–6 y	Ongoing	The University of Texas, Houston, USA NCT01700166
Multiple transplantation of BM-derived CD133 cell in cerebral palsy	April 2012–April 2014	Intrathecal injection of BM-derived CD133 cells vs subjects not receiving stem cells	4 y–12 y	Ongoing	Royan Institute, Iran NCT01763255
Autologous stem cells in newborns with oxygen deprivation	January 2012–April 2013	IV infusion of autologous stem cells within the first 48 h after birth vs control group of subjects that meet the inclusion criteria but the family does not choose intervention	37 wk–42 wk	Completed, results not available	Hospital Universitario Gonzalez Monterrey, Mexico NCT01506258
Safety and efficacy of BM-MNC for the treatment of cerebral palsy in subjects <15 y	March 2011–August 2014	Intrathecal injection of autologous MNC	3 y–15 y	Ongoing	Chaitanya Hospital, Pune, India NCT01832454

Allogenic UCB and erythropoietin combination therapy for cerebral palsy	May 2010–April 2011	Allogeneic UCB infusion under nonmyeloablative immunosuppression, plus erythropoietin twice weekly for 4 wk (two initial doses of 500 IU/kg IV, followed by 6 doses of 250 IU/kg subcutaneously) and rehabilitation vs erythropoietin plus rehabilitation vs rehabilitation only	10 mo–10 y	Completed, positive preliminary results available	Sung Kwang Medical Foundation, South Korea NCT01193660
Safety and effectiveness of cord blood stem cell infusion for the treatment of cerebral palsy in children	January 2010–February 2014	Mononuclear cell enriched cord blood unit prepared for infusion vs placebo	1 y–12 y	Ongoing	Georgia Regents University, USA NCT01072370
Intrathecal autologous stem cells for children with hypoxic or ischemic brain injury	July 2009–April 2010	Subjects stimulated with granulocyte colony-stimulating factor 5 times, BM harvest, and infused 8–10 mL of stem cells (CD34+) by intrathecal route	1 y–8 y	Completed, results not available	Hospital Universitario Gonzalez Monterrey, Mexico NCT01019733

view, in addition to the careful consideration of data from the recently completed small RCTs, several issues need to be addressed before moving toward larger-scale clinical trials:

1. What is the best type of stem cell to use in neonates? Should different types of stem cells be used according to the specific foci of the injury, the cause, and/or the age at birth? Comparing the efficacy of different types of stem cells in different animal models of neonatal brain injury should address this key question.

2. What is the best route of stem cell administration? Stem cells may be delivered either systemically into the vasculature or locally into the brain (intraparenchymally, intraventricularly, and intrathecally).[72,73] Many stem cells are capable of migration toward a focus of injury.[51] In rodent models, NSCs have generally been delivered directly into the brain, whereas MSCs have usually been given systemically or, more recently, intranasally.[55] How do these administration routes translate into clinical practice, what is ethically acceptable, and what are the potential side effects? Critically, is the elegant intranasal route applicable to the human brain in which the distances for cell migration to the site of injury are larger when compared with a rodent brain? Studies in a primate model of neonatal brain injury should allow testing of the latter question.

3. What is the optimal window for intervention and what is the therapeutic window? Should stem cells be administered as soon as possible after the insult or should treatment be delayed to provide a less deleterious environment for the transplanted cells? Should single, double, or multiple injections of stem cells be performed? Available data in rodents suggest that administration of NSCs at 4 hours or 3 days after a neonatal excitotoxic insult afford similar neuroprotection[51] and that administration MSCs at 3 and 10 days after a neonatal HI insult gives better results than a single injection at day three.[57] Despite these data encouraging the possibility of increased efficacy with an optimized treatment regime, no systematic study of the efficacy of treatment relative to timing has been reported to the authors' knowledge.

4. What are the mechanisms by which stem cells afford neuroprotection? The original hypothesis that transplanted stem cells would replace the dead brain cells and integrate into functional networks has been invalidated in most experimental paradigms.[74] Indeed, a large proportion of transplanted cells die within a few weeks. Different alternate mechanisms for neuroprotection have been proposed, including antiinflammatory effects, production of trophic factors, stimulation of proliferation, survival and differentiation of endogenous stem cells, facilitation of endogenous postlesion plasticity, and transfer of healthy mitochondria to endogenous neural cells.[74–76] Additional experimental studies are necessary to pinpoint the most relevant protective mechanisms in neonatal brain damage afforded by the different sources of stem cells. Although the identification of the precise mechanism of neuroprotection is not mandatory for using stem cells in humans, such knowledge would strengthen the rationale for translating to human neonates and might allow the identification of novel and druggable targets for neuroprotection.

5. Do in vitro–engineered stem cells provide any therapeutic advantage over naïve stem cells? In this context, a recent study showed that MSCs and Brain Derived Growth Factor (BDNF)-hypersecreting MSCs were equally effective in reducing brain damage in a model of neonatal stroke.[58]

6. Could membrane vesicles such as exosomes be used as a substitute for cell-based therapies for the treatment of neonatal brain damage?[77] Exosomes are cell-derived vesicles released in staggeringly large numbers by many cell types, including stem

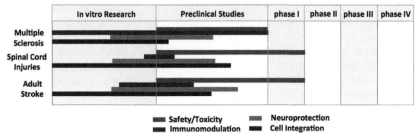

Fig. 1. Timeline of stem cell therapy development in adult neurologic injuries. (*Data from* Giusto E, Donega M, Cossetti C, et al. Neuro-immune interactions of neural stem cell transplants: From animal disease models to human trials. Exp Neurol 2013 Mar 16 [Epub ahead of print].)

cells, and contain proteins, active enzymes, mRNA, and micro-RNAs. They seem to play important roles in cell-to-cell signaling.

7. What are the short-term and long-term risks for a negative immune or inflammatory response following cell transplantation? As previously discussed, some stem cells are less immunogenic than others are (ie, MSC), potentially decreasing the risk of an immune response. This may be particularly advantageous if multiple injections of stem cells are required for efficacy.

8. What is the risk for tumor formation following cell transplantation? Is this risk limited to ESCs and iPSCs? In one study, brain tumor formation has been reported following NSC transplantation in a model of neonatal HI brain injury.[53] In addition, a report from Russia described a young patient with Ataxia telangiectasia [sic] who developed several neuroblastomas potentially derived from the donor human NSC transplants.[78] Although the risk of tumor formation is probably low with MSCs and NSCs, these studies support the need for thorough long-term safety assessment in subjects during future clinical trials.

In considering these issues, stem cell therapy for diseases of the adult nervous system has moved forward following a more systematic approach than currently used (**Fig. 1**). This type of rationalized approach should inspire perinatologists to take full advantage of the chance to demonstrate the efficacy and safety of stem cell therapy to protect and/or repair the newborn brain.

SUMMARY

Understanding of the characteristics of stem cells and, in particular, those with therapeutic potential are greatly increasing. In addition, there are strong preclinical data that stem cells are effective neurotherapies and this seems to be supported (albeit preliminarily) by small clinical trials. However, a lack of comprehensive preclinical testing of different types of cells across models means there is still a lack of information about the specific situations in which each may have greatest therapeutic efficacy. As such, there are many variables to explore to ensure perinatologists can identify the right cells for the right patients at the right time to achieve the overarching goal of improving the outcome for neonates suffering brain injury.

REFERENCES

1. Czeh M, Gressens P, Kaindl AM. The yin and yang of microglia. Dev Neurosci 2011;33(3–4):199–209.

2. Degos V, Favrais G, Kaindl AM, et al. Inflammation processes in perinatal brain damage. J Neural Transm 2010;117(8):1009–17.

3. Hagberg H, Peebles D, Mallard C. Models of white matter injury: comparison of infectious, hypoxic-ischemic, and excitotoxic insults. Ment Retard Dev Disabil Res Rev 2002;8(1):30–8.

4. Kaindl AM, Favrais G, Gressens P. Molecular mechanisms involved in injury to the preterm brain. J Child Neurol 2009;24(9):1112–8.

5. Mallard EC, Williams CE, Johnston BM, et al. Increased vulnerability to neuronal damage after umbilical cord occlusion in fetal sheep with advancing gestation. Am J Obstet Gynecol 1994;170(1 Pt 1):206–14.

6. Ireland Z, Dickinson H, Fleiss B, et al. Behavioural effects of near-term acute fetal hypoxia in a small precocial animal, the spiny mouse (*Acomys cahirinus*). Neonatology 2010;97(1):45–51.

7. Yager JY, Brucklacher RM, Vannucci RC. Cerebral energy metabolism during hypoxia-ischemia and early recovery in immature rats. Am J Phys 1992; 262(3 Pt 2):H672–7.

8. Raymond M, Li P, Mangin JM, et al. Chronic perinatal hypoxia reduces glutamate-aspartate transporter function in astrocytes through the Janus kinase/signal transducer and activator of transcription pathway. J Neurosci 2011;31(49): 17864–71.

9. Baud O, Daire JL, Dalmaz Y, et al. Gestational hypoxia induces white matter damage in neonatal rats: a new model of periventricular leukomalacia. Brain Pathol 2004;14(1):1–10.

10. Du X, Fleiss B, Li H, et al. Systemic stimulation of TLR2 impairs neonatal mouse brain development. PLoS One 2011;6(5):e19583.

11. Favrais G, van de Looij Y, Fleiss B, et al. Systemic inflammation disrupts the developmental program of white matter. Ann Neurol 2011;70(4):550–65.

12. Ramanantsoa N, Bouslama M, Matrot B, et al. Bench to cribside: the path for developing a neuroprotectant. Transl Stroke Res 2013;4(2):258–77.

13. Dommergues MA, Patkai J, Renauld JC, et al. Proinflammatory cytokines and interleukin-9 exacerbate excitotoxic lesions of the newborn murine neopallium. Ann Neurol 2000;47(1):54–63.

14. Eklind S, Mallard C, Leverin AL, et al. Bacterial endotoxin sensitizes the immature brain to hypoxic–ischaemic injury. Eur J Neurosci 2001;13(6):1101–6.

15. Bjorklund LM, Sanchez-Pernaute R, Chung S, et al. Embryonic stem cells develop into functional dopaminergic neurons after transplantation in a Parkinson rat model. Proc Natl Acad Sci U S A 2002;99(4):2344–9.

16. Carson CT, Aigner S, Gage FH. Stem cells: the good, bad and barely in control. Nat Med 2006;12(11):1237–8.

17. Takahashi K, Yamanaka S. Induction of pluripotent stem cells from mouse embryonic and adult fibroblast cultures by defined factors. Cell 2006;126(4):663–76.

18. Diecke S, Wu JC. Pushing the reset button: chemical-induced conversion of amniotic fluid stem cells into a pluripotent state. Mol Ther 2012;20(10):1839–41.

19. Kim JB, Sebastiano V, Wu G, et al. Oct4-induced pluripotency in adult neural stem cells. Cell 2009;136(3):411–9.

20. Sterneckert J, Hoing S, Scholer HR. Concise review: Oct4 and more: the reprogramming expressway. Stem Cells 2012;30(1):15–21.

21. Zhou H, Li W, Zhu S, et al. Conversion of mouse epiblast stem cells to an earlier pluripotency state by small molecules. J Biol Chem 2010;285(39):29676–80.

22. Hou P, Li Y, Zhang X, et al. Pluripotent stem cells induced from mouse somatic cells by small-molecule compounds. Science 2013;341(6146):651–4.

23. Moschidou D, Mukherjee S, Blundell MP, et al. Valproic acid confers functional pluripotency to human amniotic fluid stem cells in a transgene-free approach. Mol Ther 2012;20(10):1953–67.
24. Moschidou D, Mukherjee S, Blundell MP, et al. Human mid-trimester amniotic fluid stem cells cultured under embryonic stem cell conditions with valproic acid acquire pluripotent characteristics. Stem Cells Dev 2013;22(3):444–58.
25. Moschidou D, Drews K, Eddaoudi A, et al. Molecular signature of human amniotic fluid stem cells during fetal development. Curr Stem Cell Res Ther 2013; 8(1):73–81.
26. Alvarez-Buylla A, Temple S. Stem cells in the developing and adult nervous system. J Neurobiol 1998;36(2):105–10.
27. Gage FH. Mammalian neural stem cells. Science 2000;287(5457):1433–8.
28. Kohyama J, Abe H, Shimazaki T, et al. Brain from bone: efficient "meta-differentiation" of marrow stroma-derived mature osteoblasts to neurons with Noggin or a demethylating agent. Differentiation 2001;68(4–5):235–44.
29. Lu P, Blesch A, Tuszynski MH. Induction of bone marrow stromal cells to neurons: differentiation, transdifferentiation, or artifact? J Neurosci Res 2004; 77(2):174–91.
30. Lu P, Jones LL, Snyder EY, et al. Neural stem cells constitutively secrete neurotrophic factors and promote extensive host axonal growth after spinal cord injury. Exp Neurol 2003;181(2):115–29.
31. Montzka K, Lassonczyk N, Tschoke B, et al. Neural differentiation potential of human bone marrow-derived mesenchymal stromal cells: misleading marker gene expression. BMC Neurosci 2009;10:16.
32. Neuhuber B, Gallo G, Howard L, et al. Reevaluation of in vitro differentiation protocols for bone marrow stromal cells: disruption of actin cytoskeleton induces rapid morphological changes and mimics neuronal phenotype. J Neurosci Res 2004;77(2):192–204.
33. Pappa KI, Anagnou NP. Novel sources of fetal stem cells: where do they fit on the developmental continuum? Regen Med 2009;4(3):423–33.
34. Dezawa M, Kanno H, Hoshino M, et al. Specific induction of neuronal cells from bone marrow stromal cells and application for autologous transplantation. J Clin Invest 2004;113(12):1701–10.
35. Kaplan JM, Youd ME, Lodie TA. Immunomodulatory activity of mesenchymal stem cells. Curr Stem Cell Res Ther 2011;6(4):297–316.
36. Sato K, Ozaki K, Mori M, et al. Mesenchymal stromal cells for graft-versus-host disease: basic aspects and clinical outcomes. J Clin Exp Hematop 2010;50(2): 79–89.
37. Lee MW, Yang MS, Park JS, et al. Isolation of mesenchymal stem cells from cryopreserved human umbilical cord blood. Int J Hematol 2005;81(2): 126–30.
38. Ingram DA, Mead LE, Tanaka H, et al. Identification of a novel hierarchy of endothelial progenitor cells using human peripheral and umbilical cord blood. Blood 2004;104(9):2752–60.
39. Markov V, Kusumi K, Tadesse MG, et al. Identification of cord blood-derived mesenchymal stem/stromal cell populations with distinct growth kinetics, differentiation potentials, and gene expression profiles. Stem Cells Dev 2007;16(1): 53–73.
40. Tondreau T, Meuleman N, Delforge A, et al. Mesenchymal stem cells derived from CD133-positive cells in mobilized peripheral blood and cord blood: proliferation, Oct4 expression, and plasticity. Stem Cells 2005;23(8):1105–12.

41. Gao F, Wu DQ, Hu YH, et al. In vitro cultivation of islet-like cell clusters from human umbilical cord blood-derived mesenchymal stem cells. Transl Res 2008; 151(6):293–302.

42. Haase A, Olmer R, Schwanke K, et al. Generation of induced pluripotent stem cells from human cord blood. Cell Stem Cell 2009;5(4):434–41.

43. Das H, Abdulhameed N, Joseph M, et al. Ex vivo nanofiber expansion and genetic modification of human cord blood-derived progenitor/stem cells enhances vasculogenesis. Cell Transplant 2009;18(3):305–18.

44. Buzanska L, Jurga M, Stachowiak EK, et al. Neural stem-like cell line derived from a nonhematopoietic population of human umbilical cord blood. Stem Cells Dev 2006;15(3):391–406.

45. Kogler G, Sensken S, Airey JA, et al. A new human somatic stem cell from placental cord blood with intrinsic pluripotent differentiation potential. J Exp Med 2004;200(2):123–35.

46. Jang YK, Park JJ, Lee MC, et al. Retinoic acid-mediated induction of neurons and glial cells from human umbilical cord-derived hematopoietic stem cells. J Neurosci Res 2004;75(4):573–84.

47. Rocha V, Wagner JE Jr, Sobocinski KA, et al. Graft-versus-host disease in children who have received a cord-blood or bone marrow transplant from an HLA-identical sibling. Eurocord and International Bone Marrow Transplant Registry Working Committee on Alternative Donor and Stem Cell Sources. N Engl J Med 2000;342(25):1846–54.

48. Baksh D, Yao R, Tuan RS. Comparison of proliferative and multilineage differentiation potential of human mesenchymal stem cells derived from umbilical cord and bone marrow. Stem Cells 2007;25(6):1384–92.

49. De Coppi P, Bartsch G Jr, Siddiqui MM, et al. Isolation of amniotic stem cell lines with potential for therapy. Nat Biotechnol 2007;25(1):100–6.

50. Jones GN, Moschidou D, Puga-Iglesias TI, et al. Ontological differences in first compared to third trimester human fetal placental chorionic stem cells. PLoS One 2012;7(9):e43395.

51. Titomanlio L, Bouslama M, Le Verche V, et al. implanted neurosphere-derived precursors promote recovery after neonatal excitotoxic brain injury. Stem Cells Dev 2011;20(5):865–79.

52. Mueller D, Shamblott MJ, Fox HE, et al. Transplanted human embryonic germ cell-derived neural stem cells replace neurons and oligodendrocytes in the forebrain of neonatal mice with excitotoxic brain damage. J Neurosci Res 2005; 82(5):592–608.

53. Comi AM, Cho E, Mulholland JD, et al. Neural stem cells reduce brain injury after unilateral carotid ligation. Pediatr Neurol 2008;38(2):86–92.

54. Daadi MM, Davis AS, Arac A, et al. Human neural stem cell grafts modify microglial response and enhance axonal sprouting in neonatal hypoxic-ischemic brain injury. Stroke 2010;41(3):516–23.

55. van Velthoven CT, Kavelaars A, van Bel F, et al. Nasal administration of stem cells: a promising novel route to treat neonatal ischemic brain damage. Pediatr Res 2010;68(5):419–22.

56. van Velthoven CT, Kavelaars A, van Bel F, et al. Mesenchymal stem cell treatment after neonatal hypoxic-ischemic brain injury improves behavioral outcome and induces neuronal and oligodendrocyte regeneration. Brain Behav Immun 2010;24(3):387–93.

57. van Velthoven CT, Kavelaars A, van Bel F, et al. Repeated mesenchymal stem cell treatment after neonatal hypoxia-ischemia has distinct effects on formation

and maturation of new neurons and oligodendrocytes leading to restoration of damage, corticospinal motor tract activity, and sensorimotor function. J Neurosci 2010;30(28):9603–11.

58. van Velthoven CT, Sheldon RA, Kavelaars A, et al. Mesenchymal stem cell transplantation attenuates brain injury after neonatal stroke. Stroke 2013;44(5): 1426–32.

59. Kim ES, Ahn SY, Im GH, et al. Human umbilical cord blood-derived mesenchymal stem cell transplantation attenuates severe brain injury by permanent middle cerebral artery occlusion in newborn rats. Pediatr Res 2012;72(3):277–84.

60. Xia G, Hong X, Chen X, et al. Intracerebral transplantation of mesenchymal stem cells derived from human umbilical cord blood alleviates hypoxic ischemic brain injury in rat neonates. J Perinat Med 2010;38(2):215–21.

61. Dalous J, Pansiot J, Pham H, et al. Use of human umbilical cord blood mononuclear cells to prevent perinatal brain injury: a preclinical study. Stem Cells Dev 2013;22(1):169–79.

62. de Paula S, Vitola AS, Greggio S, et al. Hemispheric brain injury and behavioral deficits induced by severe neonatal hypoxia-ischemia in rats are not attenuated by intravenous administration of human umbilical cord blood cells. Pediatr Res 2009;65(6):631–5.

63. Meier C, Middelanis J, Wasielewski B, et al. Spastic paresis after perinatal brain damage in rats is reduced by human cord blood mononuclear cells. Pediatr Res 2006;59(2):244–9.

64. Pimentel-Coelho PM, Magalhaes ES, Lopes LM, et al. Human cord blood transplantation in a neonatal rat model of hypoxic-ischemic brain damage: functional outcome related to neuroprotection in the striatum. Stem Cells Dev 2010;19(3): 351–8.

65. Wasielewski B, Jensen A, Roth-Harer A, et al. Neuroglial activation and Cx43 expression are reduced upon transplantation of human umbilical cord blood cells after perinatal hypoxic-ischemic injury. Brain Res 2012;1487:39–53.

66. Edwards AD, Brocklehurst P, Gunn AJ, et al. Neurological outcomes at 18 months of age after moderate hypothermia for perinatal hypoxic ischaemic encephalopathy: synthesis and meta-analysis of trial data. BMJ 2010;340:c363.

67. Choi HA, Badjatia N, Mayer SA. Hypothermia for acute brain injury–mechanisms and practical aspects. Nat Rev Neurol 2012;8(4):214–22.

68. de Haan TR, Bijleveld YA, van der Lee JH, et al. Pharmacokinetics and pharmacodynamics of medication in asphyxiated newborns during controlled hypothermia. The PharmaCool multicenter study. BMC Pediatr 2012;12:45.

69. van den Broek MP, Groenendaal F, Egberts AC, et al. Effects of hypothermia on pharmacokinetics and pharmacodynamics: a systematic review of preclinical and clinical studies. Clin Pharm 2010;49(5):277–94.

70. Sun J, Allison J, McLaughlin C, et al. Differences in quality between privately and publicly banked umbilical cord blood units: a pilot study of autologous cord blood infusion in children with acquired neurologic disorders. Transfusion 2010;50(9):1980–7.

71. Trials.gov C. Allogenic Umbilical Cord Blood and Erythropoietin Combination Therapy for Cerebral Palsy. 2013 [cited 2013 01.08.2013]; Available at.

72. Corti S, Locatelli F, Papadimitriou D, et al. Multipotentiality, homing properties, and pyramidal neurogenesis of CNS-derived LeX(ssea-1)+/CXCR4+ stem cells. FASEB J 2005;19(13):1860–2.

73. Fujiwara Y, Tanaka N, Ishida O, et al. Intravenously injected neural progenitor cells of transgenic rats can migrate to the injured spinal cord and differentiate

into neurons, astrocytes and oligodendrocytes. Neurosci Lett 2004;366(3): 287–91.

74. Titomanlio L, Kavelaars A, Dalous J, et al. Stem cell therapy for neonatal brain injury: perspectives and challenges. Ann Neurol 2011;70(5):698–712.

75. Donega V, van Velthoven CT, Nijboer CH, et al. The endogenous regenerative capacity of the damaged newborn brain: boosting neurogenesis with mesenchymal stem cell treatment. J Cereb Blood Flow Metab 2013;33(5):625–34.

76. Islam MN, Das SR, Emin MT, et al. Mitochondrial transfer from bone-marrow-derived stromal cells to pulmonary alveoli protects against acute lung injury. Nat Med 2012;18(5):759–65.

77. Braccioli L, van Velthoven C, Heijnen CJ. Exosomes: a new weapon to treat the central nervous system. Mol Neurobiol 2013. [Epub ahead of print].

78. Amariglio N, Hirshberg A, Scheithauer BW, et al. Donor-derived brain tumor following neural stem cell transplantation in an ataxia telangiectasia patient. PLoS Med 2009;6(2):e1000029.

Outcomes of Hypoxic-Ischemic Encephalopathy in Neonates Treated with Hypothermia

Seetha Shankaran, MD

KEYWORDS

- Encephalopathy • Neonatal • Hypothermia • Outcome • Predictors

KEY POINTS

- Hypothermia for neonatal hypoxic-ischemic encephalopathy is safe and effective in reducing death and disability at 18 months of age.
- This neuroprotection continues into childhood, as demonstrated by a reduction in mortality and major disability at 6 to 7 years of age.
- Outcome at 18 months of age is a good predictor of childhood outcome.

OUTCOMES OF CHILDREN WITH BIRTH DEPRESSION/ENCEPHALOPATHY BEFORE HYPOTHERMIA THERAPY

Before the advent of neuroprotective therapy with hypothermia, studies evaluating outcomes of children born at term with birth depression or encephalopathy were generally cohort studies, each having unique inclusion criteria, evaluation methods, and duration of follow-up. Among these studies, the outcome of children with acute perinatal asphyxia and/or neonatal encephalopathy was a disability rate of 6% to 21% in children with moderate encephalopathy and 42% to 100% in those with severe encephalopathy.[1–5] Among nondisabled children who were able to undergo psychometric and behavioral testing, lower executive function and delays in school readiness (reading, spelling, and arithmetic) and lower scores in language, memory, and sensorimotor perception have been noted.[1,3,6] The possibility of an increase in the rate of symptoms associated with attention-deficit/hyperactivity disorder, including anxiety, depression, attention regulation, time perception, and thought problems, as well as an increased risk of autism has been noted in children with encephalopathy or depression at birth.[6–9] A recent systematic review of long-term neurodevelopmental outcomes after intrauterine and neonatal insults, especially in low- and middle-income countries (LMIC), noted that the 27 studies evaluating 2708 infants reported sequelae

The author has no financial disclosures.
Division of Neonatal/Perinatal Medicine, Children's Hospital of Michigan, 3901 Beaubien, Detroit, MI, USA
E-mail address: sshankar@med.wayne.edu

in 1002 (37%) children. Cognitive, general developmental delay or learning difficulties were noted in 45%, cerebral palsy (CP) in 29%, deafness/hearing loss in 9%, impaired vision/blindness in 26%, gross motor coordination problems in 17%, epilepsy in 12%, and behavioral problems in 1% of children. Multiple impairments were reported in 20.5% of children while at least 1 impairment was noted in 44%, and severe sequelae in at least 1 domain in 27%.[10]

OUTCOMES OF CHILDREN WITH MODERATE OR SEVERE ENCEPHALOPATHY AT 18 MONTHS OF AGE FOLLOWING HYPOTHERMIA THERAPY

All of the randomized controlled trials (RCTs) of neuroprotection with hypothermia for neonatal hypoxic-ischemic encephalopathy (HIE) have had very similar inclusion criteria ($\geq$36 weeks gestational age, severe acidosis or birth depression, moderate or severe encephalopathy with or without an abnormal amplitude-integrated electro-encephalogram [aEEG]) and cooling initiated within 6 hours of age. The exclusion criteria were infants of age greater than 6 hours, those with major congenital or chromosomal abnormalities, or those with severe intrauterine growth restriction. The neurodevelopmental assessment tools evaluating 18-month outcome were similar and comparable between trials. Details of the results of the primary outcomes, components of the primary outcome, and predefined secondary outcomes are summarized herein. Predictors of 18-month outcomes are also presented, as this information may be helpful in discussions with families of infants with HIE.

CoolCap Trial

The CoolCap Trial was the first large RCT of hypothermia to be published.[11] Selective head cooling to a target temperature of 34° to 35° for 72 hours, or intensive care alone following moderate or severe encephalopathy and an abnormal aEEG or seizures, was compared among 234 neonates, 116 infants assigned to cooling and 118 to conventional care. Eight infants were lost to follow-up in each group. The primary outcome was mortality or severe neurodevelopmental disability at 18 months. Severe disability was defined as gross motor function level (GMF) of 3 to 5, Bayley Scales of Infant Development (BSID II) with either Mental Development Index (MDI) or a Psychomotor Development Index (PDI) less than 70 (2 standard deviations [SD] below normal), or bilateral cortical visual impairment. Nine survivors did not have MDI scores and 4 of 9 were missing visual outcome data, but all had GMF scores of 3 or higher. Death or severe disability was noted in 59 of 108 (55%) cooled infants versus 73 of 110 (66%) control-group infants, odds ratio (OR) 0.61 (95% confidence interval [CI] 0.34–1.09); with mortality rates of 33% versus 38%, OR 0.81 (0.47–1.41) and severe disability in 14 of 72 (19%) versus 21 of 68 (31%), OR 0.54 (0.25–1.17) in the cooled and control groups, respectively. A Bayley MDI score of lower than 70 occurred in 21 of 70 (30%) versus 24 of 61 (39%), and visual impairment in 7 of 72 (10%) versus 11 of 64 (17%) cooled and control infants (P not significant).

Predictors of 18-month outcome in the CoolCap RCT[12]:

1. The primary outcome was lower among infants who received hypothermia.
2. Primary outcome was also lower among infants with a less severe aEEG pattern at study intervention.
3. A worse outcome was noted among infants with severe HIE in comparison with infants with moderate HIE.
4. The absence of seizures by aEEG was associated with better outcome.
5. Elevated temperature in control-group infants was associated with worse outcomes.

6. Age at randomization of study infants within 6 hours did not influence the outcome.
7. Hypothermia altered the accuracy of the neuroexamination after cooling.[13]

The National Institute of Child Health and Human Development (NICHD) RCT

Whole-body hypothermia to a target temperature of 33° to 34°C or usual care was assigned randomly following moderate or severe HIE.[14] There were 102 infants in the hypothermia group and 106 in the control group. The primary outcome was death or moderate or severe disability at 18 months. Severe disability was defined as Bayley II MDI less than 70, Gross Motor Function Classification System (GMFCS) level 3 to 5, or hearing impairment requiring aids or blindness. Moderate disability was defined as MDI 70 to 84 and GMFCS level 2, hearing impairment without amplification, or a persistent seizure disorder. Data were unavailable for 3 infants. The primary outcome was seen in 45 of 102 (44%) hypothermia and 64 of 103 (62%) control infants. Risk ratio (RR) adjusted for center was 0.72 (95% CI 0.54–0.95). Death occurred in 24 of 102 (24%) and 38 of 106 (37%) infants, RR 0.68 (0.44–1.05), in the hypothermia and control groups, respectively. Moderate/severe CP occurred in 15 of 78 (19%) and 19 of 68 (30%), blindness in 7% and 14%, and hearing impairment in 4% and 6% of infants in the hypothermia and control groups, respectively. Moderate disability occurred in 3 infants, 2 in the hypothermia group and 1 in the control group.[15] The treatment was reported to be safe, and was associated with a consistent trend for decreasing frequency in each of the components of disability.[15]

Predictors of 18-month outcome in the NICHD whole-body hypothermia trial with secondary analyses of data from the NICHD trial data have found the following:

1. An elevated temperature (in the control group of infants) was associated with an increase in the risk of death or disability at 18 months.[16]
2. An elevated urinary lactate to creatinine ratio was associated with poor outcome.[17]
3. Classification and regression-tree analysis revealed that cord pH, spontaneous activity of the infants, base deficit of the first postnatal blood gas, and the level of partial pressure of carbon dioxide (Pco_2) in the cord gas was useful in predicting outcome.[18]
4. Death or moderate severe HIE was noted to be common among infants with a persistently low 10-minute Apgar score; however, not all infants with an Apgar score lower than 3 at 10 minutes had a uniformly poor outcome.[19]
5. Persistence of severe encephalopathy at 72 hours increased the risk of death or disability, as did the presence of an abnormal neurologic examination at neonatal hospital discharge.[20]
6. Clinical seizures were not associated with outcome when adjusted for confounding variables.[21]
7. Location of birth (inborn vs outborn) did not influence outcome.[22]
8. Smaller, sicker infants had more decreases in temperature, both during induction and maintenance phase of cooling.[23]
9. Time to initiation of cooling did not influence outcome.[15]
10. In a subset of trial infants and prospectively cooled infants (after trial accrual closed), the aEEG was noted to add minimally to predictive value of stage of encephalopathy.[24]
11. The administration of phenobarbital for seizures before the onset of initiation of cooling was associated with a lower temperature during the induction phase of cooling.[25]

12. Both minimum Pco_2 and cumulative Pco_2 lower than 35 mm Hg from birth to 12 hours of age were associated with poor outcome.[26]
13. The 18- to 22-month outcome was not associated with the APOE genotype among survivors.[27]

TOBY Trial

The TOBY Trial inclusion criteria involved both the presence of moderate or severe HIE and an abnormal aEEG.[28] Whole-body hypothermia to a target of 33.5°C for 72 hours or intensive care alone was compared between the 2 study arms. Primary outcome was death or severe disability, defined as BSID II MDI lower than 70, GMFCS level 3 to 5, or bilateral cortical visual impairment. The study is the largest to date, with 325 (163 hypothermia and 162 control) infants enrolled. In both groups, 1 infant was lost to follow-up. The primary outcome was noted in 74 of 163 (45%) cooled versus 86 of 162 (53%) control, RR 0.86 (95% CI 0.68–1.07). Results were unchanged when adjusted for severity of aEEG background, sex, or age at randomization. Survivors with severe disability were 32 of 120 (27%) hypothermia and 42 of 117 (36%) control, RR 0.74 (0.51–1.09). The predefined secondary outcome of survival free of neurologic abnormalities was 71 of 163 (44%) hypothermia and 45 of 162 (28%) control, RR 1.57 (1.16–2.12). Among hypothermia and control-group infants, higher rates of BSID MDI of 85 or higher (70% vs 55%) and PDI of 85 or higher (68% vs 53%), normal neurologic examination (71% vs 54%), and lower rates of CP (28 vs 41%) and multiple disabilities (19% and 30%) were noted in the hypothermia group (all $P<.05$).

Predictors of 18-month outcome in the TOBY trial:

1. More infants with a severe abnormal aEEG background died in comparison with those with a moderate background.
2. The effect of cooling did not vary according to the severity of abnormality on the aEEG.
3. Time to randomization did not influence outcome.

nEURO.Network RCT

This trial used both aEEG and moderate or severe HIE criteria and whole-body cooling to 33° to 34°C with cotreatment of morphine.[29] The primary outcome was death or severe disability at 15 months with severe disability defined as GMFCS 3 to 5, Griffith Developmental Quotient less than 2 SD below normal of 100, or severe cortical visual deficit. The sample size was 150, but the trial was stopped early because of lack of equipoise among investigators. There were 64 infants assigned to the hypothermia group and 65 to the control group; data at 18 months were available for 53 and 58 infants in the hypothermia and control groups, respectively. Death or severe disability occurred in 27 of 53 (51%) in the hypothermia group versus 48 of 58 (83%) in the control group; OR adjusted for severity of HIE was 0.21 (95% CI 0.09–0.54). CP occurred in 4 of 32 (12%) versus 10 of 21 (48%), OR 0.15 (0.04–0.60), in the hypothermia and control groups, respectively.

Predictors of Outcome of nEURO RCT: In this study, the severity of encephalopathy significantly affected the outcome.

ICE Trial

The ICE Trial involved cooling initiated at the birth hospital for outborn infants by dedicated neonatal retrieval teams, using gel packs on the chest and shoulder and discontinuing the overhead warmer and temperature in the transport incubator.[30] Clinical eligibility criteria were moderate or severe HIE, and target temperature was 33° to 34°C. Infants who required more than 80% oxygen therapy were also excluded. The primary outcome was death or sensorineural disability at 24 months, defined as moderate or severe CP, GMFCS 2 to 5, BSID II MDI or PDI less than 2 SD below normal, or BSID III cognitive, language, or motor score less than 2 SD below normal, blindness, or deafness. The sample size was 150 per group, but recruitment stopped early because of publication of earlier RCTs and loss of equipoise by investigators. The hypothermia and control groups had 110 and 111 infants assigned; data were available for the primary outcome for 107 and 101 infants, respectively. Mild HIE was noted in 42 infants. Death or disability occurred in 55 of 107 (51%) hypothermia infants versus 67 of 101 (66%) control infants, RR 0.77 (95% CI 0.62–0.98); the effect persisted after excluding the infants with mild HIE. Severe disability was seen in 28 of 80 (35%) hypothermia versus 25 of 59 (42%) control infants (P not significant). Survival free of disability was 40% hypothermia versus 23% control (P = .01).

Trials in Low-Income and Middle-Income Countries

Seven RCTs with a total of 567 infants are included in a recent meta-analysis of hypothermia for HIE in LMIC.[31] The largest study from China enrolled 100 hypothermia and 94 control-group infants while another from India enrolled 62 infants in each group. Three studies involved head cooling, 4 involved whole-body cooling using water bottles, 1 study each used phase-changing materials or gel packs, and 1 study did not specify the method of cooling. Follow-up data are not available from all the studies, and the overall mortality was RR 0.74 (95% CI 0.44–1.25). The study by Zhou and colleagues[32] excluded infants with infection and anemia as eligibility criteria. In this study, head cooling to a target of 34° to 35°C was used. Primary outcome was death or disability at 18 months. Of the 256 infants recruited there were 21 postrandomization exclusions, and 41 infants did not have follow-up data. Death or severe disability defined as GMFCS 3 to 5 or developmental quotient less than 70 on the Gesell Child Development Age Scale was noted in 31% and 49%, OR 0.47 (0.26–0.84), and severe disability in 11 of 80 (14%) versus 19 of 67 (28%) infants, OR 0.40 (0.17–0.92), among the hypothermia and control groups, respectively. The inadequate quality of the LMIC trials, including lack of comprehensive follow-up of trial subjects, currently provides neither evidence of safety nor efficacy of hypothermia as neuroprotection for neonatal HIE. Prospective, well-designed RCTs are needed in LMIC; one such trial is evaluating feasibility (Hypothermia for Encephalopathy in Low Income Countries, the HELIX trial; NCT01760629).

META-ANALYSIS OF TRIALS WITH 18 MONTHS' OUTCOME

The analysis by Edwards and colleagues[33] after evaluation of the CoolCap, NICHD, and TOBY trials (all in high-income countries) clearly demonstrated with a sample of 767 trial participants that hypothermia was neuroprotective, with a reduction in mortality and disability and an increase in survival free of disability (**Table 1**); lack of benefit was noted in infants with severe HIE. The recent meta-analysis by Tagin and colleagues[34] of 7 studies, including the aforementioned trial by Zhou and colleagues,[32] notes that cooling is effective in reducing death and all components of disability among survivors, and increasing the rate of normal survivors. In addition, cooling is effective in infants with severe HIE in addition to those with moderate HIE. Both approaches to cooling, either head or whole-body hypothermia, are neuroprotective (**Table 2**).[34]

Table 1
Meta-analysis of CoolCap, NICHD, and TOBY trials

767 Participants	RR (95% CI)
Death and disability	0.81 (0.71–0.93)
Mortality	0.78 (0.66–0.93)
Severe disability	0.71 (0.56–0.91)
Cerebral palsy	0.69 (0.54–0.89)
PDI <70	0.73 (0.56–0.95)
MDI <70	0.71 (0.54–0.92)
Blindness	0.57 (0.33–0.96)
Deafness	0.76 (0.36–1.62)
Normal survivors	1.53 (1.22–1.93)
Moderate HIE	0.73 (0.58–0.92)
Severe HIE	0.87 (0.75–1.01)

Abbreviations: CI, confidence interval; HIE, hypoxic-ischemic encephalopathy; MDI, mental developmental index; PDI, psychomotor developmental index; RR, risk ratio.

Data from Edwards AD, Brocklehurst P, Gunn AJ, et al. Neurological outcomes at 18 months of age after moderate hypothermia for perinatal hypoxic ischaemic encephalopathy: synthesis and meta-analysis of trial data. BMJ 2010;340:c363.

OUTCOMES IN CHILDHOOD OF NEONATES WITH HYPOTHERMIA FOR MODERATE OR SEVERE HIE
Seven- to 8-Year Follow-Up of the CoolCap Trial

The CoolCap trial evaluated whether 18- to 22-month outcome predicted functional outcomes at 7 to 8 years of age among survivors by evaluating WeeFIM rating measuring self-care, mobility, and cognitive functions by telephone interviews.[35] There was 1 parent refusal, 14 of the CoolCap centers did not participate, and 58 children were lost to follow-up among participating centers. The demographic data of

Table 2
Meta-analysis of trials by Gunn, CoolCap, NICHD, TOBY, nEURO, China, and ICE

1214 Participants	RR (95% CI)
Death and disability	0.76 (0.69–0.84)
Death	0.75 (0.63–0.88)
Major disability	0.68 (0.56–0.83)
Cerebral palsy	0.62 (0.49–0.78)
Developmental delay	0.66 (0.52–0.82)
Blindness	0.56 (0.33–0.94)
Deafness	0.64 (0.32–1.27)
Normal survivors	1.63 (1.36–1.95)
Moderate HIE	0.67 (0.56–0.81)
Severe HIE	0.83 (0.74–0.92)
Whole-body cooling	0.75 (0.66–0.85)
Head cooling	0.77 (0.65–0.93)

Data from Tagin MA, Woolcott CG, Vincer MJ, et al. Hypothermia for neonatal hypoxic ischemic encephalopathy: an updated systematic review and meta-analysis. Arch Pediatr Adolesc Med 2012;166(6):558–66.

children assessed (62 children) were similar to those not evaluated (73 children), hence the study cohort was considered to be representative of the trial. The characteristics between cooled (n = 32) and control (n = 30) children were also comparable. Status at 18 months was associated with status at 7 to 8 years (P<.001) with a rating of 115 ± 19 (mean ± SD) in those with a favorable 18-month outcome and 67 ± 42 in those with an adverse outcome. Adjustment for confounding variables and treatment did not affect the association. CP diagnosed at 18 months was highly associated with WeeFIM mobility score at 7 to 8 years.

Childhood Outcomes at 6 to 7 Years in the NICHD Trial

The primary outcome at 6- to 7-year outcome in the NICHD Trial was death or IQ of less than 70 while secondary outcomes included death, severe disability, components of disability, higher cognitive function, and psychosocial health.[36] Assessment tools included the evaluation of IQ with the Wechsler Preschool and Primary Scale of Intelligence III (WPPSI) (n = 96) and the Wechsler Intelligence Scale for Children IV (WAIS) (n = 18). Verbal comprehension, perceptual organization, and processing speed were assessed yielding a verbal IQ and performance IQ, which were combined to give a full-scale IQ (normal value 100 ± 15). Higher cognitive function was assessed by subtests of attention, executive function, and visuospatial reasoning using the Developmental Neuropsychological Assessment (NEPSY) (mean 100 ± 15). Lastly, the Child Health Questionnaire assessed physical, emotional, and social well-being of the child and the effects of the child's health on the parents. All testing was conducted by examiners trained to reliability and unaware of the treatment assignment. The neurologic functional assessment was evaluated using the GMFCS for 6- to 7-year-old children: GMFCS level 1, walking without restriction; II, walking without assisted device; III, walking with an assistive device; IV, self-mobility with limitation; and V, severe limitation of mobility. Severe disability was defined as IQ less than 3 SD below the mean (<55), GMFCS level IV or V, or bilateral blindness. Moderate disability was IQ less than 2 to 3 SD below the mean (55–69), a GMFCS level of III, bilateral deafness, or refractory epilepsy. Mild disability was IQ 1 to 2 SD below the mean (70–84) and a GMFCS level I or II. No disability was IQ greater than 1 SD below the mean (>85) with no CP, hearing, or vision deficit, or epilepsy. Among nondisabled survivors, everyday motor function was tested by the heel-to-toe test, ability to hop, standing on one foot, or Romberg test, while fine motor function tests of coordination included finger-nose, rapid alteration of hands, thumb–index finger apposition, thumb–4-finger apposition sequentially, heel-to-shin test, and foot tapping. The primary outcome was adjusted for center and level of HIE.

Primary outcome data were available for 190 of 208 (91% of participants): 97 of 100 (97%) in the hypothermia group and 93 of 106 (88%) in the control group; 5 hypothermia and 3 control-group children were lost to follow-up. The primary outcome was seen in 46 of 97 (47%) hypothermia and 58 of 93 (62%) control children; RR 0.78 (95% CI 0.61–1.01) adjusted for center. The mortality rate was 27 of 97 (28%) hypothermia versus 41 of 93 (44%) control, RR 0.66 (0.45–0.97); 3 in each group died after the 18-month visit. Death or severe disability was 41% versus 60% (P = .03), death or IQ less than 55 was 41% versus 60% (P = .03), and death or CP 41% versus 60%, P = .02 in the hypothermia and control groups, respectively. Among survivors, IQ less than 70 occurred in 27% versus 33%, and CP in 17% versus 29% (both P not significant). Attention and executive function scores lower than 70 occurred in 2 of 48 and 4 of 32 children, and visuospatial scores lower than 70 in 2 of 53 and 1 of 36 children who could be tested in the hypothermia and control group (P not significant). There were no differences between groups when parental assessment of child's esteem was evaluated; the emotional impact of the child's well-being on parents was also similar between groups. There were no differences between groups in the assessment of the child's physical health.

Predictors of Outcome at 6 to 7 Years in the NICHD Trial

Among children in the trial who had moderate or severe disability at 18 months, the corresponding rates at 6 to 7 years was 15 of 17 (88%) in the hypothermia group and 18 of 19 (95%) in the control group. All children with CP at 18 months had CP at 6 to 7 years; among those with seizures at 18 months, the corresponding rates at 6 to 7 years were 4 of 10 (40%) in the hypothermia group and 5 of 10 (50%) in the control group. The predictive value of moderate or severe disability at 6 to 7 years for children disabled at 18 months in the hypothermia group was sensitivity 63%, specificity 96%, positive predictive value (PPV) 88%, and negative predictive value (NPV) 83%, whereas the corresponding rates in the control group were 95%, 97%, 95%, and 97%, respectively. The predictive value of moderate or severe CP at 6 to 7 years for children with moderate or severe CP at 18 months had sensitivity of 100%, specificity 100%, PPV 100%, and NPV 100% in the hypothermia group and 93%, 100%, 100%, and 97% in the control group, respectively. The odds of disability at 6 to 7 years for an infant disabled at an earlier age, compared with one not disabled, was 37 times higher (95% CI 7–189) in the hypothermia group and 576 times higher in the control group (34–9774). Thus, a high concordance was noted between assessment of moderate or severe disability at 18 to 22 months and similar assessments at 6 to 7 years or age.[36]

Secondary analysis of the 6- to 7-year outcome following hypothermia for neonatal HIE has yielded useful information.

1. The growth of children with HIE treated with hypothermia is similar to that of control-group children; growth failure seen in children with CP, irrespective of intervention, presents to childhood.[37]
2. Control-group infants who had elevated temperatures during the study intervention in the neonatal course continued to have an increased risk of death or disability at 6 to 7 years.[38]
3. Among trial participants, 10-minute Apgar scores were associated with school-age outcomes. However, one-fifth of the children with 10-minute Apgar scores of 0 survived without disability to school age.[39]

THE FUTURE OF HYPOTHERMIA THERAPY

Hypothermia therapy for neonatal HIE has demonstrated neuroprotection; however, mortality rates and disability rates continue to be high. The future of hypothermia therapy will include adjunctive therapy with hypothermia.[40] The following adjunctive therapies are being examined in trials: xenon (NCT01545271 and NCT00934700), erythropoietin (NCT00719407), darbepoetin (NCT0147105), and topiramate (NCT01241019). The use of human cord blood for the hypoxic-ischemic neonate is also being investigated. It remains to be seen whether early accurate neonatal biomarkers of neurologic and developmental assessments at follow-up will become available. The TOBY, NICHD, and ICE trials have noted that brain injury on neonatal magnetic resonance imaging in subsets of trial subjects is associated with 18-month outcome.[41–43] Two ongoing trials, one of the optimum depth of temperature and duration of cooling (NCT01192776) in term infants and the other evaluating neuroprotection with cooling of infants of 34 to 35 weeks gestational age (NCT00620711), will also yield useful information in this evolving and exciting field.

SUMMARY

Hypothermia is a safe and effective treatment for neonatal HIE. The data from childhood outcomes have shown that the benefits seen at 18 months continue to childhood, without an increase in survivors with disabilities. Outcome at 18 months correlates well with that at 6 to 7 years of age, hence new innovative trials of hypothermia plus therapies can continue to follow infants to 18 months of age. The search for an early neonatal biomarker for 18-month outcome should continue.

REFERENCES

1. Shankaran S, Woldt E, Koepke T, et al. Acute neonatal morbidity and long-term central nervous system sequelae of perinatal asphyxia in term infants. Early Hum Dev 1991;25:135–48.
2. Robertson CM. Long term follow-up of term infants with perinatal asphyxia. In: Stevenson DK, Benitz WE, Sunshine P, editors. Fetal and neonatal brain injury. 3rd edition. Cambridge: Cambridge University; 2003. p. 829–58.
3. Marlow N, Rose AS, Rands CE, et al. Neuropsychological and educational problems at school age associated with neonatal encephalopathy. Arch Dis Child Fetal Neonatal Ed 2005;90:F380–7.
4. Gonzalez FF, Miller SP. Does perinatal asphyxia impair cognitive function without cerebral palsy? Arch Dis Child Fetal Neonatal Ed 2006;91(6):F454–9.
5. de Vries LS, Jongmans MJ. Long-term outcome after neonatal hypoxic-ischaemic encephalopathy. Arch Dis Child Fetal Neonatal Ed 2010;95(3):F220–4.
6. Odd DE, Whitelaw A, Gunnell D, et al. The association between birth condition and neuropsychological functioning and educational attainment at school age: a cohort study. Arch Dis Child 2011;96(1):30–7.
7. van Handel M, Swaab H, de Vries LS, et al. Behavioral outcome in children with a history of neonatal encephalopathy following perinatal asphyxia. J Pediatr Psychol 2010;35(3):286–95.
8. Lindström K, Lagerroos P, Gillberg C, et al. Teenage outcome after being born at term with moderate neonatal encephalopathy. Pediatr Neurol 2006;35(4): 268–74.
9. Badawi N, Dixon G, Felix JF, et al. Autism following a history of newborn encephalopathy: more than a coincidence? Dev Med Child Neurol 2006;48(2):85–9.
10. Mwaniki MK, Atieno M, Lawn JE, et al. Long-term neurodevelopmental outcomes after intrauterine and neonatal insults: a systematic review. Lancet 2012; 379(9814):445–52.
11. Gluckman PD, Wyatt J, Azzopardi DV, et al, on the behalf of the Cool Cap Study Group. Selective head cooling with mild systemic hypothermia after neonatal encephalopathy: multicenter randomised trial. Lancet 2005;365:663–70.
12. Wyatt JS, Gluckman PD, Liu PY, et al. Determinants of outcomes after head cooling for Neonatal Encephalopathy. Pediatrics 2007;119(5):912–21.
13. Gunn AJ, Wyatt JS, Whitelaw A, et al. Therapeutic hypothermia changes the prognostic value of clinical evaluation of neonatal encephalopathy. J Pediatr 2008;152(1):55–8, 58.e1.
14. Shankaran S, Laptook AR, Ehrenkranz RA, et al. Whole-body hypothermia for neonates with hypoxic-ischemic encephalopathy. N Engl J Med 2005;353: 1574–84.
15. Shankaran S, Pappas A, Laptook AR, et al. Outcomes of safety and effectiveness in a multicenter randomized, controlled trial of whole-body hypothermia for neonatal hypoxic-ischemic encephalopathy. Pediatrics 2008;122(4):e791–8.

16. Laptook A, Tyson J, Shankaran S, et al. Elevated temperature after hypoxic-ischemic encephalopathy: a risk factor for adverse outcome. Pediatrics 2008; 122(3):491–9.

17. Oh W, Perritt R, Shankaran S, et al. Association between urinary lactate to creatinine ratio and neurodevelopmental outcome in term infants with hypoxic-ischemic encephalopathy. J Pediatr 2008;153(3):375–8.

18. Ambalavanan N, Carlo WA, Shankaran S, et al. Predicting outcomes of neonates diagnosed with hypoxemic-ischemic encephalopathy. Pediatrics 2006;118: 2084–93.

19. Laptook AR, Shankaran S, Ambalavanan N, et al. Outcome of term infants using Apgar scores at 10 minutes following hypoxic-ischemic encephalopathy. Pediatrics 2009;124(6):1619–26.

20. Shankaran S, Laptook AR, Tyson JE, et al. Evolution of encephalopathy during whole body hypothermia for neonatal hypoxic-ischemic encephalopathy. J Pediatr 2012;160(4):567–72.e3.

21. Kwon JM, Guillet R, Shankaran S, et al. Clinical seizures in neonatal hypoxic-ischemic encephalopathy have no independent impact on neurodevelopmental outcome: secondary analyses of data from the neonatal research network hypothermia trial. J Child Neurol 2011;26(3):322–8.

22. Natarajan G, Pappas A, Shankaran S, et al. Effect of inborn vs. outborn delivery on neurodevelopmental outcomes in infants with hypoxic-ischemic encephalopathy: secondary analyses of the NICHD whole-body cooling trial. Pediatr Res 2012;72(4):414–9.

23. Shankaran S, Laptook AR, McDonald SA, et al. Temperature profile and outcomes of neonates undergoing whole body hypothermia for neonatal hypoxic-ischemic encephalopathy. Pediatr Crit Care Med 2012;13(1):53.

24. Shankaran S, Pappas A, McDonald SA, et al. Predictive value of an early amplitude integrated electroencephalogram and neurologic examination. Pediatrics 2011;128(1):e112–20.

25. Sant'Anna G, Laptook AR, Shankaran S, et al. Phenobarbital and temperature profile during hypothermia for hypoxic-ischemic encephalopathy. J Child Neurol 2012;27(4):451–7.

26. Pappas A, Shankaran S, Laptook AR, et al. Hypocarbia and adverse outcome in neonatal hypoxic-ischemic encephalopathy. J Pediatr 2011;158(5):752–8.e1.

27. Cotton CM, Goldstein RF, McDonald SA, et al. Apolipoprotein E (APOE) geneotype and outcome in infants with hypoxic ischemic encephalopathy. Pediatr Res 2013. in press.

28. Azzopardi DV, Strohm B, Edwards AD, et al. Moderate hypothermia to treat perinatal asphyxial encephalopathy. N Engl J Med 2009;361(14):1349–58.

29. Simbruner G, Mittal RA, Rohlmann F, et al, neo.nEURO.network Trial Participants. Systemic hypothermia after neonatal encephalopathy: outcomes of neo.nEURO.-network RCT. Pediatrics 2010;126(4):e771–8.

30. Jacobs SE, Morley CJ, Inder TE, et al. Whole-body hypothermia for term and near-term newborns with hypoxic-ischemic encephalopathy: a randomized controlled trial. Arch Pediatr Adolesc Med 2011;165(8):692–700.

31. Pauliah SS, Shankaran S, Wade A, et al. Therapeutic hypothermia for neonatal encephalopathy in low- and middle-income countries: a systematic review and meta-analysis. PLoS One 2013;8(3):e58834.

32. Zhou WH, Cheng GQ, Shao XM, et al. Selective head cooling with mild systemic hypothermia after neonatal hypoxic-ischemic encephalopathy: a multicenter randomized controlled trial in China. J Pediatr 2010;157(3):367–72, 372.e1–3.

33. Edwards AD, Brocklehurst P, Gunn AJ, et al. Neurological outcomes at 18 months of age after moderate hypothermia for perinatal hypoxic ischaemic encephalopathy: synthesis and meta-analysis of trial data. BMJ 2010;340:c363.

34. Tagin MA, Woolcott CG, Vincer MJ, et al. Hypothermia for neonatal hypoxic ischemic encephalopathy: an updated systematic review and meta-analysis. Arch Pediatr Adolesc Med 2012;166(6):558–66.

35. Guillet R, Edwards AD, Thoresen M, et al. Seven- to eight-year follow-up of the CoolCap trial of head cooling for neonatal encephalopathy. Pediatr Res 2012; 71(2):205–9.

36. Shankaran S, Pappas A, McDonald SA, et al. Childhood outcomes after hypothermia for neonatal encephalopathy. N Engl J Med 2012;366(22):2085–92.

37. Vohr BR, Stephens BE, McDonald SA, et al. Cerebral palsy and growth failure at 6 to 7 years. Pediatrics 2013;132(4):e905–14.

38. Laptook AR, McDonald SA, Shankaran S, et al. Elevated temperature and 6- to 7-year outcome of neonatal encephalopathy. Ann Neurol 2013;73:520–8.

39. Natarajan G, Shankaran S, Laptook AR, et al. Apgar scores at 10 min and outcomes at 6-7 years following hypoxic-ischaemic encephalopathy. Arch Dis Child Fetal Neonatal Ed 2013;98(6):F473–9.

40. Robertson NJ, Tan S, Groenendaal F, et al. Which neuroprotective agents are ready for bench to bedside translation in the newborn infant? J Pediatr 2012; 160:544–52.e4.

41. Rutherford M, Ramenghi LA, Edwards AD, et al. Assessment of brain tissue injury after moderate hypothermia in neonates with hypoxic-ischaemic encephalopathy: a nested sub-study of a randomised controlled trial. Lancet Neurol 2010; 9(1):39–45.

42. Shankaran S, Barnes PD, Hintz SR, et al. Brain injury following trial of hypothermia for neonatal hypoxic-ischaemic encephalopathy. Arch Dis Child Fetal Neonatal Ed 2012;97(6):F398–404.

43. Cheong JL, Coleman L, Hunt RW, et al. Prognostic utility of magnetic resonance imaging in neonatal hypoxic-ischemic encephalopathy: substudy of a randomized trial. Arch Pediatr Adolesc Med 2012;166(7):634–40.

Mechanisms of Hypothermic Neuroprotection

Paul P. Drury, BSc, Eleanor R. Gunn, MBChB, Laura Bennet, PhD,
Alistair J. Gunn, MBChB, PhD*

KEYWORDS

- Therapeutic hypothermia • Neuroprotection • Fetal sheep • Mechanisms
- Hypoxia-ischemia • Newborn infant • Neonatal encephalopathy

KEY POINTS

- Prolonged, mild hypothermia can improve outcomes from neonatal hypoxic-ischemic encephalopathy.
- Hypothermia during hypoxia-ischemia/reperfusion helps reduce anoxic depolarization, excitotoxicity, free radical exposure, and blood-brain barrier dysfunction.
- The latent phase of recovery, before delayed deterioration after hypoxia-ischemia, represents the window of opportunity for hypothermic neuroprotection.
- Key targets of delayed hypothermia in the latent phase include programmed cell death, microglial activation, and abnormal excitatory receptor activity.
- Hypothermia is not generally protective after the onset of the secondary mitochondrial failure, but may help reduce secondary, seizure-mediated, extension of injury.
- We hypothesize that overall, mild hypothermia suppresses secondary injury processes without impairing recovery of normal brain homeostasis.

INTRODUCTION

There is now compelling clinical evidence from meta-analyses of large randomized controlled trials that in term infants with moderate to severe hypoxia-ischemia (HI) encephalopathy, prolonged, moderate cerebral hypothermia initiated within a few hours after birth and continued until resolution of the acute phase of delayed cell death reduces neural injury[1,2] and improves neurodevelopmental outcome in the medium to long term.[3–5] The specific mechanisms of this protection remain surprisingly unclear,

Disclosure/Conflict of Interest: All authors report no conflict of interest.

This work was supported by grants from the Health Research Council of New Zealand, the Auckland Medical Research Foundation, and Lottery Health Grants Board New Zealand. P.P. Drury was supported by the New Zealand Neurologic Foundation W&B Miller Doctoral Scholarship.

Department of Physiology, Faculty of Medical and Health Sciences, University of Auckland, Private Bag 92019, Auckland 1023, New Zealand

* Corresponding author.

E-mail address: aj.gunn@auckland.ac.nz

in part paradoxically because a wide range of potentially deleterious mechanisms are suppressed, making it difficult to distinguish between changes during cooling that are critically beneficial, compared with those that are indifferent or even deleterious. In this article we critically assess potential mechanisms of hypothermic neuroprotection in relation to the window of opportunity for cooling after severe HI.

THE EVOLUTION OF HI INJURY

The central insight that underpinned development of therapeutic hypothermia was that HI injury evolves over time. It is now known that although neurons may die during the actual ischemic or asphyxial event (the primary phase), many cells initially recover at least partially from the primary insult in a latent phase during which oxidative metabolism is at least partially restored despite continuing suppression of electroencephalogram activity.[6–8] After moderate to severe injury, this is typically followed by secondary deterioration, starting hours later (approximately 6–15 hours), with delayed seizures,[9] cytotoxic edema, accumulation of excitatory amino acids (EAAs), failure of mitochondrial oxidative activity,[8,10] and ultimately cell death.[11] More severe primary insults are typically associated with more severe primary damage,[12] and more rapidly developing delayed cell death.[12,13]

WHAT CAN BE LEARNED FROM THE WINDOW OF OPPORTUNITY FOR HYPOTHERMIA?

It is not completely clear when in this process evolving cell death becomes irreversible. Empirically, neuroprotection requires that hypothermia is started during the so-called latent or early recovery phase of transient restoration of cerebral oxidative metabolism, before secondary failure of oxidative metabolism, and continued until after resolution of the secondary phase.[9,13–16] Thus, pragmatically, the window for treatment seems to close after the start of secondary energy failure, corresponding with an irreversible stage in the evolution of delayed cell death.[17]

MECHANISMS OF ACTION OF HYPOTHERMIA DURING HI

At the most fundamental level, injury requires a period of insufficient delivery of oxygen and substrates, such as glucose (and lactate in the fetus), such that neurons and glia cannot maintain homeostasis. As outlined in **Fig. 1**, the key mechanism of primary injury and death includes anoxic depolarization. Once the neuron's supply of high-energy metabolites, such as ATP, can no longer be maintained during HI, the energy-dependent mechanisms of intracellular homeostasis including the Na^+/K^+ ATP-dependent pump begin to fail. Neuronal depolarization opens sodium and calcium channels, leading to rapid entry of these cations into cells (and potassium out). This creates an osmotic and electrochemical gradient that in turn favors further chloride and water entry leading to cell swelling (cytotoxic edema). If sufficiently severe, this may lead to acute cell lysis.[18]

Even after surprisingly prolonged and severe insults, however, many swollen neurons can still recover, at least temporarily, if the hypoxic insult is reversed or the osmotic environment is manipulated. Evidence suggests that several additional factors act to increase cell injury during and after depolarization. The first additional factor is extracellular accumulation of EAAs, mediated by increased release after neuronal depolarization coupled with impaired energy-dependent reuptake by astrocytes,[19] which in turn promote further receptor-mediated cell swelling and intracellular calcium entry.[18] Another additional factor is generation of oxygen free radicals, such as the highly toxic hydroxyl radical ($^•OH$), leading to lipid peroxidation and DNA/RNA

Primary Phase: Hypoxia-ischemia

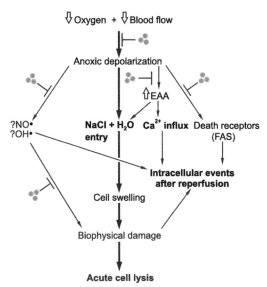

Fig. 1. Flow chart illustrating injurious events during hypoxia-ischemia and potential thera-peutic targets for hypothermia. EAAs, excitatory amino acids; NO•, nitric oxide; OH•, hydroxyl free radical.

fragmentation.[20,21] Finally, neuronal nitric oxide synthase (nNOS)–mediated release of the reactive oxygen species NO•[22] can damage key lipoproteins in cell membrane, organelles, and mitochondria.

These damaging events are partly balanced by protective responses that help reduce cell injury, including inhibitory amino acids, such as γ-aminobutyric acid, that accumulate to much greater levels in the developing brain than in adult animals,[19] and adenosine, an inhibitory neuromodulator derived from breakdown of ATP that helps delay onset and reduces the severity of energy failure during asphyxia.[23]

Hypothermia protects the brain during severe HI by a graded reduction in cerebral metabolism of about 5% for every degree of temperature reduction,[24] which delays the onset of anoxic cell depolarization. The protective effects of intrainsult hypother-mia are not simply caused by reduced metabolism, because cooling substantially re-duces damage for a given absolute duration of depolarization compared with normothermia.[25] There are two additional factors. The first is reduced accumulation of EAAs during intraischemic hypothermia in adult and newborn animals.[26,27] This is primarily caused by the delay in depolarization, although there is evidence for a reduc-tion in the rate of release even after depolarization has occurred.[28] The second is sup-pression of NO and superoxide formation, presumptively caused by slowing of chemical reactions, as shown in hippocampal slice cultures,[29] during ischemia and reperfusion in rodents,[30] cardiac arrest in young adult dogs,[31] and during and imme-diately after HI in the piglet.[27]

COOLING DURING REPERFUSION

After cerebral circulation and oxygenation are restored at the end of the insult, oxidative metabolism rapidly recovers in surviving cells and cytotoxic edema resolves over approximately 30 to 60 minutes.[7,19,32] The key events outlined in **Fig. 2** include (1) EAA levels rapidly fall in parallel with resolution of the acute cell swelling[19]; (2) the rapid restoration of tissue oxygenation is associated with a further rapid burst of NO and superoxide formation[27]; and (3) breakdown of the blood-brain barrier (BBB), allowing large proteins to leak out in the extracellular space. This may increase brain swelling and is associated with degradation of key regulatory proteins in the vascular basement membrane, at least in part mediated by induction of enzymes called metalloproteases.[33]

Hypothermia started immediately after reperfusion in newborn piglets seemed to accelerate this resolution as shown by reduced extracellular levels of EAAs and reduced NO efflux in the brain.[27] Furthermore, in adult rats, cooling after global ischemia was associated with reduced BBB leakiness and brain edema 24 hours later, provided that it was induced within 1 hour after ischemia, apparently through inhibition of metalloproteinases.[33] However, metalloproteinase inhibition after HI in neonatal rats has had inconsistent effects.[34] Taken with the observation that hypothermia is neuroprotective even when delayed by more than an hour after HI[9,13,15,35] it seems unlikely that these mechanisms are critical to its beneficial effects.

ARE EXCITOTOXICITY AND FREE RADICALS RELEVANT TO POSTINSULT COOLING?

Both extracellular accumulation of EAAs and excess free radical production largely resolve during reperfusion after the insult and seem to have returned to normal values during the latent phase of recovery from HI.[19,21,27,36] In vitro, intrainsult hypothermia did not prevent intracellular accumulation of calcium during cardiac arrest in vivo,[37] or during EAA exposure in vitro.[38] Cooling initiated after wash-out of EAAs prevented neuronal degeneration in vitro.[38]

Thus, the ability of hypothermia to reduce release of excitotoxins does not seem to be central to its neuroprotective effects even during HI, and cannot easily account for the protective effects of delayed cooling. These data suggest that the critical effect of hypothermia is to block the intracellular sequelae of depolarization and EAA exposure (**Box 1**).

CELL DEATH MECHANISMS IN THE LATENT PHASE

Although the mechanisms of delayed cell loss are clearly multifactorial, there is increasing evidence that key pathways include activation of programmed cell death

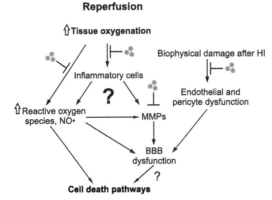

Fig. 2. Flow chart illustrating potential therapeutic targets for hypothermia during reperfusion from hypoxia-ischemia (HI). BBB, blood-brain barrier; MMPs, matrix metalloproteinases; NO•, nitric oxide.

Box 1
Therapeutic targets for hypothermia in the latent phase
Programmed cell death
Intrinsic pathway
Extrinsic pathway
Secondary inflammation
Microglial activation
Microglial chemotaxis
Cytokine release
Abnormal receptor activity
Hyperactivity
Receptor composition
Mitochondrial preservation

pathways, augmented by the inflammatory reaction and abnormal receptor activity as shown in **Fig. 3**. Programmed cell death is activated by (1) excessive calcium influx during and after HI,[39] which promotes depolarization of the mitochondria (the intrinsic pathway of apoptosis),[40] leading to permeabilization of the outer membrane of the mitochondria, with release of proapoptotic proteins, including cytochrome c; (2) abnormal excitatory receptor activity promoting further Ca^{2+} entry; (3) loss of trophic support from astrocytic growth factors[41]; and (4) secondary inflammatory reaction to HI,[42] with release of cytokines and activation of cell surface death receptors (and thus the extrinsic apoptosis pathway).[43]

Evidence that Hypothermia Can Suppress Programmed Cell Death

Postinsult hypothermia typically suppresses hypoxia-associated protein synthesis[44] and multiple gene responses to ischemia, particularly genes involved in calcium homeostasis, cellular and synaptic integrity, inflammation, cell death, and apoptosis.[45] Thus, it is plausible that hypothermia would help prevent active forms of cell death (**Box 1**). Although studies using morphologic criteria for apoptotic cell death have had inconsistent outcomes,[44] in practice posthypoxic cell death represents a continuum between apoptosis and necrosis, as recently reviewed.[46] Activation of caspase-3, the final "executioner" caspase, is a reasonable, although nonspecific, marker of activation of apoptotic pathways.

In vitro, mild hypothermia directly suppressed neuronal apoptosis induced by serum deprivation, with reduced activation of caspases-3, -8, and, -9 after 24 hours, and reduced cytochrome c translocation, consistent with suppression of the intrinsic and extrinsic pathways of apoptosis.[47] Furthermore, hypothermia during focal ischemia in adult rats reduced expression of the cell death receptor Fas and activation of caspase-8, supporting a direct effect on the extrinsic pathway of apoptosis.[48]

These studies examined forms of intrainsult cooling. However, in vivo, in the near-term fetal sheep, hypothermia delayed for 90 minutes after ischemia markedly suppressed caspase-3 activation in white matter.[14] Similarly, in postnatal day 7 rat, an age when brain development is comparable with the late preterm human infant,[49] immediate induction of hypothermia after HI reduced caspase-3 expression in the cortical infarct[50] and in preoligodendrocytes.[51] In adult rats, after transient focal or global ischemia mild hypothermia suppressed activated caspase-3 immunoreactivity,[52,53]

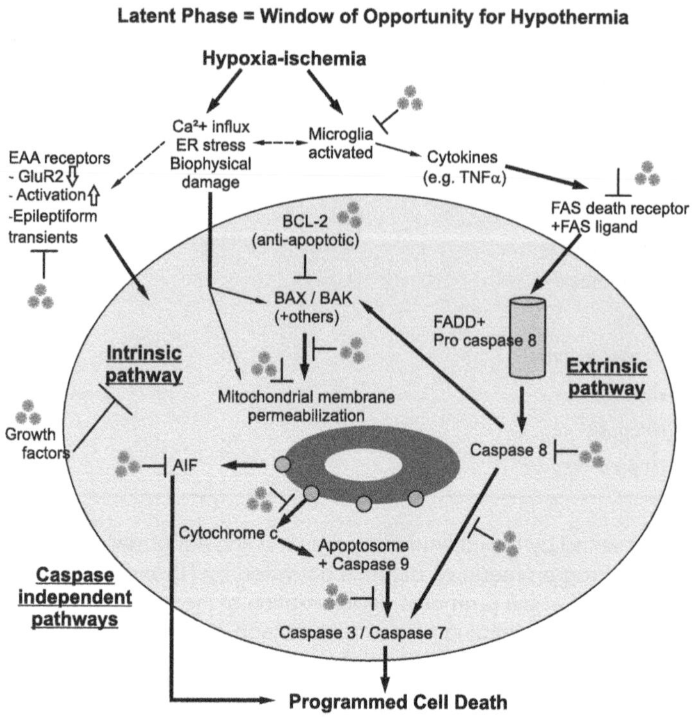

Fig. 3. Flow chart illustrating key therapeutic targets for hypothermia during the latent phase of recovery after hypoxia-ischemia. AIF, apoptosis-inducing factor; BAK, Bcl-2 antagonist/killer; BAX, Bcl-2 associated X protein; BCL-2, B-cell lymphoma 2 family of proteins; EAA, excitatory amino acid; ER, endoplasmic reticulum; FADD, Fas-associated protein with death domain; GluR2, calcium impermeable subtype of α-amino-3-hydroxy-5-methyl-4-isoxazolepropionic acid receptor; TNF-α, tumor necrosis factor-α.

upregulated the antiapoptotic protein bcl-2, reduced expression of the proapoptotic protein p53,[54] and attenuated release of cytochrome c.[53,55,56] In adult minipigs, cooling after cardiac arrest reduced opening of the mitochondrial permeability pores.[57]

Finally, combined treatment with the antiapoptotic agent, insulin-like growth factor 1, and hypothermia starting 4.5 hours after cerebral ischemia in near-term fetal sheep did not show additive neuroprotection,[58] suggesting that these treatments were working in part though overlapping mechanisms (**Box 1**).

Inflammatory Second Messengers

Brain injury leads to induction of the inflammatory cascade with increased release of cytokines and interleukins.[59] These compounds are believed to exacerbate delayed injury, whether by direct neurotoxicity and induction of the extrinsic pathway of apoptosis or by promoting leukocyte diapedesis into the ischemic brain. For example, tumor necrosis factor-α and interferon-γ mediated iNOS expression were associated with mitochondrial DNA damage and apoptosis in cultured oligodendrocytes.[60]

In vitro, hypothermia inhibits microglia proliferation, chemotaxsis, and induction of proinflammatory cytokines, and the translocation and binding of a key inflammatory signal, nuclear factor-κB, and attenuated microglia neurotoxicity, during and critically, after exposure to hypoxia and lipopolysaccharide.[61–64] In some settings, cooling may also increase release of anti-inflammatory cytokines.[65] In adult animals, hypothermia after transient focal ischemia and brief cardiac arrest attenuated subsequent increases in cytokines, such as interleukin-1β and tumor necrosis factor-α.[66] Consistent with this, postinsult hypothermia suppressed activated microglia after transient ischemia or asphyxia in fetal sheep.[14,67–69]

Intriguingly, despite potent suppression of microglia by hypothermia, it has little effect on astrocytic proliferation in vitro.[61] This raises the possibility that the hypothermic protection against postischemic neuronal damage may be, in part, the result of differential effects on glia, with suppression of microglial activation but relative sparing of restoration of the normal homeostatic environment by astrocytes.

Excitotoxicity

In contrast to their role during the primary and reperfusion phases, given that extracellular levels rapidly return to baseline values[19,27] the importance of EAAs after reperfusion is surprisingly unclear. In the temperature-controlled environment of the fetal sheep, antiexcitotoxin therapy limited to the secondary phase did not reduce neuronal injury in severely injured parasagittal cortex and had only limited neuroprotective effects in other regions.[70,71]

Nevertheless, even with normal levels of extracellular glutamate, excitotoxicity may still play an indirect role. There is evidence of pathologic hyperexcitability of glutamate receptors after HI in postnatal day 10 rats, with improved neuronal outcome after receptor blockade.[72] Consistent with this, in preterm fetal sheep, treatment with glutamate antagonist after asphyxia reduced neuronal loss,[73] although protection was much less than with hypothermia started at a similar time.[69] Furthermore, in adult animals, neuronal death after ischemia has been associated with a selective, delayed change in the composition of the α-amino-3-hydroxy-5-methyl-4-isoxazolepropionic acid receptor, with specific downregulation of GluR2, a subunit that limits Ca^{2+} influx. Hypothermia has been found to attenuate the postischemic reduction in the GluR2 subunit in adult gerbils[74] and suppress excessive transient epileptiform activity in the first 6 hours after asphyxia in preterm fetal sheep,[75] with a close correlation between suppression and neuroprotection.

Further studies are needed to confirm whether these mechanisms are important after HI injury in the term-equivalent brain.

Protection of the Mitochondria

Mitochondrial failure is a hallmark of delayed cell death.[8] Clearly, maintaining mitochondrial function is crucial in promoting survival after HI. Postischemic hypothermia maintains mitochondrial respiratory activity after 2 hours reperfusion in the adult gerbil[76] and minipig,[57] and intraischemic hypothermia has been shown to preserve activity after 4 days recovery in neonatal rats.[77] It is unclear, however, whether this reflects direct protection of the mitochondria, or whether it is secondary to suppression of inflammation and programmed cell death.

Induction of Growth Factors

Perhaps surprisingly in view of the general tendency of hypothermia to suppress new protein synthesis, there is evidence in the adult rat that mild hypothermia after cardiac arrest is associated with augmentation of the increase in levels of growth factors, such as brain-derived neurotrophic factor and others,[78,79] which might help protect injured cells. Despite this, brain-derived neurotrophic factor infusion in normothermic animals was not neuroprotective.[80] Thus, induction of these growth factors does not seem to be a major mechanism of hypothermic neuroprotection.

Box 2
Effects of hypothermia during the secondary phase

1. Possibly contributing to neuroprotection
    a. Reduced seizure burden may protect less severely injured areas of the brain by reducing anaerobic stress
2. Not contributing to neuroprotection
    a. Reduced cerebral hyperperfusion
    b. Reduced cytotoxic edema

HYPOTHERMIA IN THE SECONDARY PHASE

There is compelling evidence that hypothermia started in the latent phase must be continued for 48 hours or more to achieve optimal neuroprotection.[11] The precise reasons are unknown. The most likely explanation is that it is necessary to continue suppressing the programmed cell death and inflammatory pathways until normal homeostasis returns. However, it could in part reflect suppression of secondary events in this phase, including hyperperfusion, cytotoxic edema, and delayed seizures **(Box 2, Fig. 4)**.

Cerebral Metabolism

During the latent phase cerebral blood flow and metabolism are both suppressed. This suppression is actively mediated by multiple neuroinhibitory pathways,[81] and likely helps mitigate the effects of abnormal excitatory activity. From 6 to 8 hours, hyperperfusion develops progressively, to a maximum after 36 to 48 hours.[9,15] Hypothermia suppresses the secondary hyperperfusion after ischemia in the fetal sheep,[9,15] but late hypothermia that was not protective also effectively suppressed it.[15] Clinically, hypothermia markedly attenuated the secondary fall in the cerebral vascular resistance index, but reduced its predictive value.[82] Thus, this effect seems to be independent of neuroprotection.

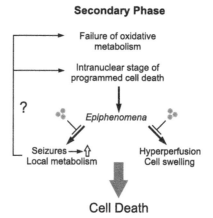

Fig. 4. Flow chart illustrating potential therapeutic targets for hypothermia, during the phase of secondary deterioration after hypoxia-ischemia.

Table 1
Potential mechanisms of hypothermic neuroprotection

Mechanism of Injury	Relevance to Therapeutic Hypothermia
Anoxic depolarization	Limited. Relevant to cooling during hypoxia-ischemia, such as during cardiac surgery.
Accumulation of EAAs/reactive oxygen species	Limited. Reduced rate of release of EAAs/reactive oxygen species by cooling during HI. Little evidence that it is affected by delayed cooling.
Prevention of BBB breakdown	Limited. Early induction of hypothermia after ischemia can prevent BBB breakdown; however, hypothermia is neuroprotective when delayed after the apparent critical window for protecting the BBB.
Programmed cell death	Strong. Hypothermia is associated with suppression of caspase-3, hypoxia-associated protein synthesis, the mitochondrial permeability transition, and components of the intrinsic and extrinsic pathways.
Secondary inflammation	Strong. Mild hypothermia potently suppresses microglial activation, production of inflammatory cytokines, and other neurotoxins.
Abnormal glutamate receptor activation	Moderate. Hypothermia reduces adverse changes in composition of the α-amino-3-hydroxy-5-methyl-4-isoxazolepropionic acid receptor and suppresses epileptiform transients/abnormal receptor activation in the latent phase. The effect correlates with neuroprotection, but more studies are needed to determine the role of these effects in term infants.
Cerebral hyperperfusion	Unlikely. Hypothermia extends the phase of cerebral hypoperfusion and reduces hyperperfusion independently of neuroprotection.
Cytotoxic edema	Unlikely. Hypothermia potently suppressed delayed cytotoxic edema, but independently of neuroprotection.
Induction of growth factors	Limited. In some settings hypothermia can augment the increase in some growth factors after HI, but not clear whether this is a significant contributor to neuroprotection.
Electrographic seizures	Limited. Potentially, hypothermia may reduce injury in penumbral, more mildly affected regions by reduced neural metabolism or antiexcitotoxicity effects; however, the neuroprotective effects of delayed hypothermia are much greater than anticonvulsants alone.

Secondary Cytotoxic Edema

Similarly, neuroprotection with delayed cerebral cooling started 90 minutes after cerebral ischemia potently suppresses secondary cytotoxic edema in near-term fetal sheep.[9] However, strikingly, late induction of hypothermia (8.5 hours after ischemia) also completely prevented secondary cytotoxic edema in the same paradigm, despite no significant neuroprotection.[16] These findings are highly consistent with the ability of hypothermia to reduce brain swelling after brain trauma and in other clinical settings[83] and suggest that it is not a direct mechanism of neuroprotection.

Seizures

Intense, difficult-to-treat seizures are one of the defining characteristics of neonatal encephalopathy.[84] Intense excitation during seizures leads to excessive local metabolic demand, which can potentially cause local neuronal death.[85] In near-term fetal sheep, treatment with MK-801, a highly potent, selective glutamate antagonist, between 6 and 24 hours after cerebral ischemia prevented delayed postischemic seizures.[70] Despite this, there was no improvement in parasagittal neuronal loss, and only a modest improvement in less damaged regions, such as the temporal lobe. These data suggest that severe seizure activity in the secondary phase can contribute to spreading of injury from the core area of damage to more mildly affected regions. Clinically and experimentally, there is evidence of reduced seizure burden and reduced intensity of seizures during cooling.[75,86,87] Thus, the reduced metabolic demand associated with hypothermia in this phase might help to protect less severely injured regions from further injury.[16]

SUMMARY

The mechanisms underlying hypothermic neuroprotection are multifactorial, as summarized in **Table 1**. Suppression of excitotoxicity, oxidative stress, inflammation, intracellular signaling, and programmed cell death are all effects of hypothermia at different times. Critically, it is suppression of downstream events after anoxic depolarization and excitotoxity that seems to be critical to hypothermic neuroprotection. We speculate that the differential effects of mild hypothermia to suppress programmed cell death and microglial activation without suppressing the recovery of normal homeostasis is central to long-term brain recovery. Further elucidation of these downstream pathways, particularly in the latent phase and during long-term recovery, will help clinicians to design effective combination therapies.

REFERENCES

1. Rutherford M, Ramenghi LA, Edwards AD, et al. Assessment of brain tissue injury after moderate hypothermia in neonates with hypoxic-ischaemic encephalopathy: a nested substudy of a randomised controlled trial. Lancet Neurol 2010;9:39–45.
2. Shankaran S, Barnes PD, Hintz SR, et al. Brain injury following trial of hypothermia for neonatal hypoxic-ischaemic encephalopathy. Arch Dis Child Fetal Neonatal Ed 2012;97:F398–404.
3. Edwards AD, Brocklehurst P, Gunn AJ, et al. Neurological outcomes at 18 months of age after moderate hypothermia for perinatal hypoxic ischaemic encephalopathy: synthesis and meta-analysis of trial data. BMJ 2010;340:C363.
4. Guillet R, Edwards AD, Thoresen M, et al. Seven- to eight-year follow-up of the CoolCap trial of head cooling for neonatal encephalopathy. Pediatr Res 2012; 71:205–9.
5. Shankaran S, Pappas A, McDonald SA, et al. Childhood outcomes after hypothermia for neonatal encephalopathy. N Engl J Med 2012;366:2085–92.
6. Azzopardi D, Wyatt JS, Cady EB, et al. Prognosis of newborn infants with hypoxic-ischemic brain injury assessed by phosphorus magnetic resonance spectroscopy. Pediatr Res 1989;25:445–51.
7. Iwata O, Iwata S, Bainbridge A, et al. Supra- and sub-baseline phosphocreatine recovery in developing brain after transient hypoxia-ischaemia: relation to baseline energetics, insult severity and outcome. Brain 2008;131:2220–6.
8. Bennet L, Roelfsema V, Pathipati P, et al. Relationship between evolving epileptiform activity and delayed loss of mitochondrial activity after asphyxia measured by near-infrared spectroscopy in preterm fetal sheep. J Physiol 2006;572:141–54.

9. Gunn AJ, Gunn TR, de Haan HH, et al. Dramatic neuronal rescue with prolonged selective head cooling after ischemia in fetal lambs. J Clin Invest 1997;99: 248–56.

10. Lorek A, Takei Y, Cady EB, et al. Delayed ("secondary") cerebral energy failure after acute hypoxia-ischemia in the newborn piglet: continuous 48-hour studies by phosphorus magnetic resonance spectroscopy. Pediatr Res 1994;36:699–706.

11. Gunn AJ, Thoresen M. Hypothermic neuroprotection. NeuroRx 2006;3:154–69.

12. Williams CE, Gunn AJ, Mallard C, et al. Outcome after ischemia in the developing sheep brain: an electroencephalographic and histological study. Ann Neurol 1992;31:14–21.

13. Sabir H, Scull-Brown E, Liu X, et al. Immediate hypothermia is not neuroprotective after severe hypoxia-ischemia and is deleterious when delayed by 12 hours in neonatal rats. Stroke 2012;43:3364–70.

14. Roelfsema V, Bennet L, George S, et al. The window of opportunity for cerebral hypothermia and white matter injury after cerebral ischemia in near-term fetal sheep. J Cereb Blood Flow Metab 2004;24:877–86.

15. Gunn AJ, Gunn TR, Gunning MI, et al. Neuroprotection with prolonged head cooling started before postischemic seizures in fetal sheep. Pediatrics 1998; 102:1098–106.

16. Gunn AJ, Bennet L, Gunning MI, et al. Cerebral hypothermia is not neuroprotective when started after postischemic seizures in fetal sheep. Pediatr Res 1999; 46:274–80.

17. Gunn AJ, Gluckman PD. Head cooling for neonatal encephalopathy: the state of the art. Clin Obstet Gynecol 2007;50:636–51.

18. Rothman SM, Olney JW. Excitotoxicity and the NMDA receptor: still lethal after eight years. Trends Neurosci 1995;18:57–8.

19. Tan WK, Williams CE, During MJ, et al. Accumulation of cytotoxins during the development of seizures and edema after hypoxic-ischemic injury in late gestation fetal sheep. Pediatr Res 1996;39:791–7.

20. Bagenholm R, Nilsson UA, Gotborg CW, et al. Free radicals are formed in the brain of fetal sheep during reperfusion after cerebral ischemia. Pediatr Res 1998;43:271–5.

21. Fraser M, Bennet L, van Zijl PL, et al. Extracellular amino acids and peroxidation products in the periventricular white matter during and after cerebral ischemia in preterm fetal sheep. J Neurochem 2008;105:2214–23.

22. Wei G, Dawson VL, Zweier JL. Role of neuronal and endothelial nitric oxide synthase in nitric oxide generation in the brain following cerebral ischemia. Biochim Biophys Acta 1999;1455:23–34.

23. Hunter CJ, Bennet L, Power GG, et al. Key neuroprotective role for endogenous adenosine A1 receptor activation during asphyxia in the fetal sheep. Stroke 2003;34:2240–5.

24. Laptook AR, Corbett RJ, Sterett R, et al. Quantitative relationship between brain temperature and energy utilization rate measured in vivo using 31P and 1H magnetic resonance spectroscopy. Pediatr Res 1995;38:919–25.

25. Bart RD, Takaoka S, Pearlstein RD, et al. Interactions between hypothermia and the latency to ischemic depolarization: implications for neuroprotection. Anesthesiology 1998;88:1266–73.

26. Nakashima K, Todd MM. Effects of hypothermia on the rate of excitatory amino acid release after ischemic depolarization. Stroke 1996;27:913–8.

27. Thoresen M, Satas S, Puka-Sundvall M, et al. Post-hypoxic hypothermia reduces cerebrocortical release of NO and excitotoxins. Neuroreport 1997;8:3359–62.

28. Nakashima K, Todd MM. Effects of hypothermia, pentobarbital, and isoflurane on postdepolarization amino acid release during complete global cerebral ischemia. Anesthesiology 1996;85:161–8.

29. McManus T, Sadgrove M, Pringle AK, et al. Intraischaemic hypothermia reduces free radical production and protects against ischaemic insults in cultured hippocampal slices. J Neurochem 2004;91:327–36.

30. Lei B, Adachi N, Arai T. The effect of hypothermia on H2O2 production during ischemia and reperfusion: a microdialysis study in the gerbil hippocampus. Neurosci Lett 1997;222:91–4.

31. Lei B, Tan X, Cai H, et al. Effect of moderate hypothermia on lipid peroxidation in canine brain tissue after cardiac arrest and resuscitation. Stroke 1994;25:147–52.

32. Bennet L, Roelfsema V, Dean J, et al. Regulation of cytochrome oxidase redox state during umbilical cord occlusion in preterm fetal sheep. Am J Physiol Regul Integr Comp Physiol 2007;292:R1569–76.

33. Nagel S, Su Y, Horstmann S, et al. Minocycline and hypothermia for reperfusion injury after focal cerebral ischemia in the rat: effects on BBB breakdown and MMP expression in the acute and subacute phase. Brain Res 2008;1188:198–206.

34. Ranasinghe HS, Scheepens A, Sirimanne E, et al. Inhibition of MMP-9 activity following hypoxic ischemia in the developing brain using a highly specific inhibitor. Dev Neurosci 2012;34:417–27.

35. Colbourne F, Corbett D, Zhao Z, et al. Prolonged but delayed postischemic hypothermia: a long-term outcome study in the rat middle cerebral artery occlusion model. J Cereb Blood Flow Metab 2000;20:1702–8.

36. Bagenholm R, Nilsson UA, Kjellmer I. Formation of free radicals in hypoxic ischemic brain damage in the neonatal rat, assessed by an endogenous spin trap and lipid peroxidation. Brain Res 1997;773:132–8.

37. Kristian T, Katsura K, Siesjo BK. The influence of moderate hypothermia on cellular calcium uptake in complete ischaemia: implications for the excitotoxic hypothesis. Acta Physiol Scand 1992;146:531–2.

38. Bruno VM, Goldberg MP, Dugan LL, et al. Neuroprotective effect of hypothermia in cortical cultures exposed to oxygen-glucose deprivation or excitatory amino acids. J Neurochem 1994;63:1398–406.

39. Zipfel GJ, Babcock DJ, Lee JM, et al. Neuronal apoptosis after CNS injury: the roles of glutamate and calcium. J Neurotrauma 2000;17:857–69.

40. Schild L, Keilhoff G, Augustin W, et al. Distinct Ca2+ thresholds determine cytochrome c release or permeability transition pore opening in brain mitochondria. FASEB J 2001;15:565–7.

41. Clawson TF, Vannucci SJ, Wang GM, et al. Hypoxia-ischemia-induced apoptotic cell death correlates with IGF-I mRNA decrease in neonatal rat brain. Biol Signals Recept 1999;8:281–93.

42. Giulian D, Vaca K. Inflammatory glia mediate delayed neuronal damage after ischemia in the central nervous system. Stroke 1993;24:I84–90.

43. Graham EM, Sheldon RA, Flock DL, et al. Neonatal mice lacking functional Fas death receptors are resistant to hypoxic-ischemic brain injury. Neurobiol Dis 2004;17:89–98.

44. Bossenmeyer-Pourie C, Koziel V, Daval JL. Effects of hypothermia on hypoxia-induced apoptosis in cultured neurons from developing rat forebrain: comparison with preconditioning. Pediatr Res 2000;47:385–91.

45. Nagel S, Papadakis M, Pfleger K, et al. Microarray analysis of the global gene expression profile following hypothermia and transient focal cerebral ischemia. Neuroscience 2012;208:109–22.

46. Northington FJ, Chavez-Valdez R, Martin LJ. Neuronal cell death in neonatal hypoxia-ischemia. Ann Neurol 2011;69:743–58.
47. Xu L, Yenari MA, Steinberg GK, et al. Mild hypothermia reduces apoptosis of mouse neurons in vitro early in the cascade. J Cereb Blood Flow Metab 2002; 22:21–8.
48. Liu L, Kim JY, Koike MA, et al. FasL shedding is reduced by hypothermia in experimental stroke. J Neurochem 2008;106:541–50.
49. Rice JEIII, Vannucci RC, Brierley JB. The influence of immaturity on hypoxic-ischemic brain damage in the rat. Ann Neurol 1981;9:131–41.
50. Askalan R, Wang C, Shi H, et al. The effect of postischemic hypothermia on apoptotic cell death in the neonatal rat brain. Dev Neurosci 2011;33:320–9.
51. Xiong M, Chen LX, Ma SM, et al. Short-term effects of hypothermia on axonal injury, preoligodendrocyte accumulation and oligodendrocyte myelination after hypoxia-ischemia in the hippocampus of immature rat brain. Dev Neurosci 2013;35:17–27.
52. Zgavc T, De Geyter D, Ceulemans AG, et al. Mild hypothermia reduces activated caspase-3 up to 1 week after a focal cerebral ischemia induced by endothelin-1 in rats. Brain Res 2013;1501:81–8.
53. Zhao H, Yenari MA, Cheng D, et al. Biphasic cytochrome *c* release after transient global ischemia and its inhibition by hypothermia. J Cereb Blood Flow Metab 2005;25:1119–29.
54. Zhang H, Xu G, Zhang J, et al. Mild hypothermia reduces ischemic neuron death via altering the expression of p53 and bcl-2. Neurol Res 2010;32:384–9.
55. Yenari MA, Iwayama S, Cheng D, et al. Mild hypothermia attenuates cytochrome *c* release but does not alter Bcl-2 expression or caspase activation after experimental stroke. J Cereb Blood Flow Metab 2002;22:29–38.
56. Zhao H, Yenari MA, Sapolsky RM, et al. Mild postischemic hypothermia prolongs the time window for gene therapy by inhibiting cytochrome *c* release. Stroke 2004;35:572–7.
57. Gong P, Hua R, Zhang Y, et al. Hypothermia-induced neuroprotection is associated with reduced mitochondrial membrane permeability in a swine model of cardiac arrest. J Cereb Blood Flow Metab 2013;33:928–34.
58. George SA, Bennet L, Weaver-Mikaere L, et al. White matter protection with insulin like-growth factor 1 (IGF-1) and hypothermia is not additive after severe reversible cerebral ischemia in term fetal sheep. Dev Neurosci 2011;33:280–7.
59. Hagberg H, Mallard C, Jacobsson B. Role of cytokines in preterm labour and brain injury. BJOG 2005;112(Suppl 1):16–8.
60. Druzhyna NM, Musiyenko SI, Wilson GL, et al. Cytokines induce nitric oxide-mediated mtDNA damage and apoptosis in oligodendrocytes. Protective role of targeting 8-oxoguanine glycosylase to mitochondria. J Biol Chem 2005;280: 21673–9.
61. Si QS, Nakamura Y, Kataoka K. Hypothermic suppression of microglial activation in culture: inhibition of cell proliferation and production of nitric oxide and superoxide. Neuroscience 1997;81:223–9.
62. Seo JW, Kim JH, Seo M, et al. Time-dependent effects of hypothermia on microglial activation and migration. J Neuroinflammation 2012;9:164.
63. Schmitt KR, Diestel A, Lehnardt S, et al. Hypothermia suppresses inflammation via ERK signaling pathway in stimulated microglial cells. J Neuroimmunol 2007; 189:7–16.
64. Yenari MA, Han HS. Influence of hypothermia on post-ischemic inflammation: role of nuclear factor kappa B (NFkappaB). Neurochem Int 2006;49:164–9.

65. Diestel A, Troeller S, Billecke N, et al. Mechanisms of hypothermia-induced cell protection mediated by microglial cells in vitro. Eur J Neurosci 2010;31:779–87.
66. Meybohm P, Gruenewald M, Zacharowski KD, et al. Mild hypothermia alone or in combination with anesthetic post-conditioning reduces expression of inflammatory cytokines in the cerebral cortex of pigs after cardiopulmonary resuscitation. Critica 2010;14:R21.
67. George SA, Barrett RD, Bennet L, et al. Nonadditive neuroprotection with early glutamate receptor blockade and delayed hypothermia after asphyxia in preterm fetal sheep. Stroke 2012;43:3114–7.
68. Barrett RD, Bennet L, Naylor A, et al. Effect of cerebral hypothermia and asphyxia on the subventricular zone and white matter tracts in preterm fetal sheep. Brain Res 2012;1469:35–42.
69. Bennet L, Roelfsema V, George S, et al. The effect of cerebral hypothermia on white and grey matter injury induced by severe hypoxia in preterm fetal sheep. J Physiol 2007;578:491–506.
70. Tan WK, Williams CE, Gunn AJ, et al. Suppression of postischemic epileptiform activity with MK-801 improves neural outcome in fetal sheep. Ann Neurol 1992; 32:677–82.
71. Gressens P, Le Verche V, Fraser M, et al. Pitfalls in the quest of neuroprotectants for the perinatal brain. Dev Neurosci 2011;33:189–98.
72. Jensen FE, Wang C, Stafstrom CE, et al. Acute and chronic increases in excitability in rat hippocampal slices after perinatal hypoxia in vivo. J Neurophysiol 1998;79:73–81.
73. Dean JM, George SA, Wassink G, et al. Suppression of post hypoxic-ischemic EEG transients with dizocilpine is associated with partial striatal protection in the preterm fetal sheep. Neuropharmacology 2006;50:491–503.
74. Colbourne F, Grooms SY, Zukin RS, et al. Hypothermia rescues hippocampal CA1 neurons and attenuates down-regulation of the AMPA receptor GluR2 subunit after forebrain ischemia. Proc Natl Acad Sci U S A 2003;100(5): 2906–10.
75. Bennet L, Dean JM, Wassink G, et al. Differential effects of hypothermia on early and late epileptiform events after severe hypoxia in preterm fetal sheep. J Neurophysiol 2007;97:572–8.
76. Canevari L, Console A, Tendi EA, et al. Effect of postischaemic hypothermia on the mitochondrial damage induced by ischaemia and reperfusion in the gerbil. Brain Res 1999;817:241–5.
77. Nakai A, Shibazaki Y, Taniuchi Y, et al. Influence of mild hypothermia on delayed mitochondrial dysfunction after transient intrauterine ischemia in the immature rat brain. Brain Res Dev Brain Res 2001;128:1–7.
78. D'Cruz BJ, Fertig KC, Filiano AJ, et al. Hypothermic reperfusion after cardiac arrest augments brain-derived neurotrophic factor activation. J Cereb Blood Flow Metab 2002;22:843–51.
79. Schmidt KM, D'Cruz BJ, DeFranco DB, et al. Cardiac arrest and hypothermia increase GDNF in brain. Acad Emerg Med 2003;10:480.
80. Callaway CW, Ramos R, Logue ES, et al. Brain-derived neurotrophic factor does not improve recovery after cardiac arrest in rats. Neurosci Lett 2008;445:103–7.
81. Jensen EC, Bennet L, Hunter CJ, et al. Post-hypoxic hypoperfusion is associated with suppression of cerebral metabolism and increased tissue oxygenation in near-term fetal sheep. J Physiol 2006;572:131–9.
82. Elstad M, Whitelaw A, Thoresen M. Cerebral Resistance Index is less predictive in hypothermic encephalopathic newborns. Acta Paediatr 2011;100:1344–9.

83. Sadaka F, Veremakis C. Therapeutic hypothermia for the management of intracranial hypertension in severe traumatic brain injury: a systematic review. Brain Inj 2012;26:899–908.
84. Williams CE, Gunn AJ, Synek B, et al. Delayed seizures occurring with hypoxic-ischemic encephalopathy in the fetal sheep. Pediatr Res 1990;27:561–5.
85. Miller SP, Weiss J, Barnwell A, et al. Seizure-associated brain injury in term newborns with perinatal asphyxia. Neurology 2002;58:542–8.
86. Srinivasakumar P, Zempel J, Wallendorf M, et al. Therapeutic hypothermia in neonatal hypoxic ischemic encephalopathy: electrographic seizures and magnetic resonance imaging evidence of injury. J Pediatr 2013;163:465–70.
87. Glass HC, Nash KB, Bonifacio SL, et al. Seizures and magnetic resonance imaging-detected brain injury in newborns cooled for hypoxic-ischemic encephalopathy. J Pediatr 2011;159:731–5.e1.

Neonatal Seizures
Advances in Mechanisms and Management

Hannah C. Glass, MDCM, MAS

KEYWORDS

- Brain injury • Developmental disability • Infant, newborn • Electroencephalography
- Epilepsy • Magnetic resonance imaging • Neurocritical care • Seizures

KEY POINTS

- Seizures occur in 1 to 5 per 1000 live births and are among the most common neurologic conditions managed by a neonatal neurocritical care service.
- The high rate of seizures in the neonatal period reflects age-specific developmental mechanisms that lead to relative excitability.
- Neonatal seizures are often caused by serious underlying brain injury such as hypoxia-ischemia, stroke, or hemorrhage.
- Clinical detection is unreliable; continuous video electroencephalogram is the gold standard for monitoring presence and burden of neonatal seizures.
- Seizures are refractory to first-line medications in approximately 50% of cases; expert opinion supports rapid treatment to abolish acute symptomatic seizures and early discontinuation of medication.

INTRODUCTION

Neonates are at especially high risk for seizures as compared to other age groups.[1] The high risk for seizures—and especially acute symptomatic seizures—is likely multifactorial and often caused due to the relative excitability of the developing neonatal brain as well as the high risk for brain injury due to global hypoxia-ischemia, stroke, and intracranial hemorrhage.[2] The estimated rate of seizures in term newborns is said to be approximately 1 to 5 per 1000 live births.[3–5] However, population-based studies do not take into account the low diagnostic accuracy of diagnosis by clinical

Financial Disclosure: Nothing to disclose.
Disclosures: None.
Project Support: H.C. Glass is supported by the NINDS K23NS066137, the Pediatric Epilepsy Research Foundation, and the Neonatal Brain Research Institute.
Departments of Neurology and Pediatrics, University of California, 505 Parnassus Avenue, M793, Box 0114, San Francisco, CA 94143-0114, USA
E-mail address: Hannah.Glass@ucsf.edu

observation alone,[6,7] and gold standard prolonged, continuous video electroencephalogram (cEEG) monitoring is not widely available enough to make population-based predictions; therefore the true incidence remains unknown.

The differential diagnosis for neonatal seizures is broad and includes structural, metabolic, and genetic causes (**Box 1**). Seizures that arise from an acute symptomatic cause, such as hypoxic-ischemic encephalopathy, transient metabolic disturbance, infection, stroke, or intracranial hemorrhage, are much more common than neonatal onset epilepsies, which may be due to malformation, prior injury, or genetic causes. Rare conditions such as inborn errors of metabolism, vitamin-responsive epilepsies, and neonatal epilepsy syndromes must be considered in the setting of refractory seizures.[8,9]

Neonatal seizures carry a high risk for early death. Among survivors, motor and cognitive disabilities, as well as epilepsy are common.[10] The outcome depends largely on the underlying disease process and severity of underlying brain injury. The impact of the seizures themselves is not known, although studies in animal models suggest that seizures can alter brain development, leading to deficits in learning, memory, and behavior.[11]

Box 1
Cause of neonatal seizures

Differential Diagnosis of Acute Symptomatic Seizures

Global hypoxia-ischemia (hypoxic-ischemic encephalopathy)

Focal hypoxia-ischemia

  Arterial stroke

  Venous stroke

Intracranial hemorrhage

  Intraventricular

  Parenchymal

  Subarachnoid

  Subdural

Transient metabolic deficit

  Hypoglycemia

  Hypocalcemia and hypomagnesemia

  Hyponatremia

Acute infection

Differential Diagnosis of Neonatal Onset Epilepsy

Brain malformation

Intrauterine injury or congenital infection

Inborn error of metabolism and vitamin-responsive epilepsies

Neonatal Onset Epilepsy Syndromes

  Benign familial neonatal seizures (eg., KCNQ2, KCNQ3)

  Neonatal epileptic encephalopathies

    Early myoclonic epilepsy

    Early infantile epileptic encephalopathy (Ohtahara syndrome)

PATHOPHYSIOLOGY

There are several, age-specific factors that are particular to the neonatal brain that lead to enhanced excitability and seizure generation, poor response to conventional medications, and adverse impact on brain development.[12]

Enhanced Excitability of the Neonatal Brain

There are numerous mechanisms that render the immature brain hyperexcitable as compared to the adult brain.[12,13] First, the neonatal period is a time of physiologic, use-dependent synaptogenesis, and both synapse and dendritic spine density are at their peak.[14,15] Second, glutamatergic neurons—the primary excitatory mechanism of both the developing and adult brain—are overabundant, and their receptors are configured with subunits that allow relative hyperexcitability.[16,17] Third, gamma-aminobutyric acid (GABA)—the primary inhibitory mechanism of the adult brain—can exert a paradoxic excitatory action in the developing brain due to the preponderance of the NKCC1 and delayed expression of the KCC2 chloride cotransporters, which lead to a high intracellular chloride concentration and *depolarization* in response to GABAergic agents.[18–20]

Anticonvulsants and the Developing Brain

Immature development of the excitatory and inhibitory neurotransmitter systems leads to a lack of good targets for conventional antiseizure medications, which makes neonatal seizures particularly difficult to treat. The immature brain may be resistant to medications that act as GABA agonists, not only as a result of the paradoxic chloride gradient as discussed earlier but also due to overall lower receptor expression and an immature subunit composition that is less sensitive to benzodiazepines than the adult brain.[12,13]

Seizures and Early Brain Development

Although early work with animal models demonstrated that the developing brain is more resistant to seizure-induced necrosis than the adult brain, more recent work has shown that early-life seizures can affect the developing brain nonetheless by altering neuronal circuitry, which can result in impaired learning and memory and enhanced susceptibility to epilepsy later in life.[11] Animal models of early-life seizures display developmental alterations that can include reduced density of dendritic spines in hippocampal pyramidal neurons; decreased neurogenesis; delayed neuronal loss; and changes in hippocampal plasticity such as decreased capacity for long-term potentiation, reduced susceptibility to kindling, and enhanced paired-pulse inhibition.[21–24] Human studies in children with hypoxic-ischemic injury show an independent association between seizures and impaired brain metabolism, as well as poor long-term neurodevelopmental outcome.[25,26]

MANAGEMENT GOALS

The overall management goal for neonatal seizures is to quickly and accurately identify, and abolish electrographic seizures, while determining the most likely underlying cause. Neonatal seizures are often the first sign of neurologic dysfunction and are frequently an indication of serious underlying brain injury.[27,28] Therefore, a suspicion of seizures in a newborn should be treated as a neurologic emergency, and prompt rapid and thorough evaluation to identify the cause, as well as emergent medical management to abolish seizures should be performed while preventing secondary injury by maintaining physiologic temperature, glucose, oxygenation, ventilation, and blood pressure.

Seizure Detection and Monitoring

Common methods for identifying neonatal seizures are outlined in **Table 1**. *Clinical evaluation* of seizures is approximately 50% accurate for events detected at the bedside. Furthermore, clinical detection requires constant observation by the bedside staff and even so will fail to detect seizures with no or very subtle clinical correlate (eg, eye deviation or subtle clonic movements that are covered by the infant's blanket). Subclinical seizures account for most seizures in neonates, especially in the setting of severe brain injury, and in children who have received seizure medications.[7,29–31]

Recent guidelines from the American Clinical Neurophysiology Society set the standard for neurophysiology monitoring in neonates.[32] cEEG, with electrodes placed according to the international 10–20 system, modified for neonates, is the gold standard for monitoring.[33–35] Barriers to implementing this technology include the need for specialized training for the application and interpretation of the recording, as well as variable access to equipment, and high cost. Once initiated, cEEG should be maintained until electrographic seizures have resolved for at least 24 hours or 3 to 4 clinical events have been captured and determined not to be seizures.[32]

Amplitude-integrated electroencephalography (aEEG; a simplified bedside neurophysiology tool that can be applied and interpreted by neonatologists, nurses, or other Intensive Care Nursery bedside staff) is used to supplement or even replace cEEG in a growing number of centers. Because aEEG uses a limited number of channels to record EEG signal that is heavily processed (filtered, rectified, and displayed on a semilogarithmic amplitude and time-compressed scale), there are several limitations to this technology that must be taken into account when it is used for management of neonatal seizures (see **Table 1**). Machines that allow for concurrent monitoring and display of aEEG (at the bedside) and cEEG (in the neurophysiology laboratory or remotely) using the same hardware have been suggested as a way to optimize use of both technologies, such that both the bedside team *and* the neurologist can be readily involved in the rapid, real-time management of electrographic seizures (**Fig. 1**).[36]

Automated seizure detection—with an alarm to alert the bedside practitioner in the case of suspected seizures—is an attractive option that may offer the most practical solution for wide-scale implementation of seizure detection and management. However, there have been several challenges that limit the development of automated detection algorithms, including highly variable nature of neonatal seizure patterns,

Table 1	
Diagnosis of neonatal seizures	
Conventional cEEG	• Gold standard for seizure detection • Recommended by the American Clinical Neurophysiology Society for monitoring neonates with paroxysmal events and/or at high risk for seizures[32]
aEEG	• Lower sensitivity and specificity than cEEG[36] • Hundred percent sensitivity for status epilepticus[37] • Lowest sensitivity for seizures that are brief, focal, and distal from recording electrodes[38,39] • Raw EEG tracing helps to distinguish artifact from seizure[40] • Experienced readers perform better than nonexperts[41]
Clinical evaluation	• Accuracy approximately 50%[6] • Will not identify most seizures (ie, subclinical or nonconvulsive seizures)[7,29–31]

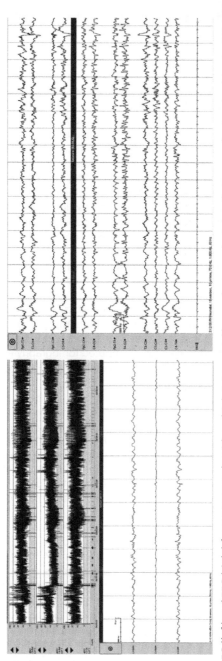

Fig. 1. aEEG (*left*) and EEG (*right*) from a term male with multiple intracranial hemorrhages and seizures that were refractory to phenobarbital, 40 mg/kg, and fosphenytoin, 30 mg/kg, and abated after 60 mg/kg levetiracetam. aEEG and EEG are recorded from a single machine at the bedside. Data are displayed differently for different users: the bedside team sees the aEEG display at left, which shows long-term trends and allows a quick review of suspicious segments of EEG. The neurophysiologist can confirm the seizures through the review of conventional, neonatal montage EEG.

high frequency of potential artifacts in the intensive care nursery, and uncertainty regarding the gold standard against which algorithms are tested given the limited information regarding inter-rater reliability among human expert readers.[42] Newer algorithms that use machine learning, as well as temporal and spatial weighting hold promise.[43–46]

Diagnostic Evaluation

Initial evaluation of a neonate with suspected seizures should also focus on rapid identification of the cause. Emergent evaluation of serum glucose and risk factors for infection is an important first step, because hypoglycemia and bacterial meningitis can lead to permanent injury if left untreated.[8] Additional bedside evaluations must include measurement and treatment of electrolyte disturbance. Comprehensive history and physical examination are important tools to assess for risk factors and signs of both common and rare causes of neonatal seizures. Further evaluation, including genetic testing, serum amino acids, ammonia, lactate, very-long-chain fatty acids, urine organic acids and sulfites, and cerebrospinal fluid studies for glucose, glycine, lactate, and neurotransmitters, as well as additional testing for inborn errors of metabolism may be warranted on a case-by-case basis, especially in the setting of medically refractory seizures of unknown cause or a burst-suppression pattern on EEG in a neonate without brain injury.

Detailed neuroimaging using magnetic resonance (MR) is essential to identify underlying injury or developmental abnormalities and to help clinicians and the family to better understand the prognosis.[47] Cranial ultrasound, which is readily available at the bedside in most units, is important for rapid initial assessment of a sick neonate to identify large space occupying lesions, such as hemorrhage, arteriovenous malformations, or hydrocephalus, but is insensitive for global and focal hypoxic-ischemic injury, especially in the days after the ictus. Computed tomography exposes the infant to ionizing radiation and provides inferior resolution to MRI in most settings, and so should be avoided.

PHARMACOLOGIC STRATEGIES

There are no evidence-based guidelines for the pharmacologic management of neonatal seizures.[48,49] Expert opinion supports use of pharmacologic treatments with a goal of abolishing electrographic seizures, even those without clinical correlate.[42] However, evidence is lacking regarding the relative benefit versus potential harm of anticonvulsants used to treat seizures in neonates, many of which can lead to neuronal apoptosis in animal models.[50]

Because seizures are refractory to initial doses of medication in approximately 50% of cases,[51] frequent reevaluation of cEEG and bedside monitoring is essential to accurately identify and treat ongoing seizures in real time. Although data are lacking regarding optimal treatment paradigms for neonatal seizures, experts advocate *rapid* administration of an adequate loading dose of medication because acute symptomatic seizure burden is highest at the onset,[52] and patients with fewer seizures are easier to treat.[51] Similarly, experts advocate treatment of both clinical *and* subclinical seizures given similar pathophysiology, and the only difference between the 2 may be slight anatomic differences in their cortical distribution.[42] Use of algorithms or guidelines to direct the treatment of neonatal seizures has gained favor, given evidence that treatment guidelines can improve outcomes in other settings.[53] As discussed later in this article, the optimal medication for seizure therapy in neonates is not known, and so guidelines should focus on an institution-specific, consensus-based protocol with input and acceptance by both neonatology and neurology services to help prevent unnecessary delays in treatment that may result from discussions over medication choice in the setting of an actively seizing neonate.

The optimal duration of pharmacologic therapy for acute symptomatic seizures is not known. Treatment practices are variable in spite of good evidence that there is no harmful effect of early discontinuation of seizure therapy and no difference in seizure recurrence risk among neonates who are maintained on therapy versus those whose medication is maintained until several months of age (**Box 2**).[54–56]

International survey data support the use of phenobarbital as the first-line medication based on expert consensus (**Table 2**).[57–59] A single randomized, controlled trial found that phenobarbital and phenytoin were equally efficacious as first-line agents for seizure cessation among term infants with seizures.[51] However, seizure control (defined by the study parameters as an 80% reduction in the severity of seizures) was achieved in fewer than half of the infants.[51] This result is supported by newer studies, which demonstrate that up to 50% of neonatal seizures are refractory to first-line medications and an additional 30% fail second-line therapy.[60]

Levetiracetam is gaining increasing support, in spite of limited efficacy data[61,62]; this is likely due to the ready availability of an intravenous formulation in the United States, as well as a favorable safety and tolerability profile among children and adults.[63] In contrast to older agents such as phenobarbital and phenytoin, levetiracetam does not appear to enhance neuronal apoptosis in animal models[64,65] and may in fact have neuroprotective and antiepileptogenic effects.[66,67] The optimal neonatal dosage of levetiracetam is not yet known: reported doses range from 5 to 60 mg/kg/d.[68] However, the high volume of distribution and rapid clearance in neonates may necessitate a higher loading dose and more frequent dosing to maintain serum concentrations in the range used for adults and children.[69,70] Published studies of the clinical efficacy of levetiracetam that report seizure reduction or resolution in 35% to 80% are limited by lack of standardized dosing, limited EEG monitoring, no placebo comparison, and/or variable timing and definition for determining the outcome.[71–73]

Common agents for refractory seizures include midazolam infusion, which may be effective for neonatal status epilepticus, and lidocaine, which is widely used for refractory neonatal seizures in Europe.[74–81] Topiramate is an antiseizure medication that has multiple mechanisms of anticonvulsant action and is an interesting option for acute symptomatic neonatal seizures because it appears to have neuroprotective effects in animal models of seizures and brain injury.[82,83] A recently developed intravenous preparation of topiramate that is well tolerated in adult volunteers and has equivalent bioavailability to the oral formulation holds promise for use in neonates.[84,85]

Bumetanide is a loop diuretic that has been proposed as an adjunct to GABAergic drugs like phenobarbital to help overcome the depolarizing action of immature neurons to GABA agonists. The mechanism of action is presumed to be through reduction in intracellular chloride concentrations, thus rendering the normally excitatory response of immature cells with high NKCC1 expression to an inhibitory response.[86] Preclinical studies demonstrate mixed effects, with reduction in seizure frequency and

---

Box 2
Principles for acute symptomatic neonatal seizure management

Rapid and accurate electrographic seizure identification

Rapid titration of medication to abolish electrographic seizures

Early discontinuation of medication once seizures have resolved

Table 2
Pharmacologic treatment of acute symptomatic neonatal seizures

Medication	Dosage	Side Effects	Notes
Levetiracetam	*Optimal dosing not known* Loading dose: 40–60 mg/kg intravenously Daily dosing: 30 mg/kg/day (target levels not known)[92]	Mild sedation/drowsiness and irritability	Limited information regarding dosing and side effects for neonatal population
Lidocaine	Loading dose: 2 mg/kg over a period of 10 min, followed by a continuous infusion of 6 mg/kg/h during the first 12 h; 4 mg/kg/h for the next 12 h, and 2 mg/kg/h for the last 12 h[a]	Arrhythmia	Should only be given in the intensive care setting with continuous cardiac monitoring. In case of cardiac arrhythmia, the infusion should be discontinued immediately. Lidocaine should not be given to patients with a congenital heart disease or to neonates who have been treated with proarrhythmic drugs like phenytoin
Lorazepam	0.05–0.1 mg/kg intravenously	Respiratory depression, depressed level of consciousness, and hypotension	May cause myoclonus in very-low-birth-weight infants
Midazolam	Loading dose: 0.2 mg/kg intravenously, followed by continuous infusion (1 mcg/kg/min) increasing by 0.5–1 mcg/kg/min every 2 min to 2–5 mcg/kg/min	Respiratory depression, depressed level of consciousness, and hypotension	
Phenobarbital	Loading dose: 20 mg/kg intravenously, repeated once as needed Daily dosing: 5 mg/kg/d (target level 40–60 mcg/mL)	Respiratory depression, depressed level of consciousness, hypotension, and hypotonia Idiosyncratic skin rash, hepatotoxicity, and blood dyscrasia	Prolonged half-life in first week of life (43–217 hours) limits need for weaning phenobarbital in the case of short-term therapy
Phenytoin and fosphenytoin	Loading dose: 20 mg/kg intravenously Daily dosing: 5 mg/kg/d (target level 10–20 mcg/mL)	Infusion site reaction and arrhythmia with intravenous phenytoin Idiosyncratic skin rash, hepatotoxicity, and blood dyscrasia	Fosphenytoin has fewer cardiovascular, central nervous system, and local cutaneous side effects than phenytoin. Significant variability and changes in pharmacokinetics over the first weeks of life may lead to inconsistent drug levels

[a] NB: Lower doses recommended for neonates undergoing therapeutic hypothermia.[79]

duration, as well as enhanced neuroprotective efficacy when combined with pheno-barbital.[87–89] A single clinical study showed reduction in seizure frequency and duration following bumetanide treatment.[90] Although promising as an add-on agent for neonatal seizures, the potential for adverse effects such as ototoxicity and partial central nervous system bioavailability may ultimately limit the utility of bumetanide.[91]

Information about agents other than phenobarbital and phenytoin is largely derived from case series rather than randomized, blinded, clinical trials, and so the true efficacy of these medications is not known. Seizures due to acute symptomatic causes such as hypoxic-ischemic brain injury and stroke rarely persist beyond a few days of life, making any add-on agent appear more effective than the initial therapy.[52] Furthermore, older studies do not include prolonged, cEEG monitoring, and so non-convulsive seizures, which are very common following administration of phenobarbital, may go undetected.

If the underlying cause of medically refractory seizures is unknown after initial screening laboratory tests and imaging studies, a trial of pyridoxine, pyridoxal 5′-phosphate, and folinic acid should be considered, and a screening metabolic evaluation should be performed.[9]

SUMMARY/DISCUSSION

Neonatal seizures are common and frequently reflect serious underlying brain injury. Prolonged cEEG is the gold standard for seizure monitoring; however availability remains limited at many centers. Phenobarbital, the preferred first-choice medication internationally, is effective in only 50% of cases and may be harmful, especially when used in high doses or for prolonged periods. However, there is abundant evidence from animal models to show that seizures themselves disrupt the developing brain, and so there is urgent need for research to develop safe, accurate, and widely available methods for identifying and treating electrographic seizures.

ACKNOWLEDGMENTS

Dr H.C. Glass thanks Jessica Kan for assistance with research and Dr Dawn Gano for careful review of the article.

REFERENCES

1. Annegers JF, Hauser WA, Lee JR, et al. Incidence of acute symptomatic seizures in Rochester, Minnesota, 1935-1984. Epilepsia 1995;36(4):327–33.
2. Jensen FE. Developmental factors regulating susceptibility to perinatal brain injury and seizures. Curr Opin Pediatr 2006;18(6):628–33.
3. Glass HC, Pham TN, Danielsen B, et al. Antenatal and intrapartum risk factors for seizures in term newborns: a population-based study, California 1998-2002. J Pediatr 2009;154(1):24–8.e1.
4. Lanska MJ, Lanska DJ, Baumann RJ, et al. A population-based study of neonatal seizures in Fayette County, Kentucky. Neurology 1995;45(4):724–32.
5. Saliba RM, Annegers JF, Waller DK, et al. Incidence of neonatal seizures in Harris County, Texas, 1992-1994. Am J Epidemiol 1999;150(7):763–9.
6. Malone A, Ryan CA, Fitzgerald A, et al. Interobserver agreement in neonatal seizure identification. Epilepsia 2009;50(9):2097–101.
7. Murray DM, Boylan GB, Ali I, et al. Defining the gap between electrographic seizure burden, clinical expression and staff recognition of neonatal seizures. Arch Dis Child Fetal Neonatal Ed 2008;93(3):F187–91.

8. Volpe JJ. Neonatal seizures. In: Volpe JJ, editor. Neurology of the newborn. Philadelphia: WB Saunders; 2008. p. 203–44.
9. Rahman S, Footitt EJ, Varadkar S, et al. Inborn errors of metabolism causing epilepsy. Dev Med Child Neurol 2013;55(1):23–36.
10. Uria-Avellanal C, Marlow N, Rennie JM. Outcome following neonatal seizures. Semin Fetal Neonatal Med 2013;18(4):224–32.
11. Holmes GL. The long-term effects of neonatal seizures. Clin Perinatol 2009; 36(4):901–14, vii–viii.
12. Jensen FE. Neonatal seizures: an update on mechanisms and management. Clin Perinatol 2009;36(4):881–900, vii.
13. Dulac O, Milh M, Holmes GL. Brain maturation and epilepsy. Handb Clin Neurol 2013;111:441–6.
14. Huttenlocher PR, de Courten C, Garey LJ, et al. Synaptogenesis in human visual cortex–evidence for synapse elimination during normal development. Neurosci Lett 1982;33(3):247–52.
15. Takashima S, Chan F, Becker LE, et al. Morphology of the developing visual cortex of the human infant: a quantitative and qualitative Golgi study. J Neuropathol Exp Neurol 1980;39(4):487–501.
16. Rakhade SN, Jensen FE. Epileptogenesis in the immature brain: emerging mechanisms. Nat Rev Neurol 2009;5(7):380–91.
17. Sanchez RM, Jensen FE. Maturational aspects of epilepsy mechanisms and consequences for the immature brain. Epilepsia 2001;42(5):577–85.
18. Dzhala VI, Staley KJ. Excitatory actions of endogenously released GABA contribute to initiation of ictal epileptiform activity in the developing hippocampus. J Neurosci 2003;23(5):1840–6.
19. Dzhala VI, Talos DM, Sdrulla DA, et al. NKCC1 transporter facilitates seizures in the developing brain. Nat Med 2005;11(11):1205–13.
20. Khazipov R, Khalilov I, Tyzio R, et al. Developmental changes in GABAergic actions and seizure susceptibility in the rat hippocampus. Eur J Neurosci 2004; 19(3):590–600.
21. Jiang M, Lee CL, Smith KL, et al. Spine loss and other persistent alterations of hippocampal pyramidal cell dendrites in a model of early-onset epilepsy. J Neurosci 1998;18(20):8356–68.
22. McCabe BK, Silveira DC, Cilio MR, et al. Reduced neurogenesis after neonatal seizures. J Neurosci 2001;21(6):2094–103.
23. Montgomery EM, Bardgett ME, Lall B, et al. Delayed neuronal loss after administration of intracerebroventricular kainic acid to preweanling rats. Brain Res Dev Brain Res 1999;112(1):107–16.
24. Lynch M, Sayin U, Bownds J, et al. Long-term consequences of early postnatal seizures on hippocampal learning and plasticity. Eur J Neurosci 2000;12(7): 2252–64.
25. Miller SP, Weiss J, Barnwell A, et al. Seizure-associated brain injury in term newborns with perinatal asphyxia. Neurology 2002;58(4):542–8.
26. Glass HC, Glidden D, Jeremy RJ, et al. Clinical neonatal seizures are independently associated with outcome in infants at risk for hypoxic-ischemic brain injury. J Pediatr 2009;155(3):318–23.
27. Glass HC, Nash KB, Bonifacio SL, et al. Seizures and magnetic resonance imaging-detected brain injury in newborns cooled for hypoxic-ischemic encephalopathy. J Pediatr 2011;159(5):731–5.e1.
28. Glass HC, Bonifacio SL, Sullivan J, et al. Magnetic resonance imaging and ultrasound injury in preterm infants with seizures. J Child Neurol 2009;24(9):1105–11.

29. Wusthoff CJ, Dlugos DJ, Gutierrez-Colina A, et al. Electrographic seizures during therapeutic hypothermia for neonatal hypoxic-ischemic encephalopathy. J Child Neurol 2011;26(6):724–8.

30. Clancy RR, Legido A, Lewis D. Occult neonatal seizures. Epilepsia 1988;29(3): 256–61.

31. Bye A, Flanagan D. Electroencephalograms, clinical observations and the monitoring of neonatal seizures. J Paediatr Child Health 1995;31(6):503–7.

32. Shellhaas RA, Chang T, Tsuchida T, et al. The American Clinical Neurophysiology Society's guideline on continuous electroencephalography monitoring in neonates. J Clin Neurophysiol 2011;28(6):611–7.

33. Clancy RR. The contribution of EEG to the understanding of neonatal seizures. Epilepsia 1996;37(Suppl 1):S52–9.

34. Wusthoff CJ. Diagnosing neonatal seizures and status epilepticus. J Clin Neurophysiol 2013;30(2):115–21.

35. McCoy B, Hahn CD. Continuous EEG monitoring in the neonatal intensive care unit. J Clin Neurophysiol 2013;30(2):106–14.

36. Glass HC, Wusthoff CJ, Shellhaas RA. Amplitude-integrated electro-encephalography: the child neurologist's perspective. J Child Neurol 2013;28(10): 1342–50.

37. Mastrangelo M, Fiocchi I, Fontana P, et al. Acute neonatal encephalopathy and seizures recurrence: a combined aEEG/EEG study. Seizure 2013;22(9):703–7.

38. Hellstrom-Westas L. Comparison between tape-recorded and amplitude-integrated EEG monitoring in sick newborn infants. Acta Paediatr 1992;81(10): 812–9.

39. Toet MC, van der Mei W, de Vries LS, et al. Comparison between simultaneously recorded amplitude integrated electroencephalogram (cerebral function monitor) and standard electroencephalogram in neonates. Pediatrics 2002; 109(5):772–9.

40. Shah DK, Mackay MT, Lavery S, et al. Accuracy of bedside electroencephalographic monitoring in comparison with simultaneous continuous conventional electroencephalography for seizure detection in term infants. Pediatrics 2008; 121(6):1146–54.

41. Rennie JM, Chorley G, Boylan GB, et al. Non-expert use of the cerebral function monitor for neonatal seizure detection. Arch Dis Child Fetal Neonatal Ed 2004; 89(1):F37–40.

42. Boylan GB, Stevenson NJ, Vanhatalo S. Monitoring neonatal seizures. Semin Fetal Neonatal Med 2013;18(4):202–8.

43. Temko A, Thomas E, Marnane W, et al. Performance assessment for EEG-based neonatal seizure detectors. Clin Neurophysiol 2011;122(3):474–82.

44. Temko A, Lightbody G, Boylan G, et al. Online EEG channel weighting for detection of seizures in the neonate. Conf Proc IEEE Eng Med Biol Soc 2011;2011: 1447–50.

45. Temko A, Boylan G, Marnane W, et al. Robust neonatal EEG seizure detection through adaptive background modeling. Int J Neural Syst 2013;23(4): 1350018.

46. Temko A, Stevenson N, Marnane W, et al. Inclusion of temporal priors for automated neonatal EEG classification. J Neural Eng 2012;9(4):046002.

47. Bonifacio SL, Miller SP. Neonatal seizures and brain imaging. J Pediatr Neurol 2009;7(1):61–7.

48. Booth D, Evans DJ. Anticonvulsants for neonates with seizures. Cochrane Database Syst Rev 2004;(4):CD004218.

49. Slaughter LA, Patel AD, Slaughter JL. Pharmacological treatment of neonatal seizures: a systematic review. J Child Neurol 2013;28(3):351–64.

50. Bittigau P, Sifringer M, Genz K, et al. Antiepileptic drugs and apoptotic neurodegeneration in the developing brain. Proc Natl Acad Sci U S A 2002;99(23): 15089–94.

51. Painter MJ, Scher MS, Stein AD, et al. Phenobarbital compared with phenytoin for the treatment of neonatal seizures. N Engl J Med 1999;341(7):485–9.

52. Lynch NE, Stevenson NJ, Livingstone V, et al. The temporal evolution of electrographic seizure burden in neonatal hypoxic ischemic encephalopathy. Epilepsia 2012;53(3):549–57.

53. Grimshaw JM, Russell IT. Effect of clinical guidelines on medical practice: a systematic review of rigorous evaluations. Lancet 1993;342(8883):1317–22.

54. Guillet R, Kwon JM. Prophylactic phenobarbital administration after resolution of neonatal seizures: survey of current practice. Pediatrics 2008;122(4):731–5.

55. Hellstrom-Westas L, Blennow G, Lindroth M, et al. Low risk of seizure recurrence after early withdrawal of antiepileptic treatment in the neonatal period. Arch Dis Child Fetal Neonatal Ed 1995;72(2):F97–101.

56. Guillet R, Kwon J. Seizure recurrence and developmental disabilities after neonatal seizures: outcomes are unrelated to use of phenobarbital prophylaxis. J Child Neurol 2007;22(4):389–95.

57. Bartha AI, Shen J, Katz KH, et al. Neonatal seizures: multicenter variability in current treatment practices. Pediatr Neurol 2007;37(2):85–90.

58. Wheless JW, Clarke DF, Arzimanoglou A, et al. Treatment of pediatric epilepsy: European expert opinion, 2007. Epileptic Disord 2007;9(4):353–412.

59. Bassan H, Bental Y, Shany E, et al. Neonatal seizures: dilemmas in workup and management. Pediatr Neurol 2008;38(6):415–21.

60. Boylan GB, Rennie JM, Chorley G, et al. Second-line anticonvulsant treatment of neonatal seizures: a video-EEG monitoring study. Neurology 2004;62(3):486–8.

61. Glass HC, Kan J, Bonifacio SL, et al. Neonatal seizures: treatment practices among term and preterm infants. Pediatr Neurol 2012;46(2):111–5.

62. Silverstein FS, Ferriero DM. Off-label use of antiepileptic drugs for the treatment of neonatal seizures. Pediatr Neurol 2008;39(2):77–9.

63. Mbizvo GK, Dixon P, Hutton JL, et al. Levetiracetam add-on for drug-resistant focal epilepsy: an updated Cochrane Review. Cochrane Database Syst Rev 2012;(9):CD001901.

64. Kim JS, Kondratyev A, Tomita Y, et al. Neurodevelopmental impact of antiepileptic drugs and seizures in the immature brain. Epilepsia 2007;48(Suppl 5): 19–26.

65. Manthey D, Asimiadou S, Stefovska V, et al. Sulthiame but not levetiracetam exerts neurotoxic effect in the developing rat brain. Exp Neurol 2005;193(2): 497–503.

66. Talos DM, Chang M, Kosaras B, et al. Antiepileptic effects of levetiracetam in a rodent neonatal seizure model. Pediatr Res 2013;73(1):24–30.

67. Kilicdag H, Daglioglu K, Erdogan S, et al. The effect of levetiracetam on neuronal apoptosis in neonatal rat model of hypoxic ischemic brain injury. Early Hum Dev 2013;89(5):355–60.

68. Tulloch JK, Carr RR, Ensom MH. A systematic review of the pharmacokinetics of antiepileptic drugs in neonates with refractory seizures. J Pediatr Pharmacol Ther 2012;17(1):31–44.

69. Merhar SL, Schibler KR, Sherwin CM, et al. Pharmacokinetics of levetiracetam in neonates with seizures. J Pediatr 2011;159(1):152–4.e3.

70. Sharpe CM, Capparelli EV, Mower A, et al. A seven-day study of the pharmaco-kinetics of intravenous levetiracetam in neonates: marked changes in pharma-cokinetics occur during the first week of life. Pediatr Res 2012;72(1):43–9.
71. Abend NS, Gutierrez-Colina AM, Monk HM, et al. Levetiracetam for treatment of neonatal seizures. J Child Neurol 2011;26(4):465–70.
72. Khan O, Chang E, Cipriani C, et al. Use of intravenous levetiracetam for man-agement of acute seizures in neonates. Pediatr Neurol 2011;44(4):265–9.
73. Furwentsches A, Bussmann C, Ramantani G, et al. Levetiracetam in the treat-ment of neonatal seizures: a pilot study. Seizure 2010;19(3):185–9.
74. Sheth RD, Buckley DJ, Gutierrez AR, et al. Midazolam in the treatment of refrac-tory neonatal seizures. Clin Neuropharmacol 1996;19(2):165–70.
75. Hu KC, Chiu NC, Ho CS, et al. Continuous midazolam infusion in the treatment of uncontrollable neonatal seizures. Acta Paediatr Taiwan 2003;44(5):279–81.
76. Castro Conde JR, Hernandez Borges AA, Domenech Martinez E, et al. Midazo-lam in neonatal seizures with no response to phenobarbital. Neurology 2005; 64(5):876–9.
77. Sirsi D, Nangia S, LaMothe J, et al. Successful management of refractory neonatal seizures with midazolam. J Child Neurol 2008;23(6):706–9.
78. Lundqvist M, Agren J, Hellstrom-Westas L, et al. Efficacy and safety of lidocaine for treatment of neonatal seizures. Acta Paediatr 2013;102(9):863–7.
79. van den Broek MP, Rademaker CM, Straaten HL, et al. Anticonvulsant treatment of asphyxiated newborns under hypothermia with lidocaine: efficacy, safety and dosing. Arch Dis Child Fetal Neonatal Ed 2013;98(4):F341–5.
80. van den Broek MP, Huitema AD, van Hasselt JG, et al. Lidocaine (lignocaine) dosing regimen based upon a population pharmacokinetic model for preterm and term neonates with seizures. Clin Pharmacokinet 2011;50(7):461–9.
81. Malingre MM, Van Rooij LG, Rademaker CM, et al. Development of an optimal lidocaine infusion strategy for neonatal seizures. Eur J Pediatr 2006;165(9): 598–604.
82. Cha BH, Silveira DC, Liu X, et al. Effect of topiramate following recurrent and prolonged seizures during early development. Epilepsy Res 2002;51(3): 217–32.
83. Liu Y, Barks JD, Xu G, et al. Topiramate extends the therapeutic window for hy-pothermia-mediated neuroprotection after stroke in neonatal rats. Stroke 2004; 35(6):1460–5.
84. Clark AM, Kriel RL, Leppik IE, et al. Intravenous topiramate: comparison of phar-macokinetics and safety with the oral formulation in healthy volunteers. Epilepsia 2013;54(6):1099–105.
85. Clark AM, Kriel RL, Leppik IE, et al. Intravenous topiramate: safety and pharma-cokinetics following a single dose in patients with epilepsy or migraines taking oral topiramate. Epilepsia 2013;54(6):1106–11.
86. Khanna A, Walcott BP, Kahle KT. Limitations of current GABA agonists in neonatal seizures: toward GABA modulation via the targeting of neuronal Cl(-) transport. Front Neurol 2013;4:78.
87. Dzhala VI, Brumback AC, Staley KJ. Bumetanide enhances phenobarbital efficacy in a neonatal seizure model. Ann Neurol 2008;63(2):222–35.
88. Cleary RT, Sun H, Huynh T, et al. Bumetanide enhances phenobarbital efficacy in a rat model of hypoxic neonatal seizures. PLoS One 2013;8(3):e57148.
89. Liu Y, Shangguan Y, Barks JD, et al. Bumetanide augments the neuroprotective efficacy of phenobarbital plus hypothermia in a neonatal hypoxia-ischemia model. Pediatr Res 2012;71(5):559–65.

90. Kahle KT, Barnett SM, Sassower KC, et al. Decreased seizure activity in a human neonate treated with bumetanide, an inhibitor of the Na(+)-K(+)-2Cl(-) co-transporter NKCC1. J Child Neurol 2009;24(5):572–6.

91. Chabwine JN, Vanden Eijnden S. A claim for caution in the use of promising bumetanide to treat neonatal seizures. J Child Neurol 2011;26(5):657–8 [author reply: 658–9].

92. ClinicalTrials.gov. Identifier: NCT01720667.

Steroids and Injury to the Developing Brain
Net Harm or Net Benefit?

Shadi N. Malaeb, MD[a],*, Barbara S. Stonestreet, MD[b]

KEYWORDS

- Brain injury ● Cerebral palsy ● Controversy ● Development ● Glucocorticoids
- Infant ● Outcomes ● Premature infant

KEY POINTS

- Steroid effects on the brain mimic an inverse-U–shaped curve, because deleterious effects result from both glucocorticoid insufficiency and/or excess glucocorticoid tissue exposure.
- The effects of glucocorticoids on the developing central nervous system are a function of both the stage of development and duration of exposure.
- The beneficial effects of glucocorticoids are optimal when given to sick premature infants in a critical window before 32 weeks' postmenstrual age.
- Glucocorticoids have net beneficial effects when given shortly after the first week of life to premature infants at high risk for severe chronic lung disease.
- The challenge is to identify infants at high risk for bronchopulmonary dysplasia (BPD) early in their course and to administer a dose that attenuates the progression of BPD.

INTRODUCTION

Glucocorticoids, commonly referred to as *steroids*, are widely used in neonatal-perinatal medicine. They are prescribed to pregnant women at risk for premature birth, and sometimes to infants with significant airway or lung disease, refractory hypotension, or septic shock. Preterm infants are at high risk for brain injury, morbidity, and mortality. Steroids are thought to attenuate some of these risks.[1,2] However, steroid regimens used vary widely, from a single short course of antenatal steroids given to the mother early in the third trimester, to repeated or prolonged courses of steroids

[a] Department of Pediatrics, St. Christopher's Hospital for Children, Drexel University College of Medicine, 245 North 15th Street, New College Building, Room 7410, Mail Stop 1029, Philadelphia, PA 19102, USA; [b] Department of Pediatrics, Women & Infants Hospital of Rhode Island, The Alpert Medical School of Brown University, 101 Dudley Street, Providence, RI 02905, USA
* Corresponding author.
E-mail address: Shadi.Malaeb@drexelmed.edu

Clin Perinatol 41 (2014) 191–208
http://dx.doi.org/10.1016/j.clp.2013.09.006   **perinatology.theclinics.com**

given over weeks to the premature infant. As more data have accumulated regarding the long-term outcomes of infants exposed to steroids, concern has been increasing about neurodevelopmental impairment after exposure to steroids in certain settings. This article summarizes some of the experimental and clinical findings, and explores the complex nature of the relationship between steroids and brain injury, with a focus on the premature brain.

OVERVIEW OF BRAIN DEVELOPMENT

Normal brain development requires a well-orchestrated ontogeny of cellular proliferation, migration, differentiation, angiogenesis, synaptogenesis, myelination, and apoptosis.[3] Neurogenesis remains active well into adulthood in the subventricular zone and hippocampal dentate gyrus.[4] Neuronal progenitor cells migrate from their sites of origin and become mature integrated neurons. Early-stage neuronal progenitor cells maintain an active cell cycle and can either divide or die via apoptosis. As progenitor cells mature, they exit the cell cycle and commit to differentiate.[5] A large number of migrating neurons populate a transient subcortical layer known as the *subplate zone*. Other neurons enter the cortical plate and integrate into neuronal circuits. Synaptic connectivity is essential to maintain survival for cortical neurons. Most subplate neurons involute through apoptosis toward late gestation and in infancy. Oligodendrocyte progenitor cells follow neuronal tracts and mature to form myelin. Cerebral vascular endothelial cells, pericytes, and astrocytes promote angiogenesis to form neurovascular units that will support neurons and form the blood–brain barrier.[6,7] The ontogeny of the developing nervous system is under tight regulation by intrinsic, paracrine, endocrine, and external modulators. Perturbations in any of these factors could result in long-term consequences that affect the structure and function of the developing central nervous system (CNS).[3]

NEUROTROPHIC EFFECTS OF STEROIDS

Steroids are essential for maturation and survival of several cell types in the CNS. Adrenalectomy in adult rats results in massive cell death in the dentate gyrus and decreases the number of dendritic branch points.[8,9] Corticosterone replacement after adrenalectomy reverses these processes.[9] Corticosterone administration accelerates neuronal migration of cerebellar granule cells and enhances cerebellar Purkinje cell growth in the offspring. This treatment also accelerates the emergence of perinucleolar rosettes forming accessory nucleolar bodies of Cajal.[10] The emergence of this structure signifies increases in transcriptional activity present during the late stages of neuronal maturation.[11] Corticosterone application early in development also accelerates the differentiation of membrane electrical properties in embryonic chick neurons.[12] In addition, glucocorticoids activate brain-derived neurotrophic factor receptor (Trk) tyrosine kinases and induce the expression of thyroid hormone–dependent transcription factor Kruppel-like factor 9 gene.[13–15] These events are implicated in the plasticity of hippocampal neurons and postnatal development.[13–15] Short-term corticosterone exposure increases synaptogenesis in the developing cortex. Reducing endogenous glucocorticoid activity decreases spine process turnover, and corticosterone reverses this process.[16,17] Therefore, corticosterone seems to accelerate neuronal maturation. Glucocorticoids also induce oligodendrocyte precursor differentiation[18] and increase oligodendroglial marker expression during myelinogenesis.[19–21] In summary, steroids exert important trophic effects on cell survival, differentiation, maturation, and synaptogenesis (**Box 1**).

> **Box 1**
> **Neurotrophic effects of glucocorticoids**
>
> - Enhance survival of early-stage neuroblasts
> - Accelerate neuronal cell migration and maturation
> - Facilitate synaptogenesis, pruning, and plasticity
> - Induce oligodendrocyte precursor differentiation

NEUROPROTECTION BY STEROIDS

Steroids protect the brain acutely from neuroinflammatory damage.[22] Glucocorticoids also attenuate excitotoxic white matter injury by protecting oligodendrocytes from alpha-amino-3-hydroxy-5-methyl-4-isoxazole propionic acid (AMPA)–induced excitotoxicity through upregulating erythropoietin signaling.[23] Prenatal glucocorticoid administration enhances pericyte coverage, inhibits angiogenesis, and results in trimming of the germinal matrix neovasculature, thereby reducing the propensity for germinal matrix hemorrhage.[24]

ANTENATAL STEROIDS ACCELERATE ONTOGENIC CHANGES IN THE DEVELOPING CNS

Ontogenic decreases in blood–brain barrier permeability have been reported in ovine fetuses from 60% of gestation up to maturity in the adult.[25] Treatment of pregnant ewes with a glucocorticoid regimen similar to those used in the clinical setting was associated with decreases in blood–brain barrier permeability in fetal sheep at 60% and 80% of gestation.[26,27] Ontogenic decreases in brain water content have also been reported in fetal sheep between 60% and 90% of gestation.[28] Maternal treatment with dexamethasone resulted in decreases in regional brain water content in fetal sheep at 60% of gestation.[28] At the molecular level, Na^+/K^+-ATPase pump α1-subunit expression is lower at 60% than at 90% of gestation, and dexamethasone treatment of pregnant ewes at 60% of gestation increased the expression of this protein.[29] Therefore, antenatal steroid treatment of pregnant ewes using regimens similar to those used in the clinical setting accelerates some aspects of brain development in the immature sheep fetus.

DEVELOPMENTAL STAGE AT TIME OF EXPOSURE AND DURATION OF EXPOSURE MODULATE STEROID EFFECTS ON THE CNS

The effects of glucocorticoids on the developing CNS are a function of both the stage of development at the time of exposure and the duration of exposure. The developmental stage reflects the systemic physiology and the nature of different cellular populations within the brain, both of which are affected by postmenstrual and chronologic ages. For example, cerebral water content in the fetal brain decreased after treatment of pregnant ewes with dexamethasone at 60% of gestation, but not at 80% or 90%.[28] Similarly, aquaporin protein expression was decreased in lambs and adult sheep brains after dexamethasone treatment, but not in the fetal brain after exposure of the ewes to dexamethasone.[30] Maternal treatment with glucocorticoids was also associated with decreases in blood–brain barrier permeability in fetal sheep at 60% and 80% of gestation, but not at 90%, and not in lambs after postnatal glucocorticoids.[27,31] Dexamethasone also reduced the affinity of the N-methyl-D-aspartate (NMDA) receptor to its ligand in lambs, but not in the fetal or adult sheep brain.[32]

Maternal exposure to dexamethasone at 70% of gestation, but not at 90%, resulted in significant decreases in total and nonneuronal apoptosis in the fetal cerebral cortex.[33]

The effect of the duration of exposure to glucocorticoids was examined by comparing fetuses of ewes exposed to a single course of dexamethasone or placebo injections every 12 hours for 48 hours between 104 and 107 days of gestation versus fetuses of ewes receiving the same treatment once a week for 5 weeks between 76 and 107 days of gestation. Full-term gestation in sheep is 147 days. Maternal dexamethasone treatment at 70% of gestation was associated with decreases in water content in the fetal brain after multiple, but not after a single course of steroids.[34] Likewise, multiple courses of steroids, but not single courses, also increased myosin isoform expression in the fetal carotid arteries.[35] In contrast, apoptosis in the fetal cerebral cortex was decreased at 70% of gestation after exposure to single, but not after multiple courses of dexamethasone.[33] Even more concerning is the finding that Na^+/K^+-ATPase enzyme activity, as an index of neuronal membrane integrity in the fetal brain, was reduced after multiple courses of dexamethasone, but not after single courses.[36] Perhaps the most intriguing aspect of modulation of the steroid effects on the brain with reference to the duration of exposure stems from observations suggesting that chronic glucocorticoid exposure facilitates paradoxic proinflammatory responses to injury in the brain,[22,37] which is in direct contrast to classical anti-inflammatory responses expected after acute glucocorticoid exposure.[38]

Taken together, these findings suggest that the developmental stage at the time of exposure and the duration of exposure each have important contributions to the ultimate glucocorticoid effects on the developing CNS. Comprehension of the pharmacodynamics of steroids in the developing CNS is also necessary to understand the multifaceted effects of glucocorticoids on the brain, and these are addressed in the following sections (**Box 2**).

Box 2
Determinants of the effect of glucocorticoids on the developing CNS

- Stage of brain development at the time of exposure
- Duration of exposure
- Pharmacodynamic properties of the steroid
- Dosage used

PHARMACODYNAMICS OF NATURAL VERSUS SYNTHETIC GLUCOCORTICOIDS IN THE BRAIN

Glucocorticoids are synthesized by the fetal adrenal cortex, mostly by maternal progesterone that crosses the placenta.[39] The natural glucocorticoid in humans is cortisol and in rodents is corticosterone. Human fetal serum cortisol levels decrease from 8 ng/mL at 15 weeks to 4 ng/mL by 20 weeks. In the absence of labor and under the regulation of placental corticotropin-releasing hormone and fetal adrenocorticotrophin, a steep increase occurs in cortisol levels: to 20 ng/mL by 36 weeks of gestation and 45 ng/mL near term.[40] Glucocorticoids are approximately 75% bound to corticosteroid-binding globulins in the circulation. Both natural and synthetic steroids readily penetrate the blood–brain barrier to reach the parenchyma. However, synthetic steroids such as dexamethasone are actively pumped out of the brain by the multidrug resistance protein 1A (mrd1A) P-glycoprotein, which is highly expressed at the blood–brain barrier.[41] Hence, dexamethasone is retained less efficiently than natural glucocorticoids in brain regions possessing a functional blood–brain barrier, and more efficiently when the blood–brain barrier is injured. Dexamethasone is also effectively retained in regions devoid of a blood–brain barrier, such as the circumventricular organs, where glucocorticoids suppress the hypothalamic-pituitary-adrenal (HPA) axis. Once in the parenchyma, steroids diffuse readily across cell membranes.

Natural and related steroids such as hydrocortisone are inactivated by an intracellular glucocorticoid-metabolizing enzyme, 11β-hydroxysteroid dehydrogenase type 2 (HSD2),[42] which converts them into inactive 11-keto derivatives.[42] HSD2 significantly attenuates the actions of natural glucocorticoids on the brain.[43,44] HSD2 expression decreases with advancing gestation from fetal to newborn, and up to adulthood, concomitantly as endogenous glucocorticoid production increases. Consequently, a larger portion of endogenous cortisol or exogenous hydrocortisone that enters the brain at more mature postmenstrual ages will remain active to bind more receptors and augment their biologic actions.[45,46] On the other hand, synthetic glucocorticoids are resistant to inactivation by HSD2. The same property, which prevents their placental deactivation, exaggerates their biologic actions in the brain, even though very little is retained because of elimination by the multiple drug resistance mrd1A protein expressed at the blood–brain barrier.

GLUCOCORTICOID RECEPTORS IN THE BRAIN

Two types of glucocorticoid receptors are present in the CNS.[47,48] The type 1 receptor is a mineralocorticoid receptor (MR), which has high affinity for cortisol and corticosterone, with aldosterone and hydrocortisone as agonists, and spironolactone as an antagonist. It binds poorly to dexamethasone and betamethasone. The type 2 receptor is a *glucocorticoid receptor* (GR), which has a high affinity for dexamethasone but 10 times lower affinity for corticosterone, with methylprednisolone and betamethasone as agonists, and mifepristone (RU 38486) as an antagonist. MRs are unique in that they are highly expressed exclusively in the hippocampus and limbic brain regions, whereas GRs are expressed ubiquitously across all brain regions. The main receptor activated at physiologic cortisol levels is the MR in the hippocampus, with little to no GR activation. The MR nuclear response elements are thought to mediate neurotrophism.[47,49] At higher cortisol levels, GRs throughout the brain become activated along with the activated MRs in the limbic brain. In contrast, when pure GR agonists such as dexamethasone or betamethasone are administered, GR activation primarily occurs throughout the CNS with little or no MR activation. Prolonged dexamethasone administration suppresses the HPA axis and depletes systemic and local cortisol levels within brain tissue. Hence, prolonged administration of pure GR agonists, as opposed to mixed MR/GR agonists, paradoxically attenuates MR activation in the hippocampus and other brain structures responsible for learning and memory.[22,37,47] Local cortisol depletion, along with limited the ability of dexamethasone to be retained because of MDR1A P-glycoprotein elimination, leads to a paradoxically enhanced microglial reactivity and sustained neuroinflammation after brain injury with prolonged exposure to the supposedly "anti-inflammatory" synthetic glucocorticoid. This process results in neurodegeneration, demyelination, synaptic dysfunction, and a loss of cortisol-mediated positive trophism. Administration of a GR antagonist, such as RU 38486 or corticosterone replacement, counteracts the cortisol-depleting effects of prolonged dexamethasone exposure on the hippocampus.[50,51] Hence, the balance between MR/GR stimulation is a major determinant of the effects of glucocorticoids on the brain.

HAZARDS OF GR OCCUPANCY

Accentuated and prolonged GR occupancy underlies an array of injurious effects of glucocorticoids on the brain. Stimulation of cultured embryonic rat neural stem cells with dexamethasone or with high concentrations of corticosterone, but not low concentrations, reduces cell proliferation.[52] These effects were inhibited by specific GR, but not MR blockade. Chronic corticosterone administration reduces neurogenesis in the adult rat dental gyrus.[50] This inhibitory effect can be reversed by treatment with the GR antagonist mifepristone.[50,53,54] Proliferation of cells in the dentate gyrus also was reduced in fetuses of pregnant monkeys receiving dexamethasone both early and late in gestation.[55] Premature human neonates whose mothers were treated with synthetic glucocorticoids and died shortly after delivery exhibited lower hippocampal neuronal densities than neonates who were not exposed to glucocorticoids.[56] These findings suggest that accentuated GR stimulation mediates glucocorticoid-related cell cycle inhibition in the developing brain.[52] Excess maternal glucocorticoid administration also retarded migration of postmitotic neurons in the fetal cerebral cortex in rats.[57] Offspring of pregnant rats exposed to high-dose maternal corticosterone showed long-lasting neurobehavioral impairment.[58] Betamethasone administration to pregnant sheep reduced the number of oligodendrocytes and axons in the corpus callosum, and delayed myelination in the fetal brain.[59–61] The inhibitory effects of synthetic steroids on myelination in the sheep were dependent on the stage of development, and decreased with advancing gestational age.[60,62] Repeated administration of dexamethasone during the first week of life to rat pups resulted in prominent apoptosis, particularly in proliferating cells, and depleted the hippocampal neural precursor cell pool, resulting in sustained reductions in the volume of the dentate gyrus.[63] Therefore, accentuated GR occupancy could have adverse effect on neurons and glia in the developing brain (**Box 3**).

Box 3
Effects of MR and GR occupancy on the developing brain

- MR occupancy mediates neurotrophism by steroids.
- Accentuated or prolonged GR occupancy underlies an array of injurious effects of glucocorticoids on the brain.

GLUCOCORTICOIDS AND RECOVERY AFTER BRAIN INJURY

Cerebral hypoxia-ischemia and reperfusion induces waves of free-radical injury, excitotoxicity, neuroinflammation, and delayed cell death.[64] Induction of neural stem cell proliferation often occurs after brain injury and during the subsequent recovery and remodeling phases.[4,65] Survival of early progenitor cells requires trophism by MR occupancy, whereas their proliferation is hindered by heightened GR occupancy. In fact, maternal pretreatment with antenatal dexamethasone did not attenuate ischemic brain injury in the ovine fetus.[66] The effects of glucocorticoids on hypoxic-ischemic brain injury were elegantly summarized in a recent review by Bennet and colleagues.[67]

UNIFYING HYPOTHESIS

The emerging picture of glucocorticoid effects on the developing brain derived from mounting experimental evidence is that of an inverse-U–shaped curve, because both insufficient glucocorticoid exposure and accentuated or prolonged exposure exert an array of deleterious effects mediated by either low MR occupancy or by high GR occupancy (**Fig. 1**). Conditions associated with excessive GR relative to MR occupancy include: (1) administration of high doses or prolonged courses of hydrocortisone; (2) administration of dexamethasone at an advanced postmenstrual age, when endogenous cortisol production had increased and HSD2 protection decreased, which could exaggerate an already heightened GR occupancy by cortisol; (3) administration of prolonged courses of dexamethasone that can suppress the HPA axis and deplete local brain tissue cortisol, thereby reducing MR occupancy; (4) administration of dexamethasone during conditions that impair elimination by the multidrug resistance pump at the blood-brain barrier, such as during cerebral hypoxia/ischemia; and (5) early administration of a pure GR agonist dexamethasone when endogenous cortisol levels for effective MR occupancy are deficient. The consequent overall effects of steroids on the brain are dependent on the developmental stage, duration of exposure, and the presence or absence of other disease processes in the brain and/or body before or after the time of exposure. The effect of steroids on the brain is also dependent on the dose and type of glucocorticoid used. This concept has been proposed by many investigators, including De Kloet and colleagues,[47] Diamond and colleagues,[68] McEwen,[69] and Sousa and Almeida.[49] These concepts could provide a basis for clarifying the disparate effects of glucocorticoids observed in clinical trials, and guiding future clinical strategies to maximize the beneficial effects of steroids while minimizing the detrimental effects of glucocorticoid therapy.

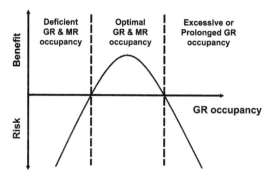

Fig. 1. Inverse-U–shaped hypothesis as a guide for risk/benefit analysis of glucocorticoid administration in experimental and clinical scenarios. Note that during the first few days of life, although a degree of MR occupancy by hydrocortisone may be neurotrophic in premature infants, systemic side effects of very early administration of hydrocortisone outweigh the potential benefits. See text for details.

CLINICAL PERSPECTIVES
Antenatal Steroids

The ability of a single antenatal course of glucocorticoids to accelerate fetal lung maturation has been extensively documented by clinical trials.[70,71] The 2 most frequently used glucocorticoids are betamethasone and dexamethasone. Betamethasone has slightly greater beneficial pulmonary effects compared with dexamethasone.[72] Antenatal administration of glucocorticoids reduces the incidence and severity of respiratory distress syndrome and decreases the incidence of intraventricular hemorrhage, necrotizing enterocolitis, and risk of mortality.[70,71] Antenatal treatment with glucocorticoids is also associated with a trend toward a lower incidence of cerebral palsy and less neurodevelopmental delays in childhood (relative risk, 0.49; 95% CI, 0.24–1.00).[70] However, when the same course of antenatal steroids was repeated weekly, head circumference at birth was smaller compared with that of infants whose mothers had received a placebo.[73] Children exposed to multiple courses of betamethasone tended to have higher incidences of cerebral palsy[74] and attention problems in later childhood.[75] In addition, multiple courses of antenatal dexamethasone were associated with an increased risk of periventricular leukomalacia and neurodevelopmental impairment at 2 years of age.[76] These findings suggest that glucocorticoids can have beneficial effects when given over short intervals, whereas prolonged GR occupancy potentially results in CNS injury and impaired development.

POSTNATAL STEROIDS: EARLY ADMINISTRATION

In several clinical trials, both hydrocortisone and dexamethasone have been administered to premature infants early in the first week of life,[1] based on the assumption by some investigators that sick premature infants could have relative adrenal insufficiency.[77–79] The existence of this condition remains controversial, and appreciation of the net benefit from this approach has been guarded at best. These studies have suggested occasional improvement and better neurologic outcomes after hydrocortisone treatment than after dexamethasone treatment, especially in infants exposed to chorioamnionitis.[80–82] However, glucocorticoid administration during the first week of life has also been associated with an increased incidence of intraventricular hemorrhage and gastrointestinal perforation.[80,83] Infants treated with dexamethasone early after birth also have been reported to have smaller head circumferences and lower weights at 36 weeks' postmenstrual age; higher incidences of cerebral palsy; and developmental delays later in life compared with placebo-treated infants.[84,85] In contrast, the risk for cerebral palsy was not increased in premature infants treated with hydrocortisone in the first week of life.[1,86] Nonetheless, these complications outweigh the neurotrophic benefits of MR occupancy by hydrocortisone, and have limited the use of glucocorticoids shortly after birth.

POSTNATAL STEROIDS: ADMINISTRATION AFTER THE FIRST WEEK OF LIFE

Glucocorticoids have also been used after the first week of life in several regimens to treat sick premature infants with pulmonary insufficiency and/or hypotensive shock.[2,87,88] Delayed administration of dexamethasone is associated with glycosuria, hypertension, and gastrointestinal bleeding, but not with perforation.[2] Moreover, an increased incidence of severe retinopathy of prematurity and abnormal neurologic examinations is seen on follow-up, warranting further scrutiny.[2,88]

POSTNATAL STEROIDS: MODERATELY EARLY VERSUS DELAYED ADMINISTRATION

A systematic review of clinical trials further compared developmental outcomes of premature infants after receiving dexamethasone courses beyond the first week of life, and focused on the timing of treatment onset.[89] Studies were stratified into trials with a moderately early onset between 1 and 2 weeks of life or delayed onset of treatment beginning after 3 weeks of life. In the trials with the moderately early treatment onset, an inverse relationship was found between the dose of dexamethasone and risk of the combined outcome of mortality and/or cerebral palsy, and of a motor developmental index less than –2 standard deviations below the mean. The negative regression correlation coefficient suggests a decreased risk for neurodevelopmental impairment with dexamethasone if treatment is started moderately early (ie, between

7 and 14 days of life). However, an increased risk for hypertension, hyperglycemia, gastrointestinal bleeding, hypertrophic cardiomyopathy, and infection was seen.[87] In contrast, delaying the initiation of therapy beyond 21 days of age was associated with a trend toward incremental increases in the risk of the combined outcome of mortality and/or cerebral palsy with increasing dexamethasone doses. Similarly, a recent large multicenter prospective cohort study of very premature infants born with birth weights less than 1000 g receiving dexamethasone starting late at 5.1 ± 2.1 weeks of life showed that an increase of each 1-mg/kg dose was associated with a 40% increase in the risk for cerebral palsy and a 2-point reduction on the mental developmental index. Treatment after 33 weeks' postmenstrual age was associated with even greater harm.[90]

In summary, these studies support the contention that the age at onset of treatment could influence the effects of steroids on the developing CNS in infants. The relationships among the dose and duration of treatment with systemic steroids and their effects on neurologic outcomes, potential beneficial effects on pulmonary outcomes, and/or systemic side effects are complex and need further investigation in large-scale randomized controlled clinical trials.[89]

POSTNATAL STEROIDS: PROLONGED TREATMENT

In one controlled trial, prolonged courses of dexamethasone were given to preterm infants born at birth weights of 1250 g or less and gestational ages of 30 weeks or less who were dependent on mechanical ventilation and oxygen at 2 weeks of age.[91] The starting dosage of 0.5 mg/kg/day was tapered over 42 days. Follow-up at 15 months of age showed normal neurologic examinations and Bayley developmental index scores greater than 83 in 7 of the 9 infants after dexamethasone, but in only 2 of 5 after placebo treatment, favoring beneficial effects for dexamethasone ($P<.05$). However, another randomized controlled trial administered a 42-day tapering course of dexamethasone to more mature preterm infants born with birth weights of 1500 g or less beginning between 15 and 25 days of age, with an initial dosage of 0.25 mg/kg/day.[92] Follow-up at 12 months of age found more abnormal neurologic findings and instances of cerebral palsy (25% vs 7%; adjusted odds ratio, 5.3; 95% CI, 1.3–21.4) in the dexamethasone-treated infants compared with those treated with placebo. Taken together, these findings suggest that the critical developmental window for optimal benefits from postnatal treatment with glucocorticoids in sick premature infants is before 32 weeks' postmenstrual age and beginning within the second week of life (**Box 4**).[90–92]

Box 4
Critical developmental window for optimal benefits from postnatal glucocorticoid administration

- Less than 32 weeks' postmenstrual age in sick premature infants
- Beginning in the second week of life

HYDROCORTISONE AND THE PREMATURE INFANT

Hydrocortisone is often prescribed for sick premature infants after the first week of life as an alternative to dexamethasone and betamethasone, with the goal of improving pulmonary outcomes and preserving neurologic function. Hydrocortisone therapy has been reported to improve severe capillary leak lung syndrome in ventilated preterm infants.[93] Extremely low-birth-weight infants receiving hydrocortisone after the second week of life had similar extubation rates and improved somatic growth compared with those receiving betamethasone.[94] Preservation of regional brain volumes at term-equivalent age was observed after treating ventilator-dependent infants with low-dose hydrocortisone for a week, suggesting the potential safety of hydrocortisone.[95–97] The effectiveness of low-dose hydrocortisone in suppressing the evolution of bronchopulmonary dysplasia (BPD) and the safety of higher doses must be confirmed in clinical trials.[86]

EFFECT MODIFICATION BY RISK OF BPD

Premature infants requiring continued respiratory support beyond 36 weeks' postmenstrual age are at high risk for developing cerebral palsy.[98] Glucocorticoids can reduce the risk of chronic lung disease. Therefore, it is reasonable to assume that steroid therapy can have indirect benefits for infants at high risk for developing BPD, by mitigating their risk of brain damage via attenuating the severity of their chronic lung disease. Occasionally, the benefits of reducing the severity of BPD could outweigh the risks of neurologic impairment resulting from the untoward effects of steroid therapy. On the other hand, the use of steroids in infants at low risk for developing BPD could unnecessarily expose infants to the adverse side effects of steroids. A meta-regression analysis conducted by Doyle and colleagues[99] found that for every 10% increase in the rate of chronic lung disease, a 2.3% decrease occurred in the risk of cerebral palsy (95% CI, 0.3%–4.3%) as a result of steroid therapy. A significant steroid-related benefit was observed only when the incidence of chronic lung disease exceeded 65%. Therefore, the challenge is to identify infants at high risk for BPD early in their course and administer a dose of glucocorticoid that can attenuate the progression of BPD (**Box 5**).

Box 5
Clinical challenges

- Identify infants at high risk for BPD early in their course
- Administer a dose of glucocorticoid that impacts BPD progression while at the same time minimizes glucocorticoid-related brain injury

---

PREDICTING RISK OF BPD

A recent large prospective cohort study of newborns of extremely low gestational age found 3 distinct patterns of respiratory disease in the first 2 postnatal weeks (see **Fig. 2**).[100] The incidence of chronic lung disease was 67% in infants with early and persistent pulmonary dysfunction. Other studies have observed that a low cortisol level in the first week of life predicts a slightly higher probability of chronic lung disease or death at 36 weeks' postmenstrual age, particularly in infants with elevated illness scores.[101–103] Hydrocortisone treatment increased survival without BPD in infants with basal serum cortisol values less than a median of 140 nmol/L.[104] When considering these findings together, one could speculate that postnatal glucocorticoid therapy may be beneficial when administered shortly after the first week of life to premature infants with early and persistent pulmonary dysfunction (**Box 6**).

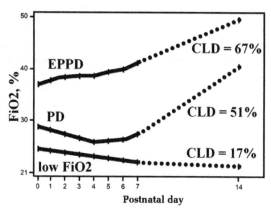

Fig. 2. Speculative predictive analysis for risk of death or cerebral palsy after postnatal gluco-corticoid therapy according to pattern of respiratory disease in premature infants. Patterns of respiratory disease during the first 2 postnatal weeks among newborns with extremely low gestational age show that the incidence of chronic lung disease was 67% in infants with early and persistent pulmonary dysfunction. Doyle et al[99] observed significant steroid-related benefit only when the incidence of chronic lung disease exceeded 65%. These data suggest that the risk of cerebral palsy may be reduced if postnatal glucocorticoids are given to sick premature infants with early and persistent pulmonary dysfunction whose risk for developing BPD may exceed 65%, particularly if they also have low basal levels of cortisol. This predictive analysis must be validated in randomized clinical trials. CLD, chronic lung disease; EPPD, early and persistent pulmonary dysfuntion; FiO₂, fraction of inspired oxygen; PD, pulmonary dysfunction. (*Adapted from* Laughon M, Allred EN, Bose C, et al. Patterns of respiratory disease during the first 2 postnatal weeks in extremely premature infants. Pediatrics 2009;123(4):1124–31; with permission.)

Box 6
Most beneficial time frame for administration of postnatal glucocorticoid therapy

- Administered shortly after first week of life to premature infants born before 30 weeks of gestation

- To infants with signs of early and persistent pulmonary dysfunction, particularly if clinical or serologic signs of relative adrenal insufficiency are evident

---

SUMMARY

The relationship between glucocorticoids and neurodevelopmental impairment is complex. A thorough understanding of the underlying physiology of the positive and negative effects of glucocorticoids on the developing brain based on the concept of the inverse-U–shaped hypothesis is essential when deciding whether to treat a sick premature infant with glucocorticoids. Clearly, steroids play a major role in supporting brain development. Most probably, some infants could benefit from antenatal and postnatal administration of steroids. Ideally, the decision to treat should ensure the maximum respiratory benefit from steroids at the lowest neurologic risk, and at the same time avoid any serious systemic complications. This article suggests the following: (1) glucocorticoid therapy should be restricted to premature infants born before 30 weeks' gestation in whom findings suggest a high risk (>65%) for developing BPD, (2) the first course of postnatal steroids should be considered at approximately day 14 of life, and

(3) the nature and dose of steroids used should be consistent with doses shown in clinical studies to be effective in improving survival and pulmonary outcomes. This approach must be validated in controlled trials. Of particular interest are 2 ongoing multicenter randomized placebo-controlled trials[105,106] investigating the use of moderately early hydrocortisone to prevent BPD in preterm infants. The results of these studies may provide a better understanding of the efficacy and safety of this approach.

REFERENCES

1. Halliday HL, Ehrenkranz RA, Doyle LW. Early (<8 days) postnatal corticosteroids for preventing chronic lung disease in preterm infants. Cochrane Database Syst Rev 2010;(1):CD001146.
2. Halliday HL, Ehrenkranz RA, Doyle LW. Late (>7 days) postnatal corticosteroids for chronic lung disease in preterm infants. Cochrane Database Syst Rev 2009;(1):CD001145.
3. Rice D, Barone S Jr. Critical periods of vulnerability for the developing nervous system: evidence from humans and animal models. Environ Health Perspect 2000;108(Suppl 3):511–33.
4. Miles DK, Kernie SG. Activation of neural stem and progenitor cells after brain injury. Prog Brain Res 2006;157:187–97.
5. Herrup K, Neve R, Ackerman SL, et al. Divide and die: cell cycle events as triggers of nerve cell death. J Neurosci 2004;24(42):9232–9.
6. Malaeb SN, Cohen SS, Virgintino D, et al. Core concepts: development of the blood-brain barrier. Neo Reviews 2012;13(4):e241–50.
7. Abbott NJ, Friedman A. Overview and introduction: the blood-brain barrier in health and disease. Epilepsia 2012;53(Suppl 6):1–6.
8. Spanswick SC, Epp JR, Sutherland RJ. Time-course of hippocampal granule cell degeneration and changes in adult neurogenesis after adrenalectomy in rats. Neuroscience 2011;190:166–76.
9. Gould E, Woolley CS, McEwen BS. Short-term glucocorticoid manipulations affect neuronal morphology and survival in the adult dentate gyrus. Neuroscience 1990;37(2):367–75.
10. Rugerio-Vargas C, Ramirez-Escoto M, DelaRosa-Rugerio C, et al. Prenatal corticosterone influences the trajectory of neuronal development, delaying or accelerating aspects of the Purkinje cell differentiation. Histol Histopathol 2007;22(9):963–9.
11. Dunn ME, Schilling K, Mugnaini E. Development and fine structure of murine Purkinje cells in dissociated cerebellar cultures: dendritic differentiation, synaptic maturation, and formation of cell-class specific features. Anat Embryol (Berl) 1998;197(1):31–50.
12. Fuentes-Pardo B, Hernandez-Falcon J, Velazquez PN, et al. Role of corticosterone on the development of passive electrical properties of cultured chick embryo neurons. J Dev Physiol 1990;13(2):67–73.
13. Numakawa T, Kumamaru E, Adachi N, et al. Glucocorticoid receptor interaction with TrkB promotes BDNF-triggered PLC-gamma signaling for glutamate release via a glutamate transporter. Proc Natl Acad Sci U S A 2009;106(2):647–52.
14. Jeanneteau F, Garabedian MJ, Chao MV. Activation of Trk neurotrophin receptors by glucocorticoids provides a neuroprotective effect. Proc Natl Acad Sci U S A 2008;105(12):4862–7.
15. Bonett RM, Hu F, Bagamasbad P, et al. Stressor and glucocorticoid-dependent induction of the immediate early gene kruppel-like factor 9: implications for neural development and plasticity. Endocrinology 2009;150(4):1757–65.

16. Liston C, Gan WB. Glucocorticoids are critical regulators of dendritic spine development and plasticity in vivo. Proc Natl Acad Sci U S A 2011;108(38): 16074–9.

17. Gray JD, Milner TA, McEwen BS. Dynamic plasticity: the role of glucocorticoids, brain-derived neurotrophic factor and other trophic factors. Neuroscience 2013; 239:214–27.

18. Joubert L, Foucault I, Sagot Y, et al. Chemical inducers and transcriptional markers of oligodendrocyte differentiation. J Neurosci Res 2010;88(12): 2546–57.

19. Campagnoni AT, Verdi JM, Verity AN, et al. Posttranscriptional regulation of myelin protein gene expression. Ann N Y Acad Sci 1991;633:178–88.

20. Cheng JD, de Vellis J. Oligodendrocytes as glucocorticoids target cells: functional analysis of the glycerol phosphate dehydrogenase gene. J Neurosci Res 2000;59(3):436–45.

21. Kumar S, Cole R, Chiappelli F, et al. Differential regulation of oligodendrocyte markers by glucocorticoids: post-transcriptional regulation of both proteolipid protein and myelin basic protein and transcriptional regulation of glycerol phosphate dehydrogenase. Proc Natl Acad Sci U S A 1989; 86(17):6807–11.

22. Bellavance MA, Rivest S. The neuroendocrine control of the innate immune system in health and brain diseases. Immunol Rev 2012;248(1):36–55.

23. Sun YY, Wang CY, Hsu MF, et al. Glucocorticoid protection of oligodendrocytes against excitotoxin involving hypoxia-inducible factor-1alpha in a cell-type-specific manner. J Neurosci 2010;30(28):9621–30.

24. Vinukonda G, Dummula K, Malik S, et al. Effect of prenatal glucocorticoids on cerebral vasculature of the developing brain. Stroke 2010;41(8):1766–73.

25. Stonestreet BS, Patlak CS, Pettigrew KD, et al. Ontogeny of blood-brain barrier function in ovine fetuses, lambs, and adults. Am J Physiol 1996;271(6 Pt 2): R1594–601.

26. Stonestreet BS, Petersson KH, Sadowska GB, et al. Antenatal steroids decrease blood-brain barrier permeability in the ovine fetus. Am J Physiol 1999;276(2 Pt 2):R283–9.

27. Stonestreet BS, Sadowska GB, McKnight AJ, et al. Exogenous and endogenous corticosteroids modulate blood-brain barrier development in the ovine fetus. Am J Physiol Regul Integr Comp Physiol 2000;279(2):R468–77.

28. Stonestreet BS, Elitt CM, Markowitz J, et al. Effects of antenatal corticosteroids on regional brain and non-neural tissue water content in the ovine fetus. J Soc Gynecol Investig 2003;10(2):59–66.

29. Kim CR, Sadowska GB, Newton SA, et al. Na+, K+-ATPase activity and subunit protein expression: ontogeny and effects of exogenous and endogenous steroids on the cerebral cortex and renal cortex of sheep. Reprod Sci 2011; 18(4):359–73.

30. Ron NP, Kazianis JA, Padbury JF, et al. Ontogeny and the effects of corticosteroid pretreatment on aquaporin water channels in the ovine cerebral cortex. Reprod Fertil Dev 2005;17(5):535–42.

31. Sysyn GD, Petersson KH, Patlak CS, et al. Effects of postnatal dexamethasone on blood-brain barrier permeability and brain water content in newborn lambs. Am J Physiol Regul Integr Comp Physiol 2001;280(2):R547–53.

32. McGowan JE, Sysyn G, Petersson KH, et al. Effect of dexamethasone treatment on maturational changes in the NMDA receptor in sheep brain. J Neurosci 2000; 20(19):7424–9.

33. Malaeb SN, Hovanesian V, Sarasin MD, et al. Effects of maternal antenatal glucocorticoid treatment on apoptosis in the ovine fetal cerebral cortex. J Neurosci Res 2009;87(1):179–89.

34. Stonestreet BS, Watkins S, Petersson KH, et al. Effects of multiple courses of antenatal corticosteroids on regional brain and somatic tissue water content in ovine fetuses. J Soc Gynecol Investig 2004;11(3):166–74.

35. Hai CM, Sadowska G, Francois L, et al. Maternal dexamethasone treatment alters myosin isoform expression and contractile dynamics in fetal arteries. Am J Physiol Heart Circ Physiol 2002;283(5):H1743–9.

36. Mehter NS, Sadowska GB, Malaeb SN, et al. Na+, K+-ATPase activity and subunit isoform protein abundance: effects of antenatal glucocorticoids in the frontal cerebral cortex and renal cortex of ovine fetuses. Reprod Sci 2009;16(3):294–307.

37. Sorrells SF, Sapolsky RM. An inflammatory review of glucocorticoid actions in the CNS. Brain Behav Immun 2007;21(3):259–72.

38. Nadeau S, Rivest S. Glucocorticoids play a fundamental role in protecting the brain during innate immune response. J Neurosci 2003;23(13):5536–44.

39. Mastorakos G, Ilias I. Maternal and fetal hypothalamic-pituitary-adrenal axes during pregnancy and postpartum. Ann N Y Acad Sci 2003;997:136–49.

40. Murphy BE. Human fetal serum cortisol levels related to gestational age: evidence of a midgestational fall and a steep late gestational rise, independent of sex or mode of delivery. Am J Obstet Gynecol 1982;144(3):276–82.

41. Meijer OC, de Lange EC, Breimer DD, et al. Penetration of dexamethasone into brain glucocorticoid targets is enhanced in mdr1A P-glycoprotein knockout mice. Endocrinology 1998;139(4):1789–93.

42. Wyrwoll CS, Holmes MC, Seckl JR. 11beta-hydroxysteroid dehydrogenases and the brain: from zero to hero, a decade of progress. Front Neuroendocrinol 2011; 32(3):265–86.

43. Holmes MC, Sangra M, French KL, et al. 11beta-Hydroxysteroid dehydrogenase type 2 protects the neonatal cerebellum from deleterious effects of glucocorticoids. Neuroscience 2006;137(3):865–73.

44. Heine VM, Rowitch DH. Hedgehog signaling has a protective effect in glucocorticoid-induced mouse neonatal brain injury through an 11betaHSD2-dependent mechanism. J Clin Invest 2009;119(2):267–77.

45. Robson AC, Leckie CM, Seckl JR, et al. 11 Beta-hydroxysteroid dehydrogenase type 2 in the postnatal and adult rat brain. Brain Res Mol Brain Res 1998; 61(1–2):1–10.

46. Noguchi KK, Lau K, Smith DJ, et al. Glucocorticoid receptor stimulation and the regulation of neonatal cerebellar neural progenitor cell apoptosis. Neurobiol Dis 2011;43(2):356–63.

47. De Kloet ER, Vreugdenhil E, Oitzl MS, et al. Brain corticosteroid receptor balance in health and disease. Endocr Rev 1998;19(3):269–301.

48. Funder JW. Glucocorticoid and mineralocorticoid receptors: biology and clinical relevance. Annu Rev Med 1997;48:231–40.

49. Sousa N, Almeida OF. Corticosteroids: sculptors of the hippocampal formation. Rev Neurosci 2002;13(1):59–84.

50. Hu P, Oomen C, van Dam AM, et al. A single-day treatment with mifepristone is sufficient to normalize chronic glucocorticoid induced suppression of hippocampal cell proliferation. PLoS One 2012;7(9):e46224.

51. Hassan AH, von Rosenstiel P, Patchev VK, et al. Exacerbation of apoptosis in the dentate gyrus of the aged rat by dexamethasone and the protective role of corticosterone. Exp Neurol 1996;140(1):43–52.

52. Sundberg M, Savola S, Hienola A, et al. Glucocorticoid hormones decrease proliferation of embryonic neural stem cells through ubiquitin-mediated degradation of cyclin D1. J Neurosci 2006;26(20):5402–10.

53. Mayer JL, Klumpers L, Maslam S, et al. Brief treatment with the glucocorticoid receptor antagonist mifepristone normalises the corticosterone-induced reduction of adult hippocampal neurogenesis. J Neuroendocrinol 2006;18(8): 629–31.

54. Claessens SE, Belanoff JK, Kanatsou S, et al. Acute effects of neonatal dexamethasone treatment on proliferation and astrocyte immunoreactivity in hippocampus and corpus callosum: towards a rescue strategy. Brain Res 2012; 1482:1–12.

55. Tauber SC, Schlumbohm C, Schilg L, et al. Intrauterine exposure to dexamethasone impairs proliferation but not neuronal differentiation in the dentate gyrus of newborn common marmoset monkeys. Brain Pathol 2006;16(3):209–17.

56. Tijsseling D, Wijnberger LD, Derks JB, et al. Effects of antenatal glucocorticoid therapy on hippocampal histology of preterm infants. PLoS One 2012;7(3): e33369.

57. Fukumoto K, Morita T, Mayanagi T, et al. Detrimental effects of glucocorticoids on neuronal migration during brain development. Mol Psychiatry 2009;14(12): 1119–31.

58. Brummelte S, Lieblich SE, Galea LA. Gestational and postpartum corticosterone exposure to the dam affects behavioral and endocrine outcome of the offspring in a sexually-dimorphic manner. Neuropharmacology 2012;62(1): 406–18.

59. Raschke C, Schmidt S, Schwab M, et al. Effects of betamethasone treatment on central myelination in fetal sheep: an electron microscopical study. Anat Histol Embryol 2008;37(2):95–100.

60. Antonow-Schlorke I, Helgert A, Gey C, et al. Adverse effects of antenatal glucocorticoids on cerebral myelination in sheep. Obstet Gynecol 2009;113(1): 142–51.

61. Dunlop SA, Archer MA, Quinlivan JA, et al. Repeated prenatal corticosteroids delay myelination in the ovine central nervous system. J Matern Fetal Med 1997;6(6):309–13.

62. Huang WL, Harper CG, Evans SF, et al. Repeated prenatal corticosteroid administration delays myelination of the corpus callosum in fetal sheep. Int J Dev Neurosci 2001;19(4):415–25.

63. Yu S, Patchev AV, Wu Y, et al. Depletion of the neural precursor cell pool by glucocorticoids. Ann Neurol 2010;67(1):21–30.

64. Ferriero DM. Neonatal brain injury. N Engl J Med 2004;351(19):1985–95.

65. Miles DK, Kernie SG. Hypoxic-ischemic brain injury activates early hippocampal stem/progenitor cells to replace vulnerable neuroblasts. Hippocampus 2008; 18(8):793–806.

66. Elitt CM, Sadowska GB, Stopa EG, et al. Effects of antenatal steroids on ischemic brain injury in near-term ovine fetuses. Early Hum Dev 2003;73(1–2): 1–15.

67. Bennet L, Davidson JO, Koome M, et al. Glucocorticoids and preterm hypoxic-ischemic brain injury: the good and the bad. J Pregnancy 2012; 2012:751694.

68. Diamond DM, Bennett MC, Fleshner M, et al. Inverted-U relationship between the level of peripheral corticosterone and the magnitude of hippocampal primed burst potentiation. Hippocampus 1992;2(4):421–30.

69. McEwen BS. Central effects of stress hormones in health and disease: understanding the protective and damaging effects of stress and stress mediators. Eur J Pharmacol 2008;583(2–3):174–85.

70. Roberts D, Dalziel S. Antenatal corticosteroids for accelerating fetal lung maturation for women at risk of preterm birth. Cochrane Database Syst Rev 2006;(3):CD004454.

71. Ment LR, Oh W, Ehrenkranz RA, et al. Antenatal steroids, delivery mode, and intraventricular hemorrhage in preterm infants. Am J Obstet Gynecol 1995; 172(3):795–800.

72. Feldman DM, Carbone J, Belden L, et al. Betamethasone vs dexamethasone for the prevention of morbidity in very-low-birthweight neonates. Am J Obstet Gynecol 2007;197(3):284.e1–4.

73. Crowther CA, Haslam RR, Hiller JE, et al. Neonatal respiratory distress syndrome after repeat exposure to antenatal corticosteroids: a randomised controlled trial. Lancet 2006;367(9526):1913–9.

74. Wapner RJ, Sorokin Y, Mele L, et al. Long-term outcomes after repeat doses of antenatal corticosteroids. N Engl J Med 2007;357(12):1190–8.

75. Crowther CA, Doyle LW, Haslam RR, et al. Outcomes at 2 years of age after repeat doses of antenatal corticosteroids. N Engl J Med 2007;357(12): 1179–89.

76. Spinillo A, Viazzo F, Colleoni R, et al. Two-year infant neurodevelopmental outcome after single or multiple antenatal courses of corticosteroids to prevent complications of prematurity. Am J Obstet Gynecol 2004;191(1):217–24.

77. Huysman MW, Hokken-Koelega AC, De Ridder MA, et al. Adrenal function in sick very preterm infants. Pediatr Res 2000;48(5):629–33.

78. Scott SM, Watterberg KL. Effect of gestational age, postnatal age, and illness on plasma cortisol concentrations in premature infants. Pediatr Res 1995;37(1): 112–6.

79. Ng PC, Lee CH, Lam CW, et al. Transient adrenocortical insufficiency of prematurity and systemic hypotension in very low birthweight infants. Arch Dis Child Fetal Neonatal Ed 2004;89(2):F119–26.

80. Watterberg KL, Gerdes JS, Cole CH, et al. Prophylaxis of early adrenal insufficiency to prevent bronchopulmonary dysplasia: a multicenter trial. Pediatrics 2004;114(6):1649–57.

81. Watterberg K. Evidence-based neonatal pharmacotherapy: postnatal corticosteroids. Clin Perinatol 2012;39(1):47–59.

82. Inder TE, Benders M. Postnatal steroids in the preterm infant-the good, the ugly, and the unknown. J Pediatr 2013;162(4):667–70.

83. Roberts RS. Early closure of the Watterberg trial. Pediatrics 2004;114(6):1670–1.

84. Stark AR, Carlo WA, Tyson JE, et al. Adverse effects of early dexamethasone in extremely-low-birth-weight infants. National Institute of Child Health and Human Development Neonatal Research Network. N Engl J Med 2001;344(2):95–101.

85. Doyle LW, Ehrenkranz RA, Halliday HL. Dexamethasone treatment in the first week of life for preventing bronchopulmonary dysplasia in preterm infants: a systematic review. Neonatology 2010;98(3):217–24.

86. Doyle LW, Ehrenkranz RA, Halliday HL. Postnatal hydrocortisone for preventing or treating bronchopulmonary dysplasia in preterm infants: a systematic review. Neonatology 2010;98(2):111–7.

87. Halliday HL, Ehrenkranz RA, Doyle LW. Moderately early (7-14 days) postnatal corticosteroids for preventing chronic lung disease in preterm infants. Cochrane Database Syst Rev 2003;(1):CD001144.

88. Halliday HL, Ehrenkranz RA, Doyle LW. Delayed (>3 weeks) postnatal cortico-steroids for chronic lung disease in preterm infants. Cochrane Database Syst Rev 2003;(1):CD001145.

89. Onland W, Offringa M, De Jaegere AP, et al. Finding the optimal postnatal dexa-methasone regimen for preterm infants at risk of bronchopulmonary dysplasia: a systematic review of placebo-controlled trials. Pediatrics 2009;123(1):367–77.

90. Wilson-Costello D, Walsh MC, Langer JC, et al. Impact of postnatal corticoste-roid use on neurodevelopment at 18 to 22 months' adjusted age: effects of dose, timing, and risk of bronchopulmonary dysplasia in extremely low birth weight infants. Pediatrics 2009;123(3):e430–7.

91. Cummings JJ, D'Eugenio DB, Gross SJ. A controlled trial of dexamethasone in preterm infants at high risk for bronchopulmonary dysplasia. N Engl J Med 1989;320(23):1505–10.

92. O'Shea TM, Kothadia JM, Klinepeter KL, et al. Randomized placebo-controlled trial of a 42-day tapering course of dexamethasone to reduce the duration of ventilator dependency in very low birth weight infants: outcome of study partic-ipants at 1-year adjusted age. Pediatrics 1999;104(1 Pt 1):15–21.

93. Mizobuchi M, Iwatani S, Sakai H, et al. Effect of hydrocortisone therapy on se-vere leaky lung syndrome in ventilated preterm infants. Pediatr Int 2012;54(5): 639–45.

94. Ben Said M, Hays S, Loys CM, et al. Postnatal steroids in extremely low birth weight infants: betamethasone or hydrocortisone? Acta Paediatr 2013;102(7): 689–94.

95. Kersbergen KJ, de Vries LS, van Kooij BJ, et al. Hydrocortisone treatment for bronchopulmonary dysplasia and brain volumes in preterm infants. J Pediatr 2013;163:666–71.e1.

96. Parikh NA, Kennedy KA, Lasky RE, et al. Pilot randomized trial of hydrocortisone in ventilator-dependent extremely preterm infants: effects on regional brain vol-umes. J Pediatr 2013;162(4):685–90.e1.

97. Benders MJ, Groenendaal F, van Bel F, et al. Brain development of the preterm neonate after neonatal hydrocortisone treatment for chronic lung disease. Pe-diatr Res 2009;66(5):555–9.

98. Van Marter LJ, Kuban KC, Allred E, et al. Does bronchopulmonary dysplasia contribute to the occurrence of cerebral palsy among infants born before 28 weeks of gestation? Arch Dis Child Fetal Neonatal Ed 2011;96(1):F20–9.

99. Doyle LW, Halliday HL, Ehrenkranz RA, et al. Impact of postnatal systemic corticosteroids on mortality and cerebral palsy in preterm infants: effect modifi-cation by risk for chronic lung disease. Pediatrics 2005;115(3):655–61.

100. Laughon M, Allred EN, Bose C, et al. Patterns of respiratory disease during the first 2 postnatal weeks in extremely premature infants. Pediatrics 2009;123(4): 1124–31.

101. Banks BA, Stouffer N, Cnaan A, et al. Association of plasma cortisol and chronic lung disease in preterm infants. Pediatrics 2001;107(3):494–8.

102. Watterberg KL, Scott SM. Evidence of early adrenal insufficiency in babies who develop bronchopulmonary dysplasia. Pediatrics 1995;95(1):120–5.

103. Watterberg KL, Scott SM, Backstrom C, et al. Links between early adrenal func-tion and respiratory outcome in preterm infants: airway inflammation and patent ductus arteriosus. Pediatrics 2000;105(2):320–4.

104. Peltoniemi O, Kari MA, Heinonen K, et al. Pretreatment cortisol values may pre-dict responses to hydrocortisone administration for the prevention of broncho-pulmonary dysplasia in high-risk infants. J Pediatr 2005;146(5):632–7.

105. Onland W, Offringa M, Cools F, et al. Systemic Hydrocortisone To Prevent Bron-chopulmonary Dysplasia in preterm infants (the SToP-BPD study); a multicenter randomized placebo controlled trial. BMC Pediatr 2011;11:102.
106. Eunice Kennedy Shriver National Institute of Child Health and Human Develop-ment (NICHD). Hydrocortisone for BPD. In: ClinicalTrials.gov [Internet]. Be-thesda (MD): National Library of Medicine (US). 2000 [cited 2013]. Available from: http://www.clinicaltrials.gov/ct2/show/NCT01353313. NLM Identifier: NCT01353313. Accessed September 26, 2013.

Neonatal Pain Control and Neurologic Effects of Anesthetics and Sedatives in Preterm Infants

Christopher McPherson, PharmD[a],*, Ruth E. Grunau, PhD[b,c]

KEYWORDS

- Pain • Newborn • Premature • Analgesia • Anesthesia • Sedation

KEY POINTS

- Optimal therapeutic approaches for the treatment of pain and agitation in the preterm infant have not been elucidated.
- Sucrose effectively reduces behavioral responses to minor procedural pain; however, the impact of repetitive dosing on long-term neurodevelopment remains unknown.
- Preterm infants often receive anesthetics during surgical procedures despite concerns about the impact of this exposure on the developing brain.
- Concerns about neurodevelopmental effects discourage chronic administration of opioids and benzodiazepines to preterm infants during mechanical ventilation, suggesting the urgent need to explore alternative agents and nonpharmacologic management.

INTRODUCTION

Historically, pain in the preterm infant has been poorly understood and often unrecognized.[1] There have been major advances in understanding the developmental physiology of nociception and responses of infants to noxious stimuli.[2] These data clearly demonstrate that nociception occurs in infants, even at the lower limit of

Dr McPherson's research program is funded by grants from the Eunice Kennedy Shriver National Institute of Child Health and Human Development (R01 HD057098; 1P30 HD062171), the Intellectual and Developmental Disabilities Research Center at Washington University (NIH/NICHD P30 HD062171), and the Doris Duke Charitable Foundation.
Dr Grunau's research program is funded by grants from the Eunice Kennedy Shriver National Institute of Child Health and Human Development (R01 HD39783), the Canadian Institutes of Health Research MOP-86489, MOP-79262, and a Senior Scientist salary award from the Child and Family Research Institute.

[a] Department of Pharmacy, St. Louis Children's Hospital, 1 Children's Place, St. Louis, MO 63110, USA; [b] Department of Pediatrics, University of British Columbia, F605B, 4480 Oak Street, Vancouver, British Columbia V6H 3V4, Canada; [c] School of Nursing and Midwifery, Queens University Belfast, 97 Lisburn Road, Belfast, BT9 7BL, Northern Ireland, UK
* Corresponding author.
E-mail address: ccm0145@bjc.org

viability. Early maturation of the ascending neural pathways responsible for nociception precedes maturation of descending inhibitory pathways, which localize and mitigate pain.[3] Additionally, the increased excitability of nociceptive neurons in the dorsal horn of the spinal cord contributes to the development of hyperalgesia and allodynia in the infant.[4] These physiologic factors create a unique susceptibility of the developing brain to both the acute and long-term adverse effects of prolonged pain exposure.[5] Greater exposure to stress and pain from procedures during neonatal intensive care is associated with decreased brain growth in the frontal and parietal lobes and alterations in organization and neuronal connections in the temporal lobes.[6,7] Additionally, greater early repetitive procedural pain-related stress in preterm infants, after adjusting for multiple clinical confounders, is associated with decreased body and brain growth from early in life to term-equivalent age, poorer cognitive and motor function at 8 and 18 months corrected chronologic ages, and altered spontaneous cortical oscillations in the resting brain at school age.[8–10]

Despite increased understanding of the developmental physiology of nociception and long-term consequences of pain and agitation in preterm infants, there is no consensus regarding safe and effective strategies for controlling pain and agitation in many clinical situations. Concern regarding the long-term neurologic impact of available interventions represents a major limitation precluding widespread utilization in clinical practice. Preterm infants experience varied forms of pain and agitation, including pain from minor procedures and major surgery and chronic agitation from life-sustaining interventions, such as mechanical ventilation. This review summarizes available data regarding the neurodevelopmental impact of agents commonly used to treat acute and chronic pain and agitation in preterm infants.

SUCROSE FOR MINOR PROCEDURAL PAIN

During neonatal intensive care, infants experience a median of 10 painful procedures per day.[11] Nonpharmacologic therapies form the foundation of pain and agitation relief for mildly painful routine procedures.[12] Therapies with evidence supporting reduction in pain scores include sucrose, nonnutritive sucking, swaddling, kangaroo care with or without breastfeeding, music therapy, and multisensorial stimulation (including massage, voice, smell, and eye contact).[13]

Clinical Data

Sucrose has widely been accepted as a nonpharmacologic intervention effective for the treatment of minor procedural pain in preterm infants.[14] Studies have extensively documented reduced crying, facial grimacing, and motor activity after oral administration of sucrose prior to minor painful procedures.[15] Recent evidence from both clinical and electroencephalography studies suggests sucrose may exert influences on the neonatal response to pain as a sedative rather than analgesic.[4,16] Further supporting this view, sucrose has variable effects on physiologic indices, such as heart rate, heart rate variability, and oxygen saturation, and no effect on cortisol.[15] There is a dearth of knowledge of the neurodevelopmental outcomes of preterm infants treated repeatedly with sucrose during a period of the most rapid brain development. To the authors' knowledge, only one study has examined repeated sucrose exposure in preterm infants, limited to the first week of life, and only examined outcomes to term-equivalent age.[17] When compared with placebo, sucrose given for invasive procedures in the first week of life in infants born at less than 31 weeks gestation had no impact on measures of motor development or attention/orientation at 36 and 40 weeks postmenstrual age. A higher number of doses of sucrose was associated, however, with poorer motor development and attention/orientation scores at 36 and 40 weeks postmenstrual age. This finding was likely not attributable to increased painful procedures, because a similar dose/outcome relationship was not observed in the placebo group. No studies (to the authors' knowledge) have assessed long-term developmental outcomes after repetitive administration of sucrose in preterm infants.

Potential Mechanisms of Neurologic Impact

Understanding the potential negative impacts of repeated sucrose administration on the developing brain requires consideration of the mechanism by which sucrose decreases the response to painful stimuli. Several potential mechanisms have been explored and include mediation of pain and/or agitation through opioid receptors, dopaminergic pathways, and cholinergic pathways. Preclinical data suggest that sucrose mediates response to pain through opioid receptors. β-endorphin levels, a marker of endogenous opioid activity, increase in response to ingestion of sweet foods in animal models.[18] Additionally, the impact of sucrose on pain threshold is reversible with coadministration of opioid receptor antagonists.[19] Considering data regarding the impact of chronic opioid administration on the developing brain (discussed later), this mechanism of action justifies concerns regarding long-term developmental impact. Sucrose administration to preterm human infants does not, however, produce a plasma β-endorphin response.[20] Also, a trial in term human newborns found no decrease in the impact of sucrose on pain-related behavior with concurrent opioid antagonist administration.[21] These results suggest additional mechanisms may be responsible for the behavioral effect of sucrose observed in infants.

The concurrent findings of pain modulation and impact on motor function and attention prompt consideration of dopaminergic and cholinergic pathways. In rodents, sucrose promotes dopamine release in the nucleus accumbens in a concentration-dependent manner.[22] Dopamine plays a central role in modulating pain perception through direct action in the descending inhibitory pathways in supraspinal regions.[23] Additionally, dopamine has antinociceptive action in the spinal cord through potassium channel activation.[24] Sucrose administration also promotes the release of acetylcholine.[25] Acetylcholine stimulates muscarinic receptors in the spinal cord reducing the release of glutamate (an excitatory neurotransmitter) and increasing the release of γ-aminobutyric acid (GABA), an inhibitory neurotransmitter acting on spinal $GABA_B$ receptors.[26] Early modulation of dopamine and acetylcholine may have an impact on attention and motor function later in life, because these neurotransmitters both play a central role in these functions.[27–29] Tolerance to the sucrose-mediated release of dopamine develops with repetitive stimulation.[30] Down-regulation of either the dopaminergic or cholinergic system secondary to early repetitive receptor stimulation may potentially have adverse consequences on neurologic function later in life.

Considering the potential adverse effects of chronic sucrose administration on the developing brain, clinicians should consider using other nonpharmacologic comfort measures for minor procedures, until evidence of long-term safety is available. For example, in general, sucrose produces a similar clinical effect to other nonpharmacologic interventions, including facilitated tucking and kangaroo care.[13] A recent study, however, suggests superior immediate pain reduction with sucrose compared with facilitated tucking.[31] These findings highlight the necessity of future studies of sucrose examining long-term neurodevelopmental and behavioral effects.

ANESTHETICS FOR MAJOR PROCEDURAL PAIN

Local anesthetics, such as lidocaine, may be useful for procedures such as chest tube insertion.[32] Topical anesthetics, such as eutectic mixture of local anesthetics (EMLA), effectively reduce pain from procedures such as lumbar puncture.[33] Systemic adverse effects seem rare, making these modalities appealing to minimize exposure to systemic agents.[34] In conjunction with local or topical anesthetics, systemic analgesia should be provided to avoid pain from major procedures. There is a paucity of clinical trials comparing different opioids for the treatment of acute pain in preterm infants. In general, agents with a rapid onset and short duration of action are preferable. On this basis, remifentanil may be the most appropriate opioid for procedural pain in preterm infants.[35] Remifentanil is metabolized by nonspecific blood and tissue esterases to an inactive form, avoiding the prolonged duration of action observed with renally eliminated opioids in preterm infants.[36] The cumulative impact of opioids on long-term outcome is discussed later. In the setting of established major procedural pain, however, the deleterious consequences of pain and ethical consideration seem to outweigh potential risks from exposure to pharmacotherapy.

To investigate the benefits of analgesia in preterm infants undergoing major surgery, Anand and colleagues[37] published a landmark randomized controlled trial in 1987 demonstrating decreased hormonal responses to patent ductus arteriosus (PDA) ligation in infants treated with high-dose fentanyl in addition to nitrous oxide and muscle relaxation. Additionally, preterm infants randomized to fentanyl experienced fewer postoperative complications. Concerns regarding the toxicity of high-dose opioids have led to the widespread utilization of balanced analgesia, an approach emphasizing concurrent administration of several agents to decrease the dosage requirement of each individual agent. Commonly used agents include volatile anesthetics, ketamine, and propofol.[38] Questions remain regarding the neurologic impact of these anesthetics in preterm infants undergoing major surgery.

Clinical Data

Complications of prematurity, including inguinal hernia, necrotizing enterocolitis (NEC), and PDA, often require surgical intervention. Approximately 20% of preterm infants undergo a surgical procedure before discharge from the neonatal intensive care unit (NICU). Several large retrospective studies have described an association between early surgical/anesthetic exposure (at <4 years of age) and learning or behavioral problems in children and adolescents.[39] Despite inconsistent findings and significant limitations, these studies have produced a strong demand for further trials exploring this association.[40,41] Smaller retrospective analyses focusing specifically on preterm infants have observed similar concerning associations. Preterm infants exposed to surgery and anesthesia have a greater incidence of moderate to severe white matter injury and smaller total brain volumes, with the greatest difference observed in the deep nuclear gray matter. These infants also exhibit poorer performance on cognitive and psychomotor assessments at 2 years of age, although importantly this finding was not significant after correction for additional risk factors.[42] Previous studies have noted, however, an association between both surgical NEC and PDA ligation and cognitive delay at 18 to 22 months of age after adjustment for confounders.[43,44] Additionally, the association between surgery requiring general anesthesia and disability persists to 5 years of age.[45]

Clinical data supporting an association between surgery/anesthesia and neurologic impact in preterm infants must be interpreted with caution. An inflammation/infection-mediated impact on brain injury, growth, and development has been demonstrated.[46]

Immature oligodendroglia in the cerebral white matter of preterm infants seem particularly vulnerable to this insult.[47] This mechanism has particular relevance to retrospective studies including bowel surgery after NEC, but does not explain associations between developmental and behavioral disorders and more minor surgical procedures, such as inguinal hernia repair.[48]

Potential Mechanism of Neurologic Impact

Preclinical evidence in newborn rodents and nonhuman primates in vivo suggests that early anesthetic exposure leads to neuroapoptosis and has an impact on long-term neurodevelopment. Cell death begins early after exposure and dramatically increases with greater doses or longer exposures.[45] Apoptosis occurs at the level of individual cells and results in rapid phagocytosis of the affected cell.[49] Vulnerability to this effect peaks during synaptogenesis.[50] Of note, widespread apoptotic cell death occurs during normal development and represents an integral aspect of central nervous system evolution.[51] Exposure to anesthetics in preclinical models, however, dramatically increases apoptosis far in excess of normal physiologic levels. The findings of decreased neuronal density and impaired cognition at maturity argue against the hypothesis that this apoptosis represents accelerated physiologic cell death rather than a pathologic reaction to anesthetic exposure.[52] Extensive debate continues regarding the applicability of this preclinical evidence to human infants. Concerns include timing of exposure relative to developmental vulnerability, the duration and degree of exposure relative to exposure in clinical practice, and the absence of surgical pain or stress in many of the preclinical models. At a minimum, however, the mechanisms of impact derived from preclinical models must be considered in the setting of retrospective clinical data in humans indicating the potential for long-term neurologic harm.

Volatile anesthetic have limited selectivity for molecular targets, acting on GABA, glutamate, nicotinic, and glycine receptors.[53] The impacts of concurrent GABA receptor agonism and N-methyl-D-aspartate (NMDA) receptor antagonism on the developing brain have been extensively explored. Concurrent GABA agonism and NMDA antagonism initially activate the intrinsic apoptotic pathway by increasing cytosolic free calcium and lowering mitochondrial transmembrane potential (**Fig. 1**).[54] This pathway commences with up-regulation of the proapoptotic bax protein and down-regulation of the counterbalancing antiapoptotic bcl-2 protein.[50,55] The bax protein translocates to mitochondrial membranes, where it disrupts membrane permeability, allowing the release of cytochrome c into the cytoplasm, triggering the caspase cascade responsible for proteolytic cleavage leading to cell death. After prolonged exposure, volatile anesthetic agents also trigger the extrinsic apoptotic pathway through up-regulation of Fas (see **Fig. 1**).[50] This death receptor on the plasma membrane initiates the caspase cascade through autocatalysis of procaspases. Finally, volatile anesthetic agents decrease levels of brain-derived neurotrophic factor (BDNF) in the thalamus. This decrease in BDNF precipitates decreased activation of tropomyosin receptor kinase (Trk) receptors, resulting in decreased release of Akt serine/threonine kinase, increasing caspase activation (**Fig. 2**). Conversely, in the cerebral cortex, volatile anesthetic agents increase levels of BDNF. However, p75 neurotrophic receptors predominate in the cortex and stimulation produces ceramide, which overrides Trk receptor–dependent production of Akt.[56]

Systemic anesthetic agents with more specific receptor selectivity may have a substantially different impact on the developing brain. Ketamine, a potent NMDA receptor antagonist, has anesthetic and analgesic properties. Prolonged, high-dose

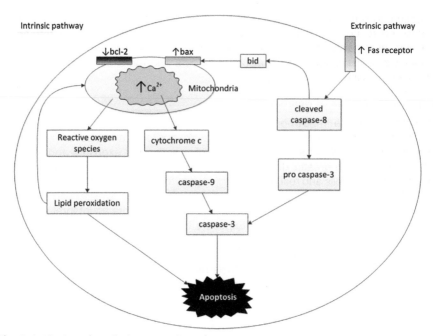

Fig. 1. Intrinsic and extrinsic apoptotic pathways.

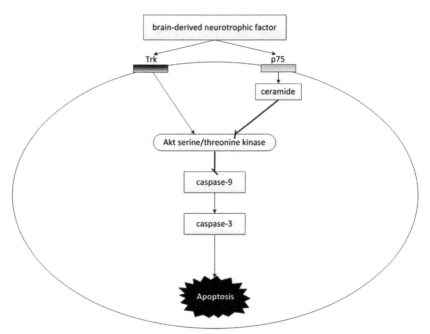

Fig. 2. Role of BDNF in regulation of apoptosis. Arrows indicate promotion; blocked connectors indicate inhibition.

exposure to ketamine in developing rodents and nonhuman primates promotes widespread neuroapoptosis.[57] NMDA receptor stimulation plays a crucial role in synaptogenesis and neuronal survival, and blockade of this stimulation may result in apoptosis of the postsynaptic neuron through the intrinsic apoptotic pathway.[58,59] However, preclinical models producing these molecular effects through relatively prolonged, high-dose ketamine exposure in the absence of surgical stress have questionable clinical relevance.[60] Preclinical models of clinically relevant doses of ketamine administered prior to inflammatory pain demonstrate amelioration of pain-induced neuroapoptosis.[61] This effect is physiologically plausible, likely resulting from a reduction in stress-induced excitotoxic cell death mediated by neuronal entry of calcium via NMDA receptors.[62] A clinical study of ketamine in infants undergoing ventricular septal defect repair with cardiopulmonary bypass demonstrated attenuation of systemic inflammation and glutamate release in the frontal white matter.[63] Considering this evidence, further investigation of the neurologic impact of ketamine in the surgical setting seems warranted.

Propofol, a potent GABA agonist, provides sedation and anesthesia with a rapid onset of action. In preclinical models, propofol induces significant apoptotic degeneration of oligodendrocytes in the developing brain.[64] These findings may be a function of the paradoxic effect of $GABA_A$ receptor stimulation in the developing brain. During synaptogenesis, $GABA_A$ receptor activation results in chloride efflux and neuronal depolarization.[65] The ensuing increase in intracellular calcium may result in neuronal injury via the intrinsic apoptotic pathway. Additionally, the paradoxically proinflammatory nature of $GABA_A$ receptors during development may activate the extrinsic apoptotic pathway.[66] The relevance of these molecular effects in preterm human infants is unknown but, taken in concert with significant hemodynamic adverse effects, discourages use of propofol in clinical practice.[67]

In summary, anesthetic agents have the potential to induce widespread neuroapoptosis through modulation of apoptotic pathways and neurotrophins. The molecular pathways by which GABA agonism and/or NMDA antagonism promote bax proteins and the Fas receptor, inhibit bcl-2 proteins, and modulate BDNF have not been elucidated. Description of these pathways will be integral to development of anesthetic agents that do not have an adverse impact on the developing neuron or protective interventions that stabilize these apoptotic pathways. Dexmedetomidine, erythropoietin, melatonin, and many other agents have been explored in preclinical studies as adjuvant therapies that may ameliorate anesthetic-induced neurotoxicity.[68] The role of these agents in neonatal anesthesia has not been studied. Intravenous acetaminophen is a promising agent that may minimize analgesic requirement in the intraoperative and postoperative periods. A recent randomized controlled trial has demonstrated a decreased opioid requirement in infants who receive intravenous acetaminophen for 48 hours after noncardiac surgery.[69] Outstanding questions include the impact on clinical outcomes and appropriate dosing in very preterm infants.[70] Future studies must establish the safety and efficacy of adjuvant therapies while ensuring continued provision of appropriate anesthesia to preterm infants undergoing major surgical procedures.

AGENTS USED FOR CHRONIC PAIN AND AGITATION

Mechanical ventilation is a common stressful experience in the management of very preterm infants during neonatal intensive care.[71] On average, preterm infants born at less than 28 weeks gestation require 2 to 4 weeks of invasive respiratory support.[72] Routine administration of pharmacologic sedation or analgesia in these preterm infants is not recommended due to concerns regarding the safety and efficacy of pharmacotherapy examined in clinical trials, specifically benzodiazepines and opioids.[32] However, the use of opioids in clinical practice remains common due to caregivers' desire to treat pain, stress, and agitation from mechanical ventilation and the lack of available alternative therapies.[73,74]

Benzodiazepines

Clinical data

Two randomized controlled trials have examined the impact of midazolam on acute brain injury in mechanically ventilated preterm infants.[75,76] The initial randomized trial of continuous infusion midazolam included a small number of preterm infants (N = 25) and avoided administration of a loading dose. This trial detected no difference in the incidence of intracranial hemorrhage or death.[75] Subsequent pharmacokinetic studies informed the design of the pilot Neonatal Outcomes and Prolonged Analgesia in Neonates (NOPAIN) trial and included a 200 mcg/kg loading dose followed by a continuous infusion.[77,78] The NOPAIN trial randomized mechanically ventilated preterm infants (N = 67) to midazolam, morphine, or placebo.[76] Infants in the midazolam group had a trend toward a higher rate of the composite outcome of severe intraventricular hemorrhage (IVH), periventricular leukomalacia (PVL), or death compared with infants receiving placebo (32% vs 24%), although the difference was not statistically significant. However, the difference in composite outcome was statistically significant when compared with morphine (32% vs 4%, $P = .03$). Clinical use of midazolam in mechanically ventilated preterm infants has declined due to the findings of the NOPAIN trial. No data exist, to the authors' knowledge, regarding the long-term neurodevelopmental impact of prolonged benzodiazepine therapy on preterm infants.

Potential mechanism of neurologic impact

The increase in brain injury observed in the NOPAIN trial likely arises from the hemodynamic adverse effects of midazolam. Midazolam boluses of 200 mcg/kg produce clinically significant hypotension in a large proportion of preterm infants (27%–45%), resulting in decreases in oxygen saturation, cerebral oxygenation index, and cerebral blood flow velocity.[79,80] Fluctuations in cerebral blood flow seem important in the pathogenesis of IVH and PVL.[81]

Benzodiazepines potentially have an impact on the developing brain beyond the initial risk of acute brain injury. Preclinical models have described widespread neuroapoptosis and suppressed neurogenesis elicited by early benzodiazepine exposure.[82,83] Additionally, prenatal benzodiazepine exposure in preclinical models produces lasting changes in hypothalamic neuron expression and delayed motor development.[84–86] Benzodiazepines provide sedation and anxiolysis by promoting the action of GABA. As described with propofol, potent stimulation of GABA receptors represents the most likely mechanism of benzodiazepine-induced neuroapoptosis.

Opioids

Clinical data

Two large randomized controlled trials have examined the impact of opioids on acute brain injury in mechanically ventilated preterm infants informed largely by the promising results of the NOPAIN trial with regard to morphine. Both trials detected no difference in the composite outcome of severe IVH, PVL, or death.[87,88] In the larger Neurologic Outcomes and Preemptive Analgesia in Neonates (NEOPAIN) trial (N = 898), subgroup analyses revealed an increase in the incidence of IVH, PVL, or death associated with randomized and open-label morphine.[88]

Conflicting results exist with regard to the long-term neurodevelopmental impact of early morphine exposure in preterm infants. Developmental follow-up of NEOPAIN infants (N = 572) at 36 weeks postmenstrual age found higher popliteal angle cluster scores, indicative of increased tone, in infants randomized to morphine.[89] This finding is corroborated by a prospective longitudinal cohort study indicating an association between greater intravenous morphine exposure and poorer motor development at 8 months of age corrected for prematurity.[9] A 5- to 7-year pilot follow-up of a small subset of NEOPAIN infants (N = 19) found no difference in overall intelligence quotient. Morphine-treated children, however, had smaller head circumference, impaired short-term memory, and social problems compared with placebo-treated children.[90] Five-year follow-up (N = 90) of participants in the randomized trial of Simons and colleagues[87] found an adverse effect of neonatal morphine on the visual analysis domain of intelligence quotient at age 5 years, indicating the importance of evaluating morphine effects on higher-order neurocognitive functions at later ages.[91] Recently, 8- to 9-year follow-up of children from the same cohort found no effects on intelligence quotient or behavior (although visual analysis was not assessed).[92] In that study, morphine exposure seemed associated with better "executive functions" assessed by parent report. Considering the high number of outcome measures tested and the lack of differences in teacher report or standardized assessment of executive functions, however, the positive association between morphine exposure and executive functions seems highly tentative. Differences in long-term outcomes of children in these 2 trials may reflect the substantially higher morphine dosing in the NEOPAIN trial[88] conducted in the United States compared with Simons and colleagues[87] conducted in Europe.

The major limitation to both these trials is the (albeit understandable) use of rescue dosing with morphine, leading to considerable crossover between randomized arms, with as much or more morphine administered to the placebo group as the morphine group in both studies. This lack of equipoise rendered the result of comparisons of the randomized group membership inconclusive, and findings were only meaningful when adjusted using propensity scores to address clinical confounders related to the decision to provide morphine beyond the confines of the trials. In 2 longitudinal clinical cohort studies statistically adjusting for key medical confounders, Grunau and colleagues[7–10,93,94] reported no evidence of protective or adverse effects of greater morphine exposure cumulatively from birth to term-equivalent age on brain development, cortisol levels, or cognitive development. However, higher morphine exposure was transiently associated with poorer motor development at 8 months but not at 18 months corrected age.[9] Moreover, in an independent cohort, higher morphine exposure across the NICU stay was associated with poorer growth of the cerebellum imaged early in life and again at term-equivalent age.[95] In summary, follow-up studies at school age of children in the NEOPAIN and the European morphine trials (after adjustment with propensity scores) suggest little evidence of major adverse relationships with psychosocial or academic functioning, although currently subtle impact on neurodevelopment cannot be ruled out.

Potential mechanism of neurologic impact

Hemodynamic effects have been identified as a contributing factor to the association between morphine and acute brain injury. Clinically significant hypotension (requiring intravenous vasopressors or fluid boluses) occurs in a large proportion of morphine-treated infants, most often following a bolus dose.[88,96] This adverse effect seems to have minimal impact on preterm infants without preexisting hypotension. In preterm infants with preexisting hypotension, however, particularly those at lower gestational ages, the hemodynamic impact of morphine is more profound and may contribute to the pathophysiology of IVH.[96]

The potential mechanism of a negative impact of opioids on the developing brain beyond the risks of acute injury has been explored extensively. Reduction of neuronal density and dendritic length as well as apoptosis has been observed in rodent models of early opioid exposure.[97–100] A similar apoptotic effect on human fetal microglia and neurons in vitro has been observed.[101] Early opioid exposure also compromises myelination.[102] The cellular etiology of these apoptotic and antiproliferative effects has been extensively explored in vitro and in preclinical models. Opioids act by agonism of the G-protein–coupled μ-opioid receptor, which produces analgesia and sedation through inhibition of ascending neural pathways in the brainstem, inhibition of neuronal firing in the dorsal horn of the spinal cord, and depression of both presynaptic and postsynaptic neuronal membrane potentials peripherally. Acute stimulation of the μ-opioid receptor decreases glutamate release reducing excitotoxic neuronal injury, potentially explaining the benefits of single, high-dose opioid administration in the surgical setting. Chronic stimulation of the μ-opioid receptor results in phosphorylation by G-protein–coupled receptor kinases (**Fig. 3**). Phosphorylation causes uncoupling of the opioid receptor from the G-protein, followed by binding of the receptor to β-arrestin. β-arrestin acts as a signal transducer, recruiting kinases including extracellular signal-regulated kinase (Erk) to the receptor. Complexing with these kinases can lead to cytosolic retention of the receptor/β-arrestin/Erk aggregate, inhibiting the growth promoting effects of Erk. Additionally, β-arrestin may scaffold with c-Jun N-terminal kinase (JNK) and apoptosis signal-regulating kinase (Ask), increasing the overall activity of this apoptosis-promoting enzyme.[103] As with anesthetic exposure in the thalamus, chronic opioid exposure results in lower levels of BDNF in the

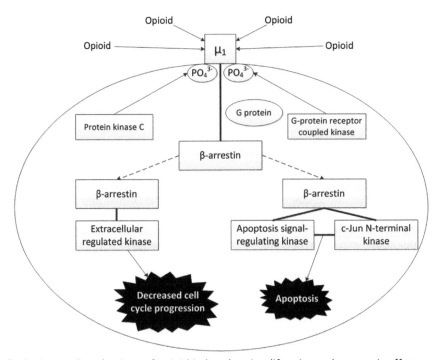

Fig. 3. Potential mechanisms of opioid-induced antiproliferative and apoptotic effects.

hippocampus, a site with high-level Trk receptor expression.[104] Cumulatively, these cellular perturbations result in reduced brain growth in preclinical models of chronic opioid exposure.[105] Furthermore, evidence suggests that these adverse effects on central nervous system development translate into abnormalities in later cognitive function and behavior. For example, rodents exposed to postnatal morphine exhibit persistently decreased motor activity and impaired learning ability.[106–109] Morphine may act differently in the brain in the presence of pain, however, compared with when pain is not present. For example, in neonatal rat pups exposed to pain induced with repeated inflammation of the paws, preemptive morphine prevented altered nociception in adulthood.[110,111] In contrast, there is preliminary evidence that early exposure to pain or morphine may have similar adverse effects on both the structure and function of the developing brain under certain circumstances.[112] In many preclinical studies, however, doses of inflammatory agents induce long-lasting tissue alterations that exceed the extent and duration of pain exposure in hospitalized preterm infants. Appropriate experimental models that examine effects of morphine combined with pain are needed, with paradigms and dosing that more closely fit the clinical experience of preterm infants.

Dexmedetomidine

Clinical data

Dexmedetomidine represents an interesting potential alternative therapy for prolonged sedation of preterm infants during mechanical ventilation. The short-term outcomes of mechanically ventilated preterm infants treated with dexmedetomidine infusion have been described in a case-control study. In this study, outcomes were compared with historical controls who received fentanyl infusion. Infants treated with dexmedetomidine required less adjunctive sedation and a shorter duration of mechanical ventilation and had a lower incidence of culture-positive sepsis.[113] These findings reflect the advantages of dexmedetomidine over standard sedative regimens demonstrated in randomized trials in adults.[114–116] In the single study in preterm infants, the incidence of severe IVH or PVL did not differ between groups.[113] No studies have reported the long-term developmental outcome of preterm infants treated with dexmedetomidine.

Potential mechanism of neurologic impact

Further studies are necessary to define the incidence of acute brain injury in preterm infants treated with dexmedetomidine. A well-described adverse effect of dexmedetomidine is hypotension, which is common with bolus doses in both adult and pediatric patients.[117,118] The incidence and degree of hypotension after bolus dosing seems similar to fentanyl and midazolam.[119,120] Avoidance of bolus doses or rapid titration of dexmedetomidine attenuates this adverse effect in adults.[121] Prospective studies of dexmedetomidine in preterm infants must include the outcome of acute brain injury as well as continuous assessment of blood pressure, heart rate, and perfusion.

The potential neuroprotective effects of dexmedetomidine on the developing brain have been explored in preclinical models. Initial models in newborn rodents examined the impact of a single bolus dose of dexmedetomidine after ibotenate-induced brain lesions (designed to mirror the pathology of PVL in the preterm human infant). Dexmedetomidine reduced the number of damaged neurons in vitro and reduced the size of the lesion in vivo.[122,123] Subsequent experiments confirming both in vitro and in vivo neuroprotection have been conducted in models of hypoxic-ischemic insult.[124] Dexmedetomidine is a highly selective agonist of the G-protein–coupled α_2-adrenergic receptor that provides analgesia, anxiolysis, and sedation via reduction in sympathetic outflow from the locus coeruleus and release of substance P from the dorsal horn of the spinal cord. Several potential molecular mechanisms may contribute to the neuroprotective actions of α_2-agonists. These agents reduce glutamate release, resulting in decreased excitotoxic damage.[125] Additionally, α_2-agonists up-regulate the bcl-2 protein and suppress bax expression,[126] contrasting directly with the actions of volatile anesthetics (discussed previously). In contrast to chronic opioid exposure, dexmedetomidine increases the expression of phosphorylated Erk through imidazoline receptor stimulation.[127] Specifically, Erk activation increases BDNF expression in cortical astrocytes, providing neuroprotection in the setting of excitotoxicity. Dexmedetomidine does not have an impact on neuronal BDNF expression.[128] The molecular effects of chronic α_2-receptor stimulation have not been explored and represent a vital need in preclinical research. The decision to pursue trials of dexmedetomidine in preterm infants must be made considering the efficacy, adverse effect profile, and potential risks and benefits of this agent with regards to neurodevelopment. When clinical trials of dexmedetomidine are undertaken in preterm infants, inclusion of advanced neuroimaging to assess brain microstructure and growth must be considered in conjunction with assessment of long-term neurodevelopmental impact.

CONCLUSIONS

Research in the developmental physiology of nociception clearly demonstrates the ability of preterm infants to perceive pain. Preclinical and clinical studies have confirmed the adverse consequences of untreated pain and stress on brain development. Based on the available evidence, treatment is indicated for acute events ranging from minor procedural pain to major surgery as well as chronic stressful experiences including mechanical ventilation. Controversy exists concerning the safety and long-term impact of interventions commonly utilized in these situations. Sucrose has widely been implemented as standard therapy for minor procedural pain. However, the mechanism of action of this therapy has not been elucidated and long-term neurodevelopmental outcomes of preterm infants after chronic exposure is unknown, with greatest concern for infants born at the lowest gestational ages. Until the long term effects of repeated sucrose exposure have been evaluated, judicious use of sucrose should be considered, as well as utilization of alternatives such as kangaroo care and facilitated tucking for humanitarian care. Anesthetics are commonly utilized during major surgery in preterm infants. Concerning preclinical and clinical data suggest these agents may promote apoptosis and impact neurodevelopment. Ongoing studies will help define the impact of these agents, fully elucidate the mechanism of impact, and identify adjuvant therapies which may ameliorate detrimental effects. Sedation is likely indicated for preterm infants requiring invasive mechanical ventilation. However, the pharmacologic agents examined in clinical trials (benzodiazepines and opioids) may have both acute and chronic adverse neurologic impacts. Dexmedetomidine represents a promising alternative, although extensive, multidisciplinary research must be completed before widespread use in preterm infants is considered.

REFERENCES

1. Anand KJ, Hickey PR. Pain and its effects in the human neonate and fetus. N Engl J Med 1987;317:1321–9.
2. Fitzgerald M. The development of nociceptive circuits. Nat Rev Neurosci 2005; 6:507–20.

3. Fitzgerald M, Koltzenburg M. The functional development of descending inhibitory pathways in the dorsolateral funiculus of the newborn rat spinal cord. Brain Res 1986;389:261–70.

4. Taddio A, Shah V, Atenafu E, et al. Influence of repeated painful procedures and sucrose analgesia on the development of hyperalgesia in newborn infants. Pain 2009;144:43–8.

5. Grunau RE, Holsti L, Peters JW. Long-term consequences of pain in human neonates. Semin Fetal Neonatal Med 2006;11:268–75.

6. Smith GC, Gutovich J, Smyser C, et al. Neonatal intensive care unit stress is associated with brain development in preterm infants. Ann Neurol 2011;70:541–9.

7. Brummelte S, Grunau RE, Chau V, et al. Procedural pain and brain development in premature newborns. Ann Neurol 2012;71:385–96.

8. Vinall J, Grunau RE, Brant R, et al. Slower postnatal growth is associated with delayed cerebral cortical maturation in preterm newborns. Sci Transl Med 2013;5:168ra8.

9. Grunau RE, Whitfield MF, Petrie-Thomas J, et al. Neonatal pain, parenting stress and interaction, in relation to cognitive and motor development at 8 and 18 months in preterm infants. Pain 2009;143:138–46.

10. Doesburg SM, Chau CM, Cheung TP, et al. Neonatal pain-related stress, functional cortical activity and visual-perceptual abilities in school-age children born at extremely low gestational age. Pain 2013;154:1946–52.

11. Carbajal R, Rousset A, Danan C, et al. Epidemiology and treatment of painful procedures in neonates in intensive care units. JAMA 2008;300:60–70.

12. Golianu B, Krane E, Seybold J, et al. Non-pharmacological techniques for pain management in neonates. Semin Perinatol 2007;31:318–22.

13. Pillai Riddell R, Racine N, Turcotte K, et al. Nonpharmacological management of procedural pain in infants and young children: an abridged Cochrane review. Pain Res Manag 2011;16:321–30.

14. Taddio A, Yiu A, Smith RW, et al. Variability in clinical practice guidelines for sweetening agents in newborn infants undergoing painful procedures. Clin J Pain 2009;25:153–5.

15. Stevens B, Yamada J, Lee GY, et al. Sucrose for analgesia in newborn infants undergoing painful procedures. Cochrane Database Syst Rev 2013;(1): CD001069.

16. Slater R, Cornelissen L, Fabrizi L, et al. Oral sucrose as an analgesic drug for procedural pain in newborn infants: a randomised controlled trial. Lancet 2010;376:1225–32.

17. Johnston CC, Filion F, Snider L, et al. Routine sucrose analgesia during the first week of life in neonates younger than 31 weeks' postconceptional age. Pediatrics 2002;110:523–8.

18. Dum J, Gramsch C, Herz A. Activation of hypothalamic beta-endorphin pools by reward induced by highly palatable food. Pharmacol Biochem Behav 1983;18: 443–7.

19. Blass E, Fitzgerald E, Kehoe P. Interactions between sucrose, pain and isolation distress. Pharmacol Biochem Behav 1987;26:483–9.

20. Taddio A, Shah V, Shah P, et al. Beta-endorphin concentration after administration of sucrose in preterm infants. Arch Pediatr Adolesc Med 2003;157:1071–4.

21. Gradin M, Schollin J. The role of endogenous opioids in mediating pain reduction by orally administered glucose among newborns. Pediatrics 2005;115:1004–7.

22. Hajnal A, Smith GP, Norgren R. Oral sucrose stimulation increases accumbens dopamine in the rat. Am J Physiol Regul Integr Comp Physiol 2004;286:R31–7.

23. Wood PB. Role of central dopamine in pain and analgesia. Expert Rev Neurother 2008;8:781–97.

24. Tamae A, Nakatsuka T, Koga K, et al. Direct inhibition of substantia gelatinosa neurones in the rat spinal cord by activation of dopamine D2-like receptors. J Physiol 2005;568:243–53.

25. Rada P, Avena NM, Hoebel BG. Daily bingeing on sugar repeatedly releases dopamine in the accumbens shell. Neuroscience 2005;134:737–44.

26. Jones PG, Dunlop J. Targeting the cholinergic system as a therapeutic strategy for the treatment of pain. Neuropharmacology 2007;53:197–206.

27. Sarter M, Gehring WJ, Kozak R. More attention must be paid: the neurobiology of attentional effort. Brain Res Rev 2006;51:145–60.

28. Pezze MA, Dalley JW, Robbins TW. Differential roles of dopamine D1 and D2 receptors in the nucleus accumbens in attentional performance on the five-choice serial reaction time task. Neuropsychopharmacology 2007;32:273–83.

29. Langguth B, Bauer E, Feix S, et al. Modulation of human motor cortex excitability by the cholinesterase inhibitor rivastigmine. Neurosci Lett 2007;415:40–4.

30. Avena NM, Rada P, Hoebel BG. Evidence for sugar addiction: behavioral and neurochemical effects of intermittent, excessive sugar intake. Neurosci Biobehav Rev 2008;32:20–39.

31. Cignacco EL, Sellam G, Stoffel L, et al. Oral sucrose and "facilitated tucking" for repeated pain relief in preterms: a randomized controlled trial. Pediatrics 2012;129:299–308.

32. Batton DG, Barrington KJ, Wallman C. Prevention and management of pain in the neonate: an update. Pediatrics 2006;118:2231–41.

33. Kaur G, Gupta P, Kumar A. A randomized trial of eutectic mixture of local anesthetics during lumbar puncture in newborns. Arch Pediatr Adolesc Med 2003;157:1065–70.

34. Lehr VT, Taddio A. Topical anesthesia in neonates: clinical practices and practical considerations. Semin Perinatol 2007;31:323–9.

35. Welzing L, Kribs A, Huenseler C, et al. Remifentanil for INSURE in preterm infants: a pilot study for evaluation of efficacy and safety aspects. Acta Paediatr 2009;98:1416–20.

36. Welzing L, Ebenfeld S, Dlugay V, et al. Remifentanil degradation in umbilical cord blood of preterm infants. Anesthesiology 2011;114:570–7.

37. Anand KJ, Sippell WG, Aynsley-Green A. Randomised trial of fentanyl anaesthesia in preterm babies undergoing surgery: effects on the stress response. Lancet 1987;1:62–6.

38. Berde CB, Jaksic T, Lynn AM, et al. Anesthesia and analgesia during and after surgery in neonates. Clin Ther 2005;27:900–21.

39. DiMaggio C, Sun LS, Ing C, et al. Pediatric anesthesia and neurodevelopmental impairments: a Bayesian meta-analysis. J Neurosurg Anesthesiol 2012;24:376–81.

40. Sun LS, Li G, DiMaggio CJ, et al. Feasibility and pilot study of the Pediatric Anesthesia NeuroDevelopment Assessment (PANDA) project. J Neurosurg Anesthesiol 2012;24:382–8.

41. Rappaport B, Mellon RD, Simone A, et al. Defining safe use of anesthesia in children. N Engl J Med 2011;364:1387–90.

42. Filan PM, Hunt RW, Anderson PJ, et al. Neurologic outcomes in very preterm infants undergoing surgery. J Pediatr 2012;160:409–14.

43. Hintz SR, Kendrick DE, Stoll BJ, et al. Neurodevelopmental and growth outcomes of extremely low birth weight infants after necrotizing enterocolitis. Pediatrics 2005;115:696–703.

44. Kabra NS, Schmidt B, Roberts RS, et al. Neurosensory impairment after surgical closure of patent ductus arteriosus in extremely low birth weight infants: results from the Trial of Indomethacin Prophylaxis in Preterms. J Pediatr 2007;150: 229–34, 234.e1.
45. Loepke AW, Soriano SG. An assessment of the effects of general anesthetics on developing brain structure and neurocognitive function. Anesth Analg 2008;106: 1681–707.
46. Adams-Chapman I, Stoll BJ. Neonatal infection and long-term neurodevelopmental outcome in the preterm infant. Curr Opin Infect Dis 2006;19:290–7.
47. Volpe JJ. Neurobiology of periventricular leukomalacia in the premature infant. Pediatr Res 2001;50:553–62.
48. DiMaggio C, Sun LS, Kakavouli A, et al. A retrospective cohort study of the association of anesthesia and hernia repair surgery with behavioral and developmental disorders in young children. J Neurosurg Anesthesiol 2009;21: 286–91.
49. Zimmermann KC, Green DR. How cells die: apoptosis pathways. J Allergy Clin Immunol 2001;108:S99–103.
50. Yon JH, Daniel-Johnson J, Carter LB, et al. Anesthesia induces neuronal cell death in the developing rat brain via the intrinsic and extrinsic apoptotic pathways. Neuroscience 2005;135:815–27.
51. Rakic S, Zecevic N. Programmed cell death in the developing human telencephalon. Eur J Neurosci 2000;12:2721–34.
52. Jevtovic-Todorovic V, Hartman RE, Izumi Y, et al. Early exposure to common anesthetic agents causes widespread neurodegeneration in the developing rat brain and persistent learning deficits. J Neurosci 2003;23:876–82.
53. Campagna JA, Miller KW, Forman SA. Mechanisms of actions of inhaled anesthetics. N Engl J Med 2003;348:2110–24.
54. Ullah I, Ullah N, Naseer MI, et al. Neuroprotection with metformin and thymoquinone against ethanol-induced apoptotic neurodegeneration in prenatal rat cortical neurons. BMC Neurosci 2012;13:11.
55. Young C, Klocke BJ, Tenkova T, et al. Ethanol-induced neuronal apoptosis in vivo requires BAX in the developing mouse brain. Cell Death Differ 2003;10:1148–55.
56. Lu LX, Yon JH, Carter LB, et al. General anesthesia activates BDNF-dependent neuroapoptosis in the developing rat brain. Apoptosis 2006;11:1603–15.
57. Brambrink AM, Evers AS, Avidan MS, et al. Ketamine-induced neuroapoptosis in the fetal and neonatal rhesus macaque brain. Anesthesiology 2012;116: 372–84.
58. Hetman M, Kharebava G. Survival signaling pathways activated by NMDA receptors. Curr Top Med Chem 2006;6:787–99.
59. Sanders RD, Hassell J, Davidson AJ, et al. Impact of anaesthetics and surgery on neurodevelopment: an update. Br J Anaesth 2013;110(Suppl 1):i53–72.
60. Bhutta AT. Ketamine: a controversial drug for neonates. Semin Perinatol 2007; 31:303–8.
61. Anand KJ, Garg S, Rovnaghi CR, et al. Ketamine reduces the cell death following inflammatory pain in newborn rat brain. Pediatr Res 2007;62:283–90.
62. Ghosh A, Greenberg ME. Calcium signaling in neurons: molecular mechanisms and cellular consequences. Science 1995;268:239–47.
63. Bhutta AT, Schmitz ML, Swearingen C, et al. Ketamine as a neuroprotective and anti-inflammatory agent in children undergoing surgery on cardiopulmonary bypass: a pilot randomized, double-blind, placebo-controlled trial. Pediatr Crit Care Med 2012;13:328–37.

64. Creeley C, Dikranian K, Dissen G, et al. Propofol-induced apoptosis of neurones and oligodendrocytes in fetal and neonatal rhesus macaque brain. Br J Anaesth 2013;110(Suppl 1):i29–38.

65. Ben-Ari Y. Excitatory actions of gaba during development: the nature of the nurture. Nat Rev Neurosci 2002;3:728–39.

66. Pesic V, Milanovic D, Tanic N, et al. Potential mechanism of cell death in the developing rat brain induced by propofol anesthesia. Int J Dev Neurosci 2009;27:279–87.

67. Welzing L, Kribs A, Eifinger F, et al. Propofol as an induction agent for endotracheal intubation can cause significant arterial hypotension in preterm neonates. Paediatr Anaesth 2010;20:605–11.

68. Lei X, Guo Q, Zhang J. Mechanistic insights into neurotoxicity induced by anesthetics in the developing brain. Int J Mol Sci 2012;13:6772–99.

69. Ceelie I, de Wildt SN, van Dijk M, et al. Effect of intravenous paracetamol on postoperative morphine requirements in neonates and infants undergoing major noncardiac surgery: a randomized controlled trial. JAMA 2013;309:149–54.

70. Allegaert K, Palmer GM, Anderson BJ. The pharmacokinetics of intravenous paracetamol in neonates: size matters most. Arch Dis Child 2011;96:575–80.

71. Hall RW, Boyle E, Young T. Do ventilated neonates require pain management? Semin Perinatol 2007;31:289–97.

72. Finer NN, Carlo WA, Walsh MC, et al. Early CPAP versus surfactant in extremely preterm infants. N Engl J Med 2010;362:1970–9.

73. Clark RH, Bloom BT, Spitzer AR, et al. Reported medication use in the neonatal intensive care unit: data from a large national data set. Pediatrics 2006;117: 1979–87.

74. Kumar P, Walker JK, Hurt KM, et al. Medication use in the neonatal intensive care unit: current patterns and off-label use of parenteral medications. J Pediatr 2008;152:412–5.

75. Jacqz-Aigrain E, Daoud P, Burtin P, et al. Placebo-controlled trial of midazolam sedation in mechanically ventilated newborn babies. Lancet 1994;344: 646–50.

76. Anand KJ, Barton BA, McIntosh N, et al. Analgesia and sedation in preterm neonates who require ventilatory support: results from the NOPAIN trial. Neonatal Outcome and Prolonged Analgesia in Neonates. Arch Pediatr Adolesc Med 1999;153:331–8.

77. Burtin P, Jacqz-Aigrain E, Girard P, et al. Population pharmacokinetics of midazolam in neonates. Clin Pharmacol Ther 1994;56:615–25.

78. Harte GJ, Gray PH, Lee TC, et al. Haemodynamic responses and population pharmacokinetics of midazolam following administration to ventilated, preterm neonates. J Paediatr Child Health 1997;33:335–8.

79. Jacqz-Aigrain E, Daoud P, Burtin P, et al. Pharmacokinetics of midazolam during continuous infusion in critically ill neonates. Eur J Clin Pharmacol 1992;42: 329–32.

80. van Alfen-van der Velden AA, Hopman JC, Klaessens JH, et al. Effects of midazolam and morphine on cerebral oxygenation and hemodynamics in ventilated premature infants. Biol Neonate 2006;90:197–202.

81. Volpe JJ. Brain injury in the premature infant. Neuropathology, clinical aspects, pathogenesis, and prevention. Clin Perinatol 1997;24:567–87.

82. Young C, Jevtovic-Todorovic V, Qin YQ, et al. Potential of ketamine and midazolam, individually or in combination, to induce apoptotic neurodegeneration in the infant mouse brain. Br J Pharmacol 2005;146:189–97.

83. Stefovska VG, Uckermann O, Czuczwar M, et al. Sedative and anticonvulsant drugs suppress postnatal neurogenesis. Ann Neurol 2008;64:434–45.

84. Kellogg C, Tervo D, Ison J, et al. Prenatal exposure to diazepam alters behavioral development in rats. Science 1980;207:205–7.

85. Simmons RD, Miller RK, Kellogg CK. Prenatal exposure to diazepam alters central and peripheral responses to stress in adult rat offspring. Brain Res 1984; 307:39–46.

86. Kellogg CK, Simmons RD, Miller RK, et al. Prenatal diazepam exposure in rats: long-lasting functional changes in the offspring. Neurobehav Toxicol Teratol 1985;7:483–8.

87. Simons SH, van Dijk M, van Lingen RA, et al. Routine morphine infusion in preterm newborns who received ventilatory support: a randomized controlled trial. JAMA 2003;290:2419–27.

88. Anand KJ, Hall RW, Desai N, et al. Effects of morphine analgesia in ventilated preterm neonates: primary outcomes from the NEOPAIN randomised trial. Lancet 2004;363:1673–82.

89. Rao R, Sampers JS, Kronsberg SS, et al. Neurobehavior of preterm infants at 36 weeks postconception as a function of morphine analgesia. Am J Perinatol 2007;24:511–7.

90. Ferguson SA, Ward WL, Paule MG, et al. A pilot study of preemptive morphine analgesia in preterm neonates: effects on head circumference, social behavior, and response latencies in early childhood. Neurotoxicol Teratol 2012;34:47–55.

91. de Graaf J, van Lingen RA, Simons SH, et al. Long-term effects of routine morphine infusion in mechanically ventilated neonates on children's functioning: five-year follow-up of a randomized controlled trial. Pain 2011;152:1391–7.

92. de Graaf J, van Lingen RA, Valkenburg AJ, et al. Does neonatal morphine use affect neuropsychological outcomes at 8 to 9 years of age? Pain 2013;154:449–58.

93. Grunau RE, Holsti L, Haley DW, et al. Neonatal procedural pain exposure predicts lower cortisol and behavioral reactivity in preterm infants in the NICU. Pain 2005;113:293–300.

94. Grunau RE, Haley DW, Whitfield MF, et al. Altered basal cortisol levels at 3, 6, 8 and 18 months in infants born at extremely low gestational age. J Pediatr 2007; 150:151–6.

95. Zwicker JG, Miller SP, Grunau RE, et al. Morphine exposure is associated with altered cerebellar growth in premature newborns. In: Pediatric Academic Societies' Abstract Archive. 2012. Available at: http://www.abstracts2view.com/pasall/view.php?nu=PAS12L1_1060. Accessed July 25, 2013.

96. Hall RW, Kronsberg SS, Barton BA, et al. Morphine, hypotension, and adverse outcomes among preterm neonates: who's to blame? Secondary results from the NEOPAIN trial. Pediatrics 2005;115:1351–9.

97. Hammer RP Jr, Ricalde AA, Seatriz JV. Effects of opiates on brain development. Neurotoxicology 1989;10:475–83.

98. Ricalde AA, Hammer RP Jr. Perinatal opiate treatment delays growth of cortical dendrites. Neurosci Lett 1990;115:137–43.

99. Seatriz JV, Hammer RP Jr. Effects of opiates on neuronal development in the rat cerebral cortex. Brain Res Bull 1993;30:523–7.

100. Atici S, Cinel L, Cinel I, et al. Opioid neurotoxicity: comparison of morphine and tramadol in an experimental rat model. Int J Neurosci 2004;114:1001–11.

101. Hu S, Sheng WS, Lokensgard JR, et al. Morphine induces apoptosis of human microglia and neurons. Neuropharmacology 2002;42:829–36.

102. Sanchez ES, Bigbee JW, Fobbs W, et al. Opioid addiction and pregnancy: perinatal exposure to buprenorphine affects myelination in the developing brain. Glia 2008;56:1017–27.

103. Tegeder I, Geisslinger G. Opioids as modulators of cell death and survival–unraveling mechanisms and revealing new indications. Pharmacol Rev 2004; 56:351–69.

104. Schrott LM, Franklin LM, Serrano PA. Prenatal opiate exposure impairs radial arm maze performance and reduces levels of BDNF precursor following training. Brain Res 2008;1198:132–40.

105. Zagon IS, McLaughlin PJ. Morphine and brain growth retardation in the rat. Pharmacology 1977;15:276–82.

106. Handelmann GE, Dow-Edwards D. Modulation of brain development by morphine: effects on central motor systems and behavior. Peptides 1985; 6(Suppl 2):29–34.

107. McPherson RJ, Gleason C, Mascher-Denen M, et al. A new model of neonatal stress which produces lasting neurobehavioral effects in adult rats. Neonatology 2007;92:33–41.

108. Ma MX, Chen YM, He J, et al. Effects of morphine and its withdrawal on Y-maze spatial recognition memory in mice. Neuroscience 2007;147:1059–65.

109. Lin CS, Tao PL, Jong YJ, et al. Prenatal morphine alters the synaptic complex of postsynaptic density 95 with N-methyl-D-aspartate receptor subunit in hippocampal CA1 subregion of rat offspring leading to long-term cognitive deficits. Neuroscience 2009;158:1326–37.

110. Bhutta AT, Rovnaghi C, Simpson PM, et al. Interactions of inflammatory pain and morphine in infant rats: long-term behavioral effects. Physiol Behav 2001;73: 51–8.

111. Laprairie JL, Johns ME, Murphy AZ. Preemptive morphine analgesia attenuates the long-term consequences of neonatal inflammation in male and female rats. Pediatr Res 2008;64:625–30.

112. Duhrsen L, Simons SH, Dzietko M, et al. Effects of repetitive exposure to pain and morphine treatment on the neonatal rat brain. Neonatology 2013;103: 35–43.

113. O'Mara K, Gal P, Wimmer J, et al. Dexmedetomidine versus standard therapy with fentanyl for sedation in mechanically ventilated premature neonates. J Pediatr Pharmacol Ther 2012;17:252–62.

114. Riker RR, Shehabi Y, Bokesch PM, et al. Dexmedetomidine vs midazolam for sedation of critically ill patients: a randomized trial. JAMA 2009;301: 489–99.

115. Pandharipande PP, Pun BT, Herr DL, et al. Effect of sedation with dexmedetomidine vs lorazepam on acute brain dysfunction in mechanically ventilated patients: the MENDS randomized controlled trial. JAMA 2007;298:2644–53.

116. Shehabi Y, Grant P, Wolfenden H, et al. Prevalence of delirium with dexmedetomidine compared with morphine based therapy after cardiac surgery: a randomized controlled trial (DEXmedetomidine COmpared to Morphine-DEXCOM Study). Anesthesiology 2009;111:1075–84.

117. Venn RM, Bradshaw CJ, Spencer R, et al. Preliminary UK experience of dexmedetomidine, a novel agent for postoperative sedation in the intensive care unit. Anaesthesia 1999;54:1136–42.

118. Petroz GC, Sikich N, James M, et al. A phase I, two-center study of the pharmacokinetics and pharmacodynamics of dexmedetomidine in children. Anesthesiology 2006;105:1098–110.

119. Erdil F, Demirbilek S, Begec Z, et al. The effects of dexmedetomidine and fentanyl on emergence characteristics after adenoidectomy in children. Anaesth Intensive Care 2009;37:571–6.
120. Koroglu A, Demirbilek S, Teksan H, et al. Sedative, haemodynamic and respiratory effects of dexmedetomidine in children undergoing magnetic resonance imaging examination: preliminary results. Br J Anaesth 2005;94:821–4.
121. Gerlach AT, Dasta JF, Steinberg S, et al. A new dosing protocol reduces dexmedetomidine-associated hypotension in critically ill surgical patients. J Crit Care 2009;24:568–74.
122. Laudenbach V, Mantz J, Lagercrantz H, et al. Effects of alpha(2)-adrenoceptor agonists on perinatal excitotoxic brain injury: comparison of clonidine and dexmedetomidine. Anesthesiology 2002;96:134–41.
123. Paris A, Mantz J, Tonner PH, et al. The effects of dexmedetomidine on perinatal excitotoxic brain injury are mediated by the alpha2A-adrenoceptor subtype. Anesth Analg 2006;102:456–61.
124. Ma D, Hossain M, Rajakumaraswamy N, et al. Dexmedetomidine produces its neuroprotective effect via the alpha 2A-adrenoceptor subtype. Eur J Pharmacol 2004;502:87–97.
125. Ma D, Rajakumaraswamy N, Maze M. alpha2-Adrenoceptor agonists: shedding light on neuroprotection? Br Med Bull 2004;71:77–92.
126. Engelhard K, Werner C, Eberspacher E, et al. The effect of the alpha 2-agonist dexmedetomidine and the N-methyl-D-aspartate antagonist S(+)-ketamine on the expression of apoptosis-regulating proteins after incomplete cerebral ischemia and reperfusion in rats. Anesth Analg 2003;96:524–31.
127. Dahmani S, Paris A, Jannier V, et al. Dexmedetomidine increases hippocampal phosphorylated extracellular signal-regulated protein kinase 1 and 2 content by an alpha 2-adrenoceptor-independent mechanism: evidence for the involvement of imidazoline I1 receptors. Anesthesiology 2008;108:457–66.
128. Degos V, Charpentier TL, Chhor V, et al. Neuroprotective effects of dexmedetomidine against glutamate agonist-induced neuronal cell death are related to increased astrocyte brain-derived neurotrophic factor expression. Anesthesiology 2013;118:1123–32.

Neurogenesis and Maturation in Neonatal Brain Injury

Natalina Salmaso, PhD[a], Simone Tomasi, MD, PhD[a],
Flora M. Vaccarino, MD[a,b],*

KEYWORDS

- Preterm birth • Neurogenesis • Neonatal brain injury • Cognitive delay

KEY POINTS

- Many human premature infants and animal models of perinatal hypoxic injury recover gross anatomic deficits, but microstructural and functional alterations persist.
- Astroglial cells are delayed in their maturation and retain stem cell properties, prolonging neurogenesis.
- A portion of PV and SST inhibitory neurons subtypes remains immature and likely function abnormally.
- There is likely aberrant connectivity and altered balance of cortical excitation/inhibition in hypoxic-reared animals.

INTRODUCTION

Approximately 1% to 2% of live births in the United States are to very low birth weight infants (VLBW), defined as weighing under 1 kg at birth, which has devastating consequences on neurologic development, including striking decreases in cortical volume, white matter abnormalities, and ventriculomegaly.[1–4] Moreover, the incidence of live preterm births continues to increase steadily in recent decades.[5] Functionally, VLBW children show increased incidence of developmental delays, motor disabilities, and psychiatric illnesses, such as anxiety disorders and autism spectrum disorders.[1,3,4,6–14] Importantly, many reports have shown that a substantial proportion of premature children recover over time. In a longitudinal study,[15] more than 50% of VLBW infants manifested no significant neuropsychological differences as compared with term-born controls by the time they reached adulthood; among these, as many as

This work was supported by NIH grants P01 NS062686, R01 MH067715, and R01 NS060750 (F.M. Vaccarino); N. Salmaso is the recipient of a Canadian Institute of Health Fellowship.
The authors declare no competing financial interests.
[a] Child Study Center, Yale University, 230 South Frontage Road, New Haven, CT 06520, USA;
[b] Department of Neurobiology, Kavli Institute for Neuroscience, Yale University, 333 Cedar Street, New Haven, CT 06520, USA
* Corresponding author. Yale Child Study Center, Yale University School of Medicine, PO Box 207900, New Haven, CT 06520.
E-mail address: flora.vaccarino@yale.edu

Clin Perinatol 41 (2014) 229–239
http://dx.doi.org/10.1016/j.clp.2013.10.007

17% surpass term control for vocabulary skills, whereas about 40% maintain mild to severe cognitive impairment.[15] With respect to the pathophysiology of abnormal neurologic development in VLBW children, a percentage of VLBW children suffer from intraventricular hemorrhage or acute brain infarcts in early postnatal life and manifest severe neurologic deficits collectively referred to as "cerebral palsy." However, the more frequent generalized neurologic and behavioral disturbances described above are seen in the absence of brain infarcts; these are thought to be due to chronic hypoxic injury suffered by VLBW children as a result of immature lung development. Indeed, using a mouse model of chronic hypoxia, induced in rodent pups during the first week after birth (an age roughly corresponding to the third trimester of pregnancy in humans), investigators have been able to recapitulate the cortical volume loss, white matter abnormalities, ventriculomegaly, and behavioral disturbances seen in the VLBW infant.[16–22] Beyond the rodent, researchers have used a range of animal models to study prematurity from baboon, sheep, to piglet and rabbit, with differing limitations and success, depending on the pathologic abnormality being studied (for reviews, see Refs.[17,23,24]); however, the capacity for transgenic manipulations in the mouse makes it an attractive model to study the basic pathologic abnormalities of prematurity as well as options for treatment.

RECOVERY FROM HYPOXIC REARING IN A MOUSE MODEL OF PREMATURITY

As in the human condition observed in clinic, substantial recovery had been documented in many of the disturbances induced by hypoxic-rearing in a mouse model of perinatal hypoxia.[19,25] Nevertheless, some abnormalities remain; for example, cognitive deficits and increased anxiety behavior persist until adulthood in this model, and the authors' research has focused on elucidating the factors involved in mediating these differential recovery trajectories. One possibility is that chronic exposure to low levels of oxygen leads to a delay in brain maturation. On the one hand, this can be conceptualized as an adaptive process that likely contributes to recovery from hypoxic injury. On the other hand, a maturation delay may also be detrimental to developmental processes that occur during specific "critical" periods or in time-sensitive sequential events that are critical to subsequent developmental stages (**Fig. 1**). Certainly, the persistence of behavioral deficits suggests that brain abnormalities related to these behaviors must exist. Abnormalities can exist on one or many levels of structure/function that are not necessarily mutually exclusive; from the integrity of cell numbers and synaptic connectivity, to large-scale structural integration of cells including intercellular architectural organization that condition neuronal network activity. This review attempts to examine perturbations at each of these levels of analysis and delineates the known underlying factors, synthesizing these data into a working hypothesis.

CORTICAL NEUROGENESIS IN PERINATAL INJURY

The decreases in cortical volume seen in VLBW children, and in response to postnatal chronic hypoxic injury in the chronic hypoxia animal model of prematurity, correspond to decreases in total number of neurons—particularly excitatory neurons, as they comprise of 90% of the neurons found in the cerebral cortex. Cortical volume following hypoxic injury in mice is decreased by approximately 24% (as compared with normoxic controls) at the end of chronic hypoxia exposure, which lasts from postnatal day 3 (P3) until P11.[16] The decreased number of neurons may be due to decreased neurogenesis or to increased cell death. Importantly, this phenomenon is not limited to rodent models of chronic hypoxia, but decreased neurogenesis has also been observed in prematurely

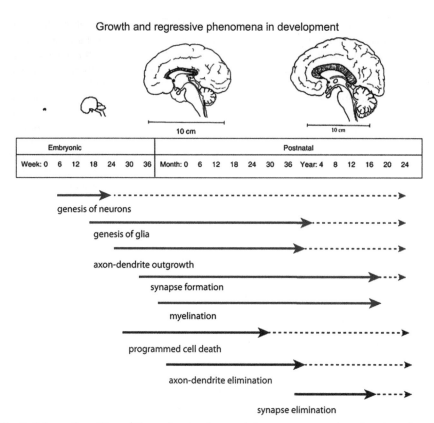

Growth and regressive phenomena in development

Fig. 1. Schematic outline of the major developmental processes occurring at embryonic and postnatal stages of human brain development. Growth processes are in red; regressive processes are in blue. Broken arrows indicate continuation of a process at reduced levels or in restricted brain areas.

delivered rabbits. Remarkably, this decrease in cortical volume and corresponding neurogenesis is partially compensated by reactive processes that begin as soon as the animals are placed in a normoxic environment. The recovery of cortical volume that occurs in the weeks following chronic hypoxia corresponds to a replenishment of the total number of excitatory neurons to those numbers seen in normoxic controls by the time mice reach early adulthood (6 weeks of age); this recovery occurs in part through an increase in cortical neurogenesis.[16] It seems that hypoxic rearing promotes an increased "stem-cell-like" capability of cortical astrocytes. It could also be that partly-damaged neurons "recover" their phenotype including marker immunoreactivity, a process that is favored by trophic factors such as fibroblast growth factor (FGF) and brain derived growth factor (BDNF) signaling. Indeed, mice with genetic deletion of FGF receptor show much worse outcome and are unable to recover total neuron number after hypoxia.[18]

Astroglia comprise stereotypic star-shaped protoplasmic astrocytes and astroglial stem cells, which exhibit a more radial-like morphology. As with all neural stem cells, this subset of astroglia can self-renew and give rise to all 3 neural lineages: astrocytes, neurons, and oligodendrocytes (microglia are thought to originate from the yolk sac). In the adult brain, stem cell activity of astroglia is restricted to the "neurogenic" regions of the brain: the dentate gyrus of the hippocampus and the subventricular zone (SVZ).

However, during the first week postnatally, parenchymal astroglia retain stem cells properties also within the neocortex, but this ability decreases in the second week and is completely abolished by P15.[26,27] Interestingly, it has been shown in mice that hypoxic-rearing extends (or reinitiates) the period during which cortical astrocytes can give rise to new neurons beyond the first postnatal week, presumably contributing to the replenishment of excitatory neurons that has been observed during the recovery from hypoxic injury.[27] Thus, the increased "stem-cell-like" capability of cortical astrocytes in hypoxic mice could be seen as a delay in the normal maturation of astrocytes, from relatively simple cellular elements with wider potential to very specialized cells with much more complex machinery. The existence of a prolonged period of cortical astroglial "stemness" is not limited to the cortex, but a similar phenomenon has been demonstrated in other regions, such as the SVZ and hippocampus.[25,27] Beyond the rodent brain, a recent study of postmortem tissue from prematurely born infants showed increased proliferation of cortical cells expressing the transcription factor Sox2.[28] Because Sox2 is typically expressed in the stem-cell-like subpopulation of astroglia, this suggests that cortical astroglial cells of premature human infants may also show increased stem-cell-like properties; however, whether this reflects a prolonged period of "stemness" as in the rodent model remains to be examined (**Table 1**).

INHIBITORY NEURON MATURATION IN PERINATAL INJURY

In rodents, cortical GABAergic neurons initially depolarize surrounding cells in early postnatal development; however, this decreases steadily until the end of the second postnatal week, when cortical GABAergic neurons make a "switch" to an inhibitory, hyperpolarizing, phenotype.[29,30] Although the details of the necessary and sufficient factors mediating this functional switch of GABAergic cells remain still largely

Table 1
Overview of cortical abnormalities in a rodent model of prematurity and VLBW infants

Cortical Unit	Rodent Hypoxia Model	Humans, VLBW
Excitatory neurons	• Reduced number early after injury[18] • Recovery by adulthood[16,18]	Unknown
Inhibitory neurons	• Persistent "immature" protein expression profile[35] • Decreased cortical GABA content[35]	• Some evidence for delayed expression of proteins associated with "developmental switch"[34] • Decreased cortical GABA signaling[34,55]
Astroglia	• Retention of stem-cell-like, early postnatal developmental properties[27] • Reduction in glutamate transport[27,56]	Unknown
Oligodendrocytes	• Increased "immature protein expression profile" • Functional abnormalities in white matter myelination[20]	• Structural and functional abnormalities in white matter[2,37,57,58]
Connectivity: synapses, networks	Unknown	Disrupted or aberrant connectivity[38–40]

unknown, it is thought to depend on local excitatory activity and involves the regulation of expression levels of the chloride transporters KCC2 and NKCC1. Both transporters colocalize with GABA$_A$ receptors, a ligand-gated ion channel that allows for chloride ion movement across the cell membrane. KCC2 moves chloride ions outside the cell, whereas NKCC1 acts in the opposite direction, increasing chloride intracellular levels. During early stages of embryogenesis, low levels of KCC2 and high levels of NKCC1 contribute to maintain high intracellular concentrations of chloride. At this time, GABA$_A$ receptor activation results in a massive outflow of chloride ions and depolarization of the cell. This mechanism of chloride homeostasis is reversed during postnatal development, because KCC2 up-regulation and NKCC1 down-regulation reverse the chloride gradient across the membrane, so that GABA$_A$ receptor activation results in chloride ion influx and hyperpolarization (for a review, see Refs.[31–33]). This "developmental switch" in GABAergic receptor function from hypo- to hyperpolarizing occurs in the first postnatal week in the rodent brain and during the last trimester of development of the human fetus. As in the rodent, this coincides with a difference in expression levels of KCC2 and NKCC1 in humans, starting at about 20 weeks of gestation and reaching peak levels at 35 weeks. The timing of the maturation of the GABAergic system occurs at precisely the period when VLBW premature infants would be born. Indeed, studies have shown significant perturbation of this developmental process in the premature infant, with decreases in GABA, KCC2, and NKCC1 within the cortex.[34] It has been suggested that these decreases in cortical GABA content and possible alterations of GABAergic function may play a causal role in the increased incidence of several disorders observed within the preterm infant population, including epilepsy, schizophrenia, and autism.[34]

Using the mouse model of postnatal chronic hypoxia, parallel changes in cortical inhibitory neurons were examined. Indeed, the authors have shown that, compared with normoxic controls, there is a significant decrease in parvalbumin (PV)+ GABAergic neurons and GABA content within the cortex of hypoxic-reared mice, and that this is attributable to long-lasting changes in their phenotype and, perhaps, functionality, although the functional question remains to be addressed (**Table 1**).[35]

Coincident with the functional maturation of cortical GABAergic neurons is the up-regulation of calcium-binding proteins, including PV, calretinin, and calbindin. PV+ cortical interneurons make up approximately 50% of the total cortical GABAergic population and are characterized by their fast-spiking capabilities. Distinct from the PV population are neurons that express the growth hormone inhibiting peptide somatostatin (SST). Like PV, SST neurons are born embryonically and migrate from the medial ganglionic eminence to the cortex, where they mature and up-regulate expression of their phenotypic protein markers, PV and SST, respectively. Raising mice under hypoxic conditions significantly decreases the number of cortical and hippocampal neurons that express PV and SST proteins, but not those that express calretinin. Given that levels of GABA, PV, and SST are all decreased in the cortex of hypoxic-reared mice, it stands to reason that there may be simply be less interneurons as compared with normoxic controls, similar to what has been observed in cortical excitatory neurons. However, the authors have not seen group differences in neuronal cell death. Furthermore, using glutamic acid decarboxylase 1 (GAD1)-green fluorescent protein (GFP) transgenic mice, no differences were found in the number of neurons marked by GFP between hypoxic- and normoxic-reared mice. Because GFP in these mice is a pan interneuron marker, allowing for the visualization of all interneurons, regardless of developmental stage, the data suggest that hypoxia did not change the number of interneurons per se, but rather the expression of phenotypic proteins associated with maturation of these cells.[35]

CONNECTIVITY AND CORTICAL NETWORK INTEGRATION IN PERINATAL INJURY

Despite the aforementioned remarkable recovery in cortical volume and excitatory neuron numbers, mice reared in hypoxic conditions continue to show behavioral disturbances on cognitive and emotional measures well into adulthood and long after excitatory neurons have been replenished to normal numbers. Therefore neurobiological perturbations must exist that account for these abnormalities. For example, the mere presence of new excitatory neurons identified through immunohistochemistry does not speak to the functionality of this newly generated cortical population. Electrophysiological recordings of these cells would be necessary to understand their capacity to function within their network. Critical relationships between cortical areas and the targets of descending or ascending connections may form aberrantly because some neurons are born after hypoxic-rearing and therefore considerably later than those born in a normoxic mouse. Moreover, because hypoxia occurs during the critical period when synaptogenesis and synaptic pruning occur in development, it is likely that neuronal connections are perturbed more generally. Disturbed connectivity in premature infants is suggested by abnormal trajectories of white matter growth and by functional connectivity studies. Although alterations in neuronal arborization and synaptic density have not yet been examined in human tissue, decreased arborization and synaptic density have been shown in a sheep model of fetal ischemia.[36–41] In hypoxic mice, connectivity has not been assessed anatomically, but a diffusion tensor imaging study showed perturbations of long-range fiber tracts.[19] Finally, beyond the physical connections themselves, altered functionality of these connections can also contribute to decreased performance; for example, delayed myelination may decrease effective and coordinated neuronal communication with their targets. Again, perturbations in myelination and connectivity may exist in VLBW infants that explain abnormalities in language brain centers and cortical and white matter connectivity observed by functional magnetic resonance imaging and diffusion tensor imaging.[36,38,39,42–44] Importantly, despite the suggestive evidence for abnormal connectivity in the VLBW infant, to date, studies have not examined whether this is also true at a microstructural and functional levels in rodent models of prematurity. Electrophysiological and structural connectivity experiments from imaging to tracing studies will be necessary to explore both connections and their functionality on a level of cell-cell interaction and within larger networks, both regional and beyond.

ABNORMAL DEVELOPMENT OF CORTICAL EXCITATORY/INHIBITORY NETWORKS IN PREMATURITY

Development of cortical connections relies heavily on interactions between excitatory and inhibitory neurons. In mice, excitatory neurons are generated starting from embryonic day 11 (E11) and in humans excitatory neurogenesis in the cerebral cortex has been reported to start around the 7th week of gestation and is completed by the 15th to 18th week of gestation (see **Fig. 1**). Although recent reports have suggested that neurogenesis arising from the SVZ may actually continue until 28 gestational weeks,[28] it is not clear whether this is cortical neurogenesis or whether these cells may migrate to the olfactory bulb. In mouse, inhibitory neurons arise from specific regions of the ventral telencephalon, namely the medial and the caudal ganglionic eminence. In humans, however, a sizable proportion of inhibitory cells may arise, like the excitatory neurons, from dorsal telencephalon.[45] After being generated, interneurons migrate to the cortical primordium, where they integrate with radially migrating excitatory neurons to form local networks, although little is known about how these two events are synchronized and reciprocally regulated.

Interneurons may be grouped into different classes according to their developmental origins, morhological features, expression of specific neuropeptides and calcium-binding proteins, mode of interaction with excitatory neurons, localization with respect to cortical layers, and electrophysiological properties. In this view, excitatory and inhibitory neurons, which are profoundly different with regard to their developmental origin and timing of differentiation, are functionally coupled together to form processing units, named cortical columns. Thus, the birth, migration, and integration of cortical pyramidal neurons and interneurons occur between E11 and E18 in mouse and the first 5 months of gestation in humans (see **Fig. 1**) (for a review, see Ref.[46]). However, neurons do continue to be generated through postnatal life in restricted niches, such as the hippocampal dentate gyrus and in the SVZ, which give rise to new granule neurons and new olfactory interneurons, respectively. Given their vulnerable timing, these processes are likely to be particularly disrupted in the premature infant.

Following neurogenesis, and during the third trimester of gestation in humans and in the first 10 days after birth in rodents, maturational processes of these newly born cells preside. As such, cortical neurons elaborate their axons and dendrites, establish synapses, and, later on, prune back these synapses, presumably to form coherent, specialized networks of activity (see **Fig. 1**). There are unique, area-specific patterns of connectivity, morphology of neurons, and electrophysiological properties. During this time, glial cells—both astrocytes and oligodendrocytes—are being generated and mature their morphology and functional properties, up-regulating proteins associated with a mature glial phenotype, such as glial fibrillary acidic protein and glutamine synthetase in astrocytes and myelin basic protein in oligodendrocytes, while down-regulating vimentin, Sox2, and NG2 (for reviews see Refs.[47–49]). As such, glia also lose their capacity for stem-cell-like activity and "retire" to their mature functional profiles, including regulating neurotransmitter turnover and providing trophic support to surrounding neurons. There is evidence that such maturational process for oligodendrocytes is irreversibly compromised in the chronic perinatak hypoxia mouse model.[20]

Furthermore, inhibitory neurons require an extended period of maturation that in rodents extends into adolescence. During this extended period, neuronal connections and synapses, which are originally produced in excess, are pruned in an activity-dependent way, to lead to mature patterns of connectivity, a process in which glial cells are also thought to substantially contribute. Because the organization of the cerebral cortex into functional modules occurs within narrow critical periods of time, it could be argued that any impairment in generation and maturation of both excitatory and inhibitory neurons as well as glia may have profound consequences on the functional outcome of a given brain region.

HYPOXIC INJURY INDUCES A DELAY IN MATURATION

In the mouse model of chronic perinatal hypoxia it was observed that (1) cortical astrocytes remain in an immature, stem-cell-like state for an extended period of time, and (2) cortical inhibitory neurons show a more immature protein expression profile. These findings might suggest that the cortical milieu of hypoxic-reared mice is developmentally stunted. Although this delay in maturation may well facilitate recovery, allowing for a prolonged period of cortical neurogenesis and synaptic plasticity, these new cells may be impaired in their ability to integrate into functional circuitry, leading to the formation of aberrant patterns of connectivity (**Box 1**).

Unfortunately, it is not yet clear whether this delay in maturation of interneurons and glial cells during the recovery process is adaptive or maladaptive. Most likely, the

---

Box 1
Evidence suggesting that chronic hypoxia induces a delay in cortical maturation

1. Cortical astroglial cells remain pluripotent, show self-renewal several days after hypoxic-rearing (P15), and express stem-cell markers; a phenotype typically restricted to the first postnatal week[26,27]

2. Oligodendrocyte progenitors increase their proliferation and show protein expression profiles that are also consistent with earlier stages of maturation following hypoxic-rearing[20]

3. Cortical interneurons fail to properly up-regulate mature protein expression markers (such as PV and SST) after hypoxic-rearing[35]

4. Interventions that increase cell maturation, such as environmental enrichment, reverse the interneuron deficits[35]

---

prolonged plasticity endangered by the maturation delay is in part beneficial by allowing alternative patterns of connectivity to emerge to compensate for lost functions, and in part deleterious, because it may cause excessive "growth" and delay the establishment of mature patterns of connectivity. Indeed, manipulations that enhance maturational processes ameliorate recovery. One such manipulation is environmental enrichment consisting of both cognitive and physical stimulation. In rodents, this is achieved through the introduction of running wheels and a changing, novel environment of toys and burrowing tubes. Environmental enrichment has been shown to enhance maturational processes (i.e., increasing the complexity of dendritic arbors of newly generated neurons).[50–53] Environmental enrichment of hypoxic-reared mice induced a more mature protein expression profile in cortical interneurons (increased PV and SST expression) and reversed cognitive deficits such that enriched, hypoxic-reared mice were no different from normoxic-reared controls.[21,25] Excitingly, the use of environmental enrichment as a therapeutic intervention also seems valuable in the clinic. Longitudinal studies have shown that environmental factors such as 2-parent households and increased maternal education predict augmented recovery in prematurely born children.[54] Nevertheless, enrichment of infants is time consuming, costly, and sometimes not entirely feasible in the premature infant. Therefore, the underlying factors involved in accelerating maturational processes need to be understood to develop novel, targeted therapeutic options that can be used to intervene early on in the developmental process.

SUMMARY

Animal models of prematurity help us understand the pathophysiology of abnormal development in children suffering from prematurity and its complications, suggesting new treatments. Important insights derived from such models are that the brain react to perinatal insults by long-lasting adaptations, which include increased neurogenesis as well as delayed neuronal and glial maturation. Delayed maturations of neurons and glial cells are thought to be responsible for most of the behavioral deficits.

ACKNOWLEDGMENTS

We acknowledge Laura Ment, Vittorio Gallo, Tamas Horvath, Michael Schwartz, and Joseph Madri for useful discussions, and Allyson Vermaak for technical assistance.

N.S. is the recipient of a postdoctoral fellowship from the Fonds de Recherche en Sante du Quebec (2009–2012) and the Canadian Institute of Health Research (2012-present).

REFERENCES

1. Volpe JJ. Brain injury in premature infants: a complex amalgam of destructive and developmental disturbances. Lancet Neurol 2009;8:110–24.
2. Volpe JJ. Cerebral white matter injury of the premature infant-more common than you think. Pediatrics 2003;112:176–80.
3. Vaccarino FM, Ment LR. Injury and repair in developing brain. Arch Dis Child Fetal Neonatal Ed 2004;89:F190–2.
4. Saigal S, Doyle LW. An overview of mortality and sequelae of preterm birth from infancy to adulthood. Lancet 2008;371:261–9.
5. Martin A, Scahill L, Kratochvil CJ. Pediatric psychopharmacology: principles and practice. 2nd edition. Oxford, New York: Oxford University Press; 2011. p. 810, xxvi.
6. Volpe JJ. Cognitive deficits in premature infants. N Engl J Med 1991;325:276–8.
7. Peterson BS, Vohr B, Staib LH, et al. Regional brain volume abnormalities and long-term cognitive outcome in preterm infants [comment]. JAMA 2000;284: 1939–47.
8. Parker J, Mitchell A, Kalpakidou A, et al. Cerebellar growth and behavioural & neuropsychological outcome in preterm adolescents. Brain 2008;131:1344–51.
9. Nosarti C, Giouroukou E, Micali N, et al. Impaired executive functioning in young adults born very preterm. J Int Neuropsychol Soc 2007;13:571–81.
10. Moore GS, Kneitel AW, Walker CK, et al. Autism risk in small- and large-for-gestational-age infants. Am J Obstet Gynecol 2012;206:314.e1–9.
11. Luu TM, Ment LR, Schneider KC, et al. Lasting effects of preterm birth and neonatal brain hemorrhage at 12 years of age. Pediatrics 2009;123:1037–44.
12. Limperopoulos C. Autism spectrum disorders in survivors of extreme prematurity. Clin Perinatol 2009;36:791–805, vi.
13. Anderson P, Doyle LW, Victorian Infant Collaborative Study Group. Neurobehavioral outcomes of school-age children born extremely low birth weight or very preterm in the 1990s. JAMA 2003;289:3264–72.
14. Allin M, Walshe M, Fern A, et al. Cognitive maturation in preterm and term born adolescents. J Neurol Neurosurg Psychiatry 2008;79:381–6.
15. Luu TM, Vohr BR, Allan W, et al. Evidence for catch-up in cognition and receptive vocabulary among adolescents born very preterm. Pediatrics 2011;128: 313–22.
16. Fagel DM, Ganat Y, Silbereis J, et al. Cortical neurogenesis enhanced by chronic perinatal hypoxia. Exp Neurol 2006;199:77–91.
17. Scafidi J, Fagel DM, Ment LR, et al. Modeling premature brain injury and recovery. Int J Dev Neurosci 2009;27:863–71.
18. Fagel DM, Ganat Y, Cheng E, et al. Fgfr1 is required for cortical regeneration and repair after perinatal hypoxia. J Neurosci 2009;29:1202–11.
19. Chahboune H, Ment LR, Stewart WB, et al. Hypoxic injury during neonatal development in murine brain: correlation between in vivo DTI findings and behavioral assessment. Cereb Cortex 2009;19(12):2891–901.
20. Jablonska B, Scafidi J, Aguirre A, et al. Oligodendrocyte regeneration after neonatal hypoxia requires FoxO1-mediated p27Kip1 expression. J Neurosci 2012;32:14775–93.

21. Douglas RM, Ryu J, Kanaan A, et al. Neuronal death during combined intermittent hypoxia/hypercapnia is due to mitochondrial dysfunction. Am J Physiol Cell Physiol 2010;298:C1594–602.

22. Cai J, Tuong CM, Zhang Y, et al. Mouse intermittent hypoxia mimicking apnoea of prematurity: effects on myelinogenesis and axonal maturation. J Pathol 2012; 226:495–508.

23. Back SA, Riddle A, Dean J, et al. The instrumented fetal sheep as a model of cerebral white matter injury in the premature infant. Neurotherapeutics 2012;9: 359–70.

24. Kinney HC, Volpe JJ. Modeling the encephalopathy of prematurity in animals: the important role of translational research. Neurol Res Int 2012;2012:295389.

25. Salmaso N, Silbereis J, Komitova M, et al. Environmental enrichment increases the GFAP+ stem cell pool and reverses hypoxia-induced cognitive deficits in juvenile mice. J Neurosci 2012;32:8930–9.

26. Laywell E, Rakic P, Kukekov VG, et al. Identification of a multipotent astrocytic stem cell in the immature and adult mouse brain. Proc Natl Acad Sci U S A 2000;97:13883–8.

27. Bi B, Salmaso N, Komitova M, et al. Cortical glial fibrillary acidic protein-positive cells generate neurons after perinatal hypoxic injury. J Neurosci 2011;31:9205–21.

28. Malik S, Vinukonda G, Vose LR, et al. Neurogenesis continues in the third trimester of pregnancy and is suppressed by premature birth. J Neurosci 2013;33:411–23.

29. Ben-Ari Y. Excitatory actions of gaba during development: the nature of the nurture. Nat Rev Neurosci 2002;3:728–39.

30. Owens DF, Kriegstein AR. Is there more to GABA than synaptic inhibition? Nat Rev Neurosci 2002;3:715–27.

31. Ben-Ari Y, Khalilov I, Kahle KT, et al. The GABA excitatory/inhibitory shift in brain maturation and neurological disorders. Neuroscientist 2012;18:467–86.

32. Fiumelli H, Woodin MA. Role of activity-dependent regulation of neuronal chloride homeostasis in development. Curr Opin Neurobiol 2007;17:81–6.

33. Kriegstein AR, Owens DF. GABA may act as a self-limiting trophic factor at developing synapses. Sci STKE 2001;2001:pe1.

34. Robinson S, Mikolaenko I, Thompson I, et al. Loss of cation-chloride cotransporter expression in preterm infants with white matter lesions: implications for the pathogenesis of epilepsy. J Neuropathol Exp Neurol 2010;69:565–72.

35. Komitova M, Xenos D, Salmaso N, et al. Hypoxia-induced developmental delays of inhibitory interneurons are reversed by environmental enrichment in the postnatal mouse forebrain. J Neurosci 2013;33:13375–87.

36. Imai M, Watanabe H, Yasui K, et al. Functional connectivity of the cortex of term and preterm infants and infants with Down's syndrome. Neuroimage 2013 [Epub ahead of print]. Available at: http://www.sciencedirect.com/science/article/pii/S1053811913004278.

37. Pavlova MA, Krageloh-Mann I. Limitations on the developing preterm brain: impact of periventricular white matter lesions on brain connectivity and cognition. Brain 2013;136:998–1011.

38. Ball G, Boardman JP, Aljabar P, et al. The influence of preterm birth on the developing thalamocortical connectome. Cortex 2013;49:1711–21.

39. Lubsen J, Vohr B, Myers E, et al. Microstructural and functional connectivity in the developing preterm brain. Semin Perinatol 2011;35:34–43.

40. Mullen KM, Vohr BR, Katz KH, et al. Preterm birth results in alterations in neural connectivity at age 16 years. Neuroimage 2011;54:2563–70.

41. Dean JM, McClendon E, Hansen K, et al. Prenatal cerebral ischemia disrupts MRI-defined cortical microstructure through disturbances in neuronal arborization. Sci Transl Med 2013;5:168ra7.

42. Smyser CD, Inder TE, Shimony JS, et al. Longitudinal analysis of neural network development in preterm infants. Cereb Cortex 2010;20:2852–62.

43. Myers EH, Hampson M, Vohr B, et al. Functional connectivity to a right hemisphere language center in prematurely born adolescents. Neuroimage 2010; 51:1445–52.

44. Constable RT, Ment LR, Vohr BR, et al. Prematurely born children demonstrate white matter microstructural differences at 12 years of age, relative to term control subjects: an investigation of group and gender effects. Pediatrics 2008;121: 306–16.

45. Letinic K, Zoncu R, Rakic P. Origin of GABAergic neurons in the human neocortex. Nature 2002;417:645–9.

46. Stevens HE, Smith KM, Rash BG, et al. Neural stem cell regulation, fibroblast growth factors, and the developmental origins of neuropsychiatric disorders. Front Neurosci 2010;4. Available at: http://www.ncbi.nlm.nih.gov/pmc/articles/PMC2944667/pdf/fnins-04-00059.pdf.

47. Molofsky AV, Krencik R, Ullian EM, et al. Astrocytes and disease: a neurodevelopmental perspective. Genes Dev 2012;26:891–907.

48. Nishiyama A, Komitova M, Suzuki R, et al. Polydendrocytes (NG2 cells): multifunctional cells with lineage plasticity. Nat Rev Neurosci 2009;10:9–22.

49. Nguyen L, Borgs L, Vandenbosch R, et al. The Yin and Yang of cell cycle progression and differentiation in the oligodendroglial lineage. Ment Retard Dev Disabil Res Rev 2006;12:85–96.

50. Liu N, He S, Yu X. Early natural stimulation through environmental enrichment accelerates neuronal development in the mouse dentate gyrus. PLoS One 2012;7:e30803.

51. Baroncelli L, Braschi C, Spolidoro M, et al. Nurturing brain plasticity: impact of environmental enrichment. Cell Death Differ 2010;17:1092–103.

52. Redila VA, Christie BR. Exercise-induced changes in dendritic structure and complexity in the adult hippocampal dentate gyrus. Neuroscience 2006;137: 1299–307.

53. Eadie BD, Redila VA, Christie BR. Voluntary exercise alters the cytoarchitecture of the adult dentate gyrus by increasing cellular proliferation, dendritic complexity, and spine density. J Comp Neurol 2005;486:39–47.

54. Ment LR, Vohr B, Allan W, et al. Change in cognitive function over time in very low-birth-weight infants. JAMA 2003;289:705–11.

55. Robinson S, Li Q, Dechant A, et al. Neonatal loss of gamma-aminobutyric acid pathway expression after human perinatal brain injury. J Neurosurg 2006;104: 396–408.

56. Raymond M, Li P, Mangin JM, et al. Chronic perinatal hypoxia reduces glutamate-aspartate transporter function in astrocytes through the Janus kinase/signal transducer and activator of transcription pathway. J Neurosci 2011;31:17864–71.

57. Nosarti C, Giouroukou E, Healy E, et al. Grey and white matter distribution in very preterm adolescents mediates neurodevelopmental outcome. Brain 2008;131:205–17.

58. Back SA. Perinatal white matter injury: the changing spectrum of pathology and emerging insights into pathogenetic mechanisms. Ment Retard Dev Disabil Res Rev 2006;12:129–40.

Neurodevelopmental Outcomes of Extremely Preterm Infants

Betty R. Vohr, MD

KEYWORDS

- Extremely preterm • Outcomes • Cognitive • Motor • Sensory

KEY POINTS

- Continued improvements in perinatal and neonatal care continue to be associated with improved survival of extremely preterm infants less than 26 weeks gestation.
- Although there has been some evidence of improvement in neurodevelopmental impairment rates since the 1990s, rates are high and are inversely related to gestational age between 22 and 25 weeks.
- There are significant differences in rates of survival and neurodevelopmental impairment by geographic region and neonatal network related to multiple factors including population characteristics, perinatal/neonatal management, follow-up protocols, assessments, and definitions.

CHALLENGES OF INTERPRETING NEURODEVELOPMENTAL OUTCOME STUDIES

When reviewing a survival or neurodevelopmental outcomes article, several factors that can impact the interpretation of the findings need to be considered. The first is the denominator for the percent of infants with a disability, which can vary from mothers presenting in labor with a live fetus, live births, infants admitted to the neonatal intensive care unit (NICU), infants discharged from the NICU, and infants seen in follow-up. For example, a hypothetical cohort of infants at 23 weeks is reported. In the first study 100 live births are reported and 10% survive, all are seen in follow-up at 24 months, and five have a major impairment. If one relates the follow-up data to live births the impairment rate is 5%, 5% have no major impairment, and 90% are deaths. The death or impairment rate is 95%. However, this may also be reported as major impairment seen in 5 (50%) of 10 of infants evaluated at 24 months. In addition, for greater generalizability, a population-based study (country, region, state) is preferable to multicenter, which is preferable to a single center study. A second variable of importance is the follow-up rate. Greater than 90% is ideal and validity of the

Disclosure Statement: B.R. Vohr has no financial interests to disclose. B.R. Vohr serves on the board of The LENA Research Foundation.

Neonatal Follow-up Program, Women and Infants Hospital, Alpert Medical School of Brown University, 101 Dudley Street, Providence, RI 02905, USA

E-mail address: bvohr@wihri.org

Clin Perinatol 41 (2014) 241–255

http://dx.doi.org/10.1016/j.clp.2013.09.003   **perinatology.theclinics.com**

outcome findings decreases as the lost-to-follow-up increases because of possible biases related to the lost cohort.[1,2] Third, is the time period because of the continually changing management of the NICU infant.[3] In addition, follow-up assessments administered may change by time period and country. Fourth, definitions, particularly of disability and impairment, and degree of severity may vary.

As an example, definitions, assessments, and protocols of neurodevelopmental outcomes for the National Institutes of Child Health and Human Development (NICHD) Neonatal Research Network (NRN) Follow-up Study have been modified between 1993 and 2013. The initial follow-up subject criteria changed from a definition based on birth weight less than 1000 g of any gestational age to a definition based on gestational age less than or equal to 26 6/7 weeks. The change was made recognizing the advantage of a defined gestational age cohort and an effort to focus on the most vulnerable preterm (PT) infants at the limits of viability. Age of evaluation of 18 to 22 months corrected age (CA) was initially chosen because Bayley testing was believed to be reliable and that prolonging the time between discharge and follow-up beyond 18 to 22 months CA would increase the lost to follow-up. As evidence began to accumulate that older age of outcome improved the predictive validity of the neurologic assessment and developmental test scores, a decision was made to change the age of outcome to 22 to 26 months CA for infants born after July 1, 2012.

The NRN used the Bayley Scales of Infant Development (Bayley II)[4] from 1993 to October 2007. A limitation of the Bayley II was that it had two developmental scores: the Mental Developmental Index, a composite of cognitive and language tasks; and the Psychomotor Developmental Index, a composite of fine and gross motor skills. The new Bayley Scales of Infant and Toddler Development, Third Edition (Bayley III),[5] consists of three separate developmental scores: a cognitive composite, a language composite (with receptive and expressive subscores), and a motor composite (with gross and fine motor subscores), in addition to social-emotional and adaptive behavior domains. Mean Bayley III cognitive scores, however, are approximately 12 points higher than mean Bayley II cognitive scores.[3,6] It is not yet entirely clear if the Bayley II underestimated scores or if the Bayley III overestimates scores. Caution is advised when comparing studies using different Bayley tests. In 2012, the NRN modified the threshold definitions for Bayley cognitive and motor impairment to moderate delay (70–84); severe delay (<70); and profound delay (≤54).

Vision and hearing have been more difficult to categorize in terms of severity within the NICHD Network because of a single follow-up visit with limited-access diagnostic tests results. This has resulted in currently categorizing the vision as bilateral blind with corrected vision of less than 20/200 and hearing impairment as permanent hearing loss that does not permit the child to understand directions of the examiner and communicate with or without amplification.

The primary focus of most published outcome reports in infancy is the incidence of moderate to severe neurodevelopmental impairment (NDI), often defined in three categories of cognition, cerebral palsy (CP), and sensory (blindness or hearing impairment). This has been the outcome of interest because of the severity of the impact of severe and combined morbidities. In the NICHD NRN, rates of NDI at 18 to 22 months during the era of testing with the Bayley II were defined as the presence of any of the following: moderate to severe CP, cognitive or motor scores more than 2 standard deviations below the mean on standardized testing, bilateral hearing impairment requiring amplification, or bilateral blindness.[7] The most current definition for NDI includes separate categories of moderate (70–84), severe (55–69 for cognitive and 47–69 for motor), and profound (<55 for cognitive and <47 for motor) impairment for Bayley III scores for infants born after July 1, 2012.

Some studies refer to impairment and some to disability for similar outcomes. Impairment is defined as the consequence of an organ-level injury (brain bleed or periventricular leukomalacia) resulting in CP (World Health Organization Model). Disability refers to the ability to carry out functional tasks (walking) and is defined as occurring at a person or societal level (National Center for Medical Rehabilitation Research). The British Association of Perinatal Medicine/Royal College of Pediatrics and Child Health working group[8] proposed a classification of degrees of disability in 2008. It incorporates motor, cognitive, and speech/language skills in addition to hearing and vision impairments. Main categories are severe and moderate neurodevelopmental disability with subcategories for hearing and vision.

Most outcome studies of premature infants in the 1980s focused on very low birth weight (VLBW) infants (<1501 g) or very PT infants (<34 weeks). However, continued advances in antenatal and perinatal medicine and enhanced neonatal interventions for management of nutrition and respiratory function have resulted in improved survival of extremely low birth weight infants (ELBW) (<1000 g) and extremely PT (EPT) infants (<28 weeks) in the past 20 years, including infants at the limits of viability (22–25 weeks).[9–14] Significant center and region variability in survival and outcome rates remain for infants at the limits of viability and are related to additional factors including the population characteristics, management style, and decisions on whether to resuscitate and initiate intensive care (**Box 1**).[15–17]

Survival and outcome data from different countries are impacted by national or regional guidelines or recommendations. The American Academy of Pediatrics published guidelines in 2010 for withholding resuscitation or discontinuing resuscitation when outcomes include almost certain death or unacceptable levels of morbidity, which includes infants less than 23 weeks or less than 400 g.[18]

SURVIVAL

Survival rates in the early 2000s were approximately 85% for VLBW ($\leq$1500 g) and 70% for ELBW infants. A 2012 NICHD[19] study of infants 404 to 1000 g between 22 weeks and 27 6/7 weeks gestation born in 2002 to 2008 reported a survival rate of 39% for infants of 22 to 24 weeks compared with 81% for infants 25 to 27 weeks gestation. The investigators reported wide center variations in obstetric and neonatal interventions among infants at 22 to 24 weeks gestation, which contributes to survival and outcome.[19,20] Center rates of use of antenatal corticosteroids ranged from 28% to 100%, cesarean section ranged from 13% to 65%, and resuscitation from 30% to 100%.[19] Centers with higher rates of antenatal corticosteroid use had lower rates of death and neonatal morbidities. Tyson and colleagues[21] identified four factors present at birth in addition to gestational age that were associated with improved survival

---

Box 1
Pitfalls in interpretation of developmental outcome studies

- Biased or nonrepresentative study sample
- Variable definitions for disability and severity of disability
- High percent lost to follow-up
- Differences in neonatal management style among centers/regions/countries
- Advances in neonatal care over time
- Revisions in standardized outcome measures

of ELBW infants within the NICHD Neonatal Network: (1) exposure to antenatal steroids, (2) female gender, (3) singleton birth, and (4) higher birth weight per 100 g increment.

There are fewer reports showing survival by week of gestational age at the limits of viability. **Table 1** shows recent reports of survival of infants of 22, 23, 24, and 25 weeks gestation from the United States and abroad with comparisons of time periods ranging for birth years 1992 to 2010. All reflect large regional, national, or multicenter populations. Trends for higher survival rates for more recent years of birth are reported particularly at 23, 24, and 25 weeks along with a survival advantage for infant girls. Survival at 22 weeks overall remains less than 10% and relatively stable except for survival reports from Japan. In a study from the Japanese NRN of infants born 2003 to 2005, 37% of infants at 22 weeks survived.[22] This study reports one death at 22 weeks in the delivery room and the remainder in the NICU. In a second study of Japanese national data for births in 2005, 34% of infants admitted to the NICU at 22 weeks survived.[23] Survival rates since the birth year 2000 range from 19% to 64.5% at 23 weeks, 40% to 77% at 24 weeks, and 66% to 85% at 25 weeks (**Box 2**).

Improvements in survival have not always been accompanied by proportional reductions in the incidence of adverse outcomes.[24] Although EPT infants are at increased risk of multiple neonatal morbidities including intraventricular hemorrhage, ventriculomegaly, and periventricular leukomalacia, these brain insults do not account for all of the impairments seen in this population or the gender disadvantage observed in boys.[25] Active brain development occurs during the second and third trimesters, with neurogenesis, neuronal migration, maturation, apoptosis, and synaptogenesis. Infants, especially EPT infants with immature brains, are at extremely high risk for brain injury during this period of active brain maturation from hypoxia, ischemia, undernutrition, and sepsis, which start a cascade of events that increase the risk of brain injuries that are associated with increased risk of NDI.[26–31]

In addition, there are major differences in rate and characteristics of brain maturation. At term age, EPT infants have reduced gray matter volume and increased cerebrospinal fluid volume when compared with term infants. Major predictors are gestational age and associated white matter injury.[31] In addition, perinatal cerebral white matter injury has deleterious effects on the development of fiber tracts in the cerebral white matter.[32] Compared with male control subjects, PT male subjects have significantly lower white matter volumes in bilateral cingulum, corpus callosum, corticospinal tract, prefrontal cortex, and superior and inferior longitudinal fasciculi; and lower gray matter volumes of prefrontal cortex, basal ganglia, and temporal lobe.[33] Decreased brain volume, microstructure abnormalities, and alterations in neural connectivity associated with low gestational age persist to school age and are associated with learning challenges.[33–37] The current status of cognitive, speech and language, motor, and neurosensory outcomes of these vulnerable EPT infants of 22 to 25 weeks gestation are discussed next.

DEVELOPMENTAL AND COGNITIVE OUTCOMES

The most common impairment seen in PT infants between 18 and 30 months is developmental- cognitive impairment, defined as scores that are more than 2 standard deviations below the mean on standardized cognitive testing. Early developmental-cognitive function of PT children, particularly in the United States, has traditionally been assessed using the Bayley.[4,5] **Table 2** shows the data of five studies with cognitive data reported at ages ranging from 18 to 22 months CA to 5 years. Follow-up rates reported range from 55 % to 92%, with only two studies achieving a follow-up rate

Table 1
Survival rates

Author	Region	Years of Birth	22 wk (%)	23 wk (%)	24 wk (%)	25 wk (%)
Wood et al,[38] 2000	United Kingdom and Ireland	1995	1	11	26	44
Bodeau-Livinec et al,[39] 2008	British Isles	1995	NA	4.2	15.7	29.4
	France	1997–1998		0	11.3	28.9
Doyle et al,[67] 2010 Victoria Infant Collaborative	Australia	1992	0	10	33	51
		1997	7	45	41	59
		2005	5	22	51	77
Field et al,[68] 2008	United Kingdom	1994–2005	0	19	24	52
		2000–2005	0	18	41	63
Mercier et al,[69] 2010	Vermont Oxford	1998–2003	4.5	38.1	63.2	76.5
Tyson et al,[21] 2008 NRN	United States	1998–2003	5	26	56	75
Fellman et al,[70] 2009 Express	Sweden	2004–2007	10	53	67	81
Hintz et al,[24] 2005 NRN	United States	2004–2005	2	22.5	53.5	NA
Ishii et al,[22] 2013 NRN	Japan	2003–2005	37.3	64.5	77.7	85.7
Itabashi et al,[23] 2009 National data	Japan	2005	34	54	77	85
Costeloe et al,[71] 2012 Epicure	United Kingdom	2006	2	19	40	66
Manktelow et al,[72] 2013	United Kingdom	1994–1997	NA	Male 20 / Female 18	Male 45 / Female 44	Male 56 / Female 65
		2008–2010		Male 29 / Female 35	Male 48 / Female 56	Male 73 / Female 67

Abbreviation: NA, not available.

Box 2
Interpreting survival rates

- Survival rates at 22 to 25 weeks vary significantly by region and country
- Survival rates overall improved for infants 23, 24, and 25 weeks gestation born between 1992 and 2012
- Survival rates at 22 weeks of large cohorts in nine studies during the same time period range from 0% to 10%
- Two studies from Japan (2003–2005 and 2005) report survival rates of 37% and 34% at 22 weeks for infants admitted to the NICU

---

greater than 90%. Three studies include both the Bayley II and Bayley III. Two studies combine data for 22 and 23 weeks because of small numbers and only the study from the Japanese NRN shows data at 22 weeks. Ishii and colleagues[22] report that 45.5% of 23-week infants tested at 36 to 42 months on the Kyoto Scale of Psychological Development had a score less than 70. Their overall NDI rate was 52% with a combined death or NDI rate of 80% (60 of 75). All studies except one[38] show decreasing rates of cognitive impairment with increasing gestational age. The highest cognitive impairment rates were reported in the NICHD Network study, which evaluated children at the youngest age (18–22 months CA) with the Bayley II and the lowest rates at 24 to 25 weeks were the children evaluated at the oldest age (6–7 years) with the Kaufman Assessment Battery for Children (K-ABC).[39] The 6 to 7 year outcome cohort, however, has a follow-up rate of 72%.

The assessment of an infant's cognitive function depends on age of the child; their motor, language, and social-emotional development; the language environment to which they are exposed; and services they receive. There are limited data on the speech and language outcomes of infants at the limits of viability. Speech and language impairments, however, are common in premature infants, with delays in the acquisition of expressive language, receptive language processing, and articulation; deficits in phonologic short-term memory; lower intelligence quotients; and lower Bayley scores.[40–45] Meta-analyses of language outcomes of PTs compared with term children have consistently identified significantly increased rates of speech and language delays and impairments.[40,45]

At school age, learning and academic disabilities and challenges are detected in 50% to 70% of children born VLBW. These include relative impairments of executive functioning, visual-motor skills, and memory, especially verbal memory.[30,46,47] In addition, former PT infants who score lower on tests of academic achievement have poor perceptual-organizational skills, difficulty with visual processing tasks, and delays in adaptive functioning compared with normal birth weight peers.[30,46,47] Studies reporting the adolescent and adult outcomes of EPT children are currently not available; however, one might predict that academic challenges will be similar or greater than those experienced by VLBW children.

High-risk infants in good environments have the potential for recovery of cognitive and academic performance with increasing age. In one cohort[48] of 330 ELBW infants, mean Bayley Mental Developmental Index at 20 months was 76 compared with a mean cognitive score of 88 at 8 years, and rate of cognitive impairment dropped from 39% at 20 months to 16% at 8 years. Luu and colleagues[46] reported that higher maternal education, and residing in a two-parent family, were associated with better cognition at age 16, whereas minority status incurred a disadvantage for PT infants less than or equal to 1250 g.

Table 2
Cognitive outcomes

Author	Region/Country	Birth Years	Age	FU Rate (%)	Outcome	22 wk (%)	23 wk (%)	24 wk (%)	25 wk (%)
Wood et al,[38] 2000	United Kingdom and Ireland	1995	30 mo	92	Bayley II 70–84 Bayley II 55–69 Bayley II <55	NA	31 0 27	40 11 19	31 13 17
Bodeau-Livinec et al,[39] 2008 EPICure and EPIPAGE	British Isles and France	1995 1997–1998	6–7 y	72	K-ABC <70 K-ABC <70	a	44.4 0[a]	14 23.1	7.2 11.9
Hintz et al,[56] 2011 NRN	United States	1999–2001 2002–2004	18–22 mo	91–92	Bayley II MDI <70 Bayley II MDI <70	b	58.4 61.8	40.7 47.2	—
Ishii et al,[22] 2013 NRN	Japan	2003–2005	36–42 mo	72	KSPD <70	45.5	32.8	36.6	33.1
Moore et al,[57] 2012 EPICure	United Kingdom	2006	36 mo	55	Bayley II and III Bayley <70	b	31	17	19

Abbreviations: K-ABC, Kaufman Assessment Battery for Children; KSPD, Kyoto Scale of Psychological Development; MDI, Mental Developmental Index; NA, not available.
[a] N, no survivors.
[b] Combined data with 23 weeks.

Table 3
Neuromotor and neurosensory outcomes

Author	Region	Years	Denominator	FU Rate (%)	Age (mo)	Outcome	22 wk (%)	23 wk (%)	24 wk (%)	25 wk (%)
Wood et al,[38] 2000	United Kingdom and Ireland	1995	Live births	92	30	Neuromotor Sev/disability	—	8	12	9
Bodeau-Livinec et al,[39] 2008 EPICure and EPIPAGE	British Isles France	1995 1997–1998	NICU admission	92	30	All CP All CP	NA	12.5 33.3	21.1 12.5	19.9 16.3
Hintz et al,[56] 2011 NRN	United States	1999–2001	NICU survival	91–93	18–22	Mod/severe CP (≥2)	15.6		9.7	—
						NDI	64		45.7	
		2002–2004				Mod/severe CP (≥2)	18.1		13.8	
						NDI	69.9		54.6	
		1999–2001				Hearing: bilateral aided	3.2		1.6	
						Vision: blind both eyes	3.1		1.6	
		2002–2004				Hearing: bilateral aided	4.9		2.9	
						Vision: blind both eyes	4		2	
Ishii et al,[22] 2013 NRN	Japan	2003–2005	NICU admission	72	36–42	All CP	21.7	17.8	8.1	15
						CP GMFCS 4–5	17.4	10.2	5.2	8.5
						NDI	52.2	57	37.3	36.8
						Hearing: bilateral amplification	0	3.4	1.2	1.3
						Vision: blind ≥1 eye	8.7	10.2	3.4	2.2

Moore et al,[57] 2012 EPICure	United Kingdom 2006	NICU survival	55	36			
Serenius et al,[55] 2013 Express	Sweden	2004–2007	Live births 94	Alive at 1 y 30.5			

Outcome				
Mod/severe Motor (≥2)	a	11	9	8
Mod/severe impairment[b]		44	25	26
Hearing severe: profound/not improved with aids	3	0	0	0
Bilateral blind	3	1		0
No disability	0	30	34	44
Mild disability	40	19	33	29
Moderate disability	20	30	21	17
Severe disability	40	21	13	9.9

Abbreviation: NA, not available.
a Combined data for infants at 22 with 23 weeks.
b Moderate = GMFCS 2 and Severe Impairment = GMFCS 3–5.

MOTOR AND CP OUTCOMES

CP is a disorder of movement and posture that involves abnormalities in tone, reflexes, coordination, and movement, delays in motor milestone achievement, and aberration in primitive reflexes that is permanent, but not unchanging and is caused by a nonprogressive interference, lesion, or abnormality of the developing immature brain.[49] It can be further categorized by type (spastic, dyskinetic, or dystonic); topography (number of limbs involved); and descriptors including monoplegia, diplegia, hemiplegia, and quadriplegia. The most common form of CP in former PT infants is spastic diplegia. One of the challenges in comparing data is the method by which examiners classify the severity of CP. Many investigators currently use the Palisano Gross Motor Classification System (GMFCS),[50] which is a functional categorization of levels of gross motor function. The United Kingdom Network of Cerebral Palsy Registers, Surveys and Databases[51,52] defines severe CP by severity of either upper extremity (unable to feed or dress selves) and lower extremity (unable to walk even with assistive aids). Investigators also use the recommendations for classification of CP developed by the British Association of Perinatal Medicine and the National Neonatal Audit Project based in the Royal College of Pediatrics and Child Health.[8]

The rate of CP among ELBW infants at 18 months CA was 15% in an NRN cohort of infants born in 1995 to 1998 with 27% in the category of moderate to severe (GMFCS 2–5).[53] The most common form of CP identified was spastic diplegia, accounting for 40% to 50% of all cases, followed by spastic quadriplegia, and hemiplegia. In a report[54] of ELBW infants less than or equal to 1000 g cared for in an NRN NICU between 1999 and 2001 the stability of a diagnosis of CP between 18 and 30 months CA was 91%.

Table 3 shows CP and motor outcome data reported by gestational age group for infants of 22 to 25 weeks gestation with dates of birth ranging from 1995 to 2007. For most studies there is an inverse relationship between gestational age and rates of CP. Outcome data for infants born at 22 weeks remain limited because of low survival and therefore numbers are frequently bundled with 23 week data. The study by the Japanese NRN[22] for infants born 2003 to 2005 has rates of severe CP (GMFCS 4–5) of 17.4% at 22 weeks with an NDI rate of 57%. The Express study[55] for birth years 2004 to 2007 for infants born at 22 weeks reports no children without disability, 40% mild disability, 20% moderate disability, and 40% severe disability. It remains challenging to make direct comparisons of CP and NDI rates because of varying definitions. The NDI rates for the seven reports[22,38,39,56,57] range from 44% to 70% at 24 weeks, 25% to 54% at 23 weeks, and 26% to 37% at 25 weeks. The findings must be evaluated with caution, noting the variability in enrollment criteria and the follow-up rates.

Although moderate to severe CP is the most disabling motor abnormality associated with prematurity it remains a relatively low incidence morbidity compared with fine and gross motor coordination deficits. Transient dystonia (increased extensor tone and atypical movements) occurs in 21% to 36% of PT infants with a peak incidence at 7 months CA. The presence of transient dystonia in the first year of life increases the risk of later motor problems including CP.[58] Overall, however, PT children have greater difficulty with motor coordination than term children.[59–61] In the past, these children were often labeled as "clumsy" but in recent years the diagnosis of developmental coordination disorder has been used for children with coordination difficulties.[61] Developmental coordination disorder is defined as impairment in motor performance sufficient to produce functional impairment that cannot be otherwise explained by the child's age, cognitive ability, or neurologic or psychiatric diagnosis. Developmental coordination disorder is found in 31% to 34% of VLBW and 50% of ELBW infants.

Box 3
Neurodevelopmental outcomes at 22 to 25 weeks

- Moderate to severe disability rates at 22 and 23 weeks remain greater than 50%
- Death or disability rates of live births at 22 weeks often approach 100%
- Rates of moderate to severe disability are high but decrease at 24 to 25 weeks
- Rates of bilateral deafness and blindness increase with decreasing gestational age at the limits of viability
- Multidisciplinary follow-up, early intervention, and education support services are indicated for all infants of 22 to 25 weeks gestation

---

HEARING AND VISION

Rates of neurosensory disabilities including hearing and impairment are low incidence but have important long-term effects. Both moderate to severe vision and hearing impairment are more common among infants with co-occurring characteristics including male gender, multiple birth, CP, hydrocephalus, and seizures.[62–66] Retinopathy remains a serious morbidity for infants of 22 to 25 weeks gestation.[22,56,57] Rates of blindness and significant hearing impairment are inversely related to gestational age with the highest rates at 22 weeks. Bilateral hearing impairment requiring amplification is reported in 1% to 9% of ELBW infants (**Box 3**).[56,57,64,67]

SUMMARY

Outcomes of EPT infants in adolescence and as adults remain unknown. Current evidence indicates this is a vulnerable population with a spectrum of neurodevelopmental morbidities. On an optimistic note, very PT infants in good environments with access to intervention and support services have the potential for recovery with increasing age. The opportunity for recovery can be facilitated by health care professionals who provide family centered multidisciplinary care and access to needed services for all high-risk PT infants.

REFERENCES

1. Vohr B, O'Shea M, Wright LL. Longitudinal multicenter follow-up of high-risk infants: why, who, when, and what to assess. Semin Perinatol 2003;27(4):333–42.
2. Castro L, Yolton K, Haberman B, et al. Bias in reported neurodevelopmental outcomes among extremely low birth weight survivors. Pediatrics 2004;114(2):404–10.
3. Vohr BR, Stephens BE, Higgins RD, et al. Are outcomes of extremely preterm infants improving? Impact of Bayley assessment on outcomes. J Pediatr 2012;161(2):222–8.e3.
4. Bayley N. Bayley Scales of infant development-II. San Antonio (TX): Psychological Corporation; 1993.
5. Bayley N. Bayley Scales of infant and toddler development. 3rd edition. San Antonio (TX): Harcourt Assessment, Inc; 2006.
6. Anderson PJ, De Luca CR, Hutchinson E, et al. Underestimation of developmental delay by the new Bayley-III Scale. Arch Pediatr Adolesc Med 2010; 164(4):352–6.

7. Vohr BR, Wright LL, Poole WK, et al. Neurodevelopmental outcomes of extremely low birth weight infants <32 weeks' gestation between 1993 and 1998. Pediatrics 2005;116(3):635–43.

8. BAPM/RCPCH. Classification of health status at 2 years as a perinatal outcome 2008. Available at: http://www.bapm.org/.

9. Fanaroff AA, Hack M, Walsh MC. The NICHD neonatal research network: changes in practice and outcomes during the first 15 years. Semin Perinatol 2003;27(4):281–7.

10. Hack M, Fanaroff AA. Outcomes of children of extremely low birthweight and gestational age in the 1990s. Semin Neonatol 2000;5(2):89–106.

11. Hintz SR, Kendrick DE, Vohr BR, et al. Changes in neurodevelopmental outcomes at 18 to 22 months' corrected age among infants of less than 25 weeks' gestational age born in 1993-1999. Pediatrics 2005;115(6):1645–51.

12. Wilson-Costello D, Friedman H, Minich N, et al. Improved survival rates with increased neurodevelopmental disability for extremely low birth weight infants in the 1990s. Pediatrics 2005;115(4):997–1003.

13. Emsley HC, Wardle SP, Sims DG, et al. Increased survival and deteriorating developmental outcome in 23 to 25 week old gestation infants, 1990-4 compared with 1984-9. Arch Dis Child Fetal Neonatal Ed 1998;78(2): F99–104.

14. O'Shea TM, Klinepeter KL, Goldstein DJ, et al. Survival and developmental disability in infants with birth weights of 501 to 800 grams, born between 1979 and 1994. Pediatrics 1997;100(6):982–6.

15. Lorenz JM, Paneth N. Treatment decisions for the extremely premature infant. J Pediatr 2000;137(5):593–5.

16. Peerzada JM, Richardson DK, Burns JP. Delivery room decision-making at the threshold of viability. J Pediatr 2004;145(4):492–8.

17. Mercurio MR. The ethics of newborn resuscitation. Semin Perinatol 2009;33(6): 354–63.

18. Kattwinkel J, Perlman JM, Aziz K, et al. Neonatal resuscitation: 2010 American Heart Association Guidelines for Cardiopulmonary Resuscitation and Emergency Cardiovascular Care. Pediatrics 2010;126(5):e1400–13.

19. Smith PB, Ambalavanan N, Li L, et al. Approach to infants born at 22 to 24 weeks' gestation: relationship to outcomes of more-mature infants. Pediatrics 2012;129(6):e1508–16.

20. Vohr BR, Wright LL, Dusick AM, et al. Center differences and outcomes of extremely low birth weight infants. Pediatrics 2004;113(4):781–9.

21. Tyson JE, Parikh NA, Langer J, et al. Intensive care for extreme prematurity: moving beyond gestational age. N Engl J Med 2008;358(16):1672–81.

22. Ishii N, Kono Y, Yonemoto N, et al. Outcomes of infants born at 22 and 23 weeks' gestation. Pediatrics 2013;132(1):62–71.

23. Itabashi K, Horiuchi T, Kusuda S, et al. Mortality rates for extremely low birth weight infants born in Japan in 2005. Pediatrics 2009;123(2):445–50.

24. Hintz SR, Poole WK, Wright LL, et al. Changes in mortality and morbidities among infants born at less than 25 weeks during the post-surfactant era. Arch Dis Child Fetal Neonatal Ed 2005;90(2):F128–33.

25. Reiss AL, Kesler SR, Vohr B, et al. Sex differences in cerebral volumes of 8-year-olds born preterm. J Pediatr 2004;145(2):242–9.

26. Ment LR, Oh W, Ehrenkranz RA, et al. Low-dose indomethacin and prevention of intraventricular hemorrhage: a multicenter randomized trial. Pediatrics 1994; 93(4):543–50.

27. Allan WC, Vohr B, Makuch RW, et al. Antecedents of cerebral palsy in a multi-center trial of indomethacin for intraventricular hemorrhage. Arch Pediatr Adolesc Med 1997;151(6):580–5.
28. Vohr B, Ment LR. Intraventricular hemorrhage in the preterm infant. Early Hum Dev 1996;44(1):1–16.
29. Ment LR, Allan WC, Makuch RW, et al. Grade 3 to 4 intraventricular hemorrhage and Bayley scores predict outcome. Pediatrics 2005;116(6):1597–8 [author reply: 1598].
30. Luu TM, Ment LR, Schneider KC, et al. Lasting effects of preterm birth and neonatal brain hemorrhage at 12 years of age. Pediatrics 2009;123(3):1037–44.
31. Inder TE, Warfield SK, Wang H, et al. Abnormal cerebral structure is present at term in premature infants. Pediatrics 2005;115(2):286–94.
32. Huppi PS, Murphy B, Maier SE, et al. Microstructural brain development after perinatal cerebral white matter injury assessed by diffusion tensor magnetic resonance imaging. Pediatrics 2001;107(3):455–60.
33. Kesler SR, Reiss AL, Vohr B, et al. Brain volume reductions within multiple cognitive systems in male preterm children at age twelve. J Pediatr 2008;152(4): 513–20, 520.e1.
34. Kesler SR, Ment LR, Vohr B, et al. Volumetric analysis of regional cerebral development in preterm children. Pediatr Neurol 2004;31(5):318–25.
35. Ment LR, Peterson BS, Vohr B, et al. Cortical recruitment patterns in children born prematurely compared with control subjects during a passive listening functional magnetic resonance imaging task. J Pediatr 2006;149(4):490–8.
36. Constable RT, Ment LR, Vohr BR, et al. Prematurely born children demonstrate white matter microstructural differences at 12 years of age, relative to term control subjects: an investigation of group and gender effects. Pediatrics 2008; 121(2):306–16.
37. Gozzo Y, Vohr B, Lacadie C, et al. Alterations in neural connectivity in preterm children at school age. Neuroimage 2009;48(2):458–63.
38. Wood NS, Marlow N, Costeloe K, et al. Neurologic and developmental disability after extremely preterm birth. EPICure Study Group. N Engl J Med 2000;343(6): 378–84.
39. Bodeau-Livinec F, Marlow N, Ancel PY, et al. Impact of intensive care practices on short-term and long-term outcomes for extremely preterm infants: comparison between the British Isles and France. Pediatrics 2008;122(5): e1014–21.
40. Barre N, Morgan A, Doyle LW, et al. Language abilities in children who were very preterm and/or very low birth weight: a meta-analysis. J Pediatr 2011;158(5): 766–74.e1.
41. Foster-Cohen SH, Friesen MD, Champion PR, et al. High prevalence/low severity language delay in preschool children born very preterm. J Dev Behav Pediatr 2010;31(8):658–67.
42. Ortiz-Mantilla S, Choudhury N, Leevers H, et al. Understanding language and cognitive deficits in very low birth weight children. Dev Psychobiol 2008;50(2): 107–26.
43. Luu TM, Vohr BR, Schneider KC, et al. Trajectories of receptive language development from 3 to 12 years of age for very preterm children. Pediatrics 2009; 124(1):333–41.
44. Luu TM, Vohr BR, Allan W, et al. Evidence for catch-up in cognition and receptive vocabulary among adolescents born very preterm. Pediatrics 2011;128(2): 313–22.

45. van Noort-van der Spek IL, Franken MC, Weisglas-Kuperus N. Language functions in preterm-born children: a systematic review and meta-analysis. Pediatrics 2012;129(4):745–54.
46. Luu TM, Ment L, Allan W, et al. Executive and memory function in adolescents born very preterm. Pediatrics 2011;127(3):e639–46.
47. Peterson J, Taylor HG, Minich N, et al. Subnormal head circumference in very low birth weight children: neonatal correlates and school-age consequences. Early Hum Dev 2006;82(5):325–34.
48. Hack M, Taylor HG, Drotar D, et al. Poor predictive validity of the Bayley Scales of infant development for cognitive function of extremely low birth weight children at school age. Pediatrics 2005;116(2):333–41.
49. Fawke J. Neurological outcomes following preterm birth. Semin Fetal Neonatal Med 2007;12(5):374–82.
50. Palisano RJ, Hanna SE, Rosenbaum PL, et al. Validation of a model of gross motor function for children with cerebral palsy. Phys Ther 2000;80(10):974–85.
51. Surman G, Bonellie S, Chalmers J, et al. UKCP: a collaborative network of cerebral palsy registers in the United Kingdom. J Public Health (Oxf) 2006;28(2):148–56.
52. Surman G, da Silva AA, Kurinczuk JJ. Cerebral palsy registers and high-quality data: an evaluation of completeness of the 4Child register using capture-recapture techniques. Child Care Health Dev 2012;38(1):98–107.
53. Vohr BR, Msall ME, Wilson D, et al. Spectrum of gross motor function in extremely low birth weight children with cerebral palsy at 18 months of age. Pediatrics 2005;116(1):123–9.
54. Peralta-Carcelen M, Moses M, Adams-Chapman I, et al. Stability of neuromotor outcomes at 18 and 30 months of age after extremely low birth weight status. Pediatrics 2009;123(5):e887–95.
55. Serenius F, Kallen K, Blennow M, et al. Neurodevelopmental outcome in extremely preterm infants at 2.5 years after active perinatal care in Sweden. JAMA 2013;309(17):1810–20.
56. Hintz SR, Kendrick DE, Wilson-Costello DE, et al. Early-childhood neurodevelopmental outcomes are not improving for infants born at <25 weeks' gestational age. Pediatrics 2011;127(1):62–70.
57. Moore T, Hennessy EM, Myles J, et al. Neurological and developmental outcome in extremely preterm children born in England in 1995 and 2006: the EPICure studies. BMJ 2012;345:e7961.
58. Pedersen SJ, Sommerfelt K, Markestad T. Early motor development of premature infants with birthweight less than 2000 grams. Acta Paediatr 2000;89(12):1456–61.
59. Burns YR, Danks M, O'Callaghan MJ, et al. Motor coordination difficulties and physical fitness of extremely-low-birthweight children. Dev Med Child Neurol 2009;51(2):136–42.
60. Marlow N, Hennessy EM, Bracewell MA, et al. Motor and executive function at 6 years of age after extremely preterm birth. Pediatrics 2007;120(4):793–804.
61. Edwards J, Berube M, Erlandson K, et al. Developmental coordination disorder in school-aged children born very preterm and/or at very low birth weight: a systematic review. J Dev Behav Pediatr 2011;32(9):678–87.
62. Vohr BR, Tyson JE, Wright LL, et al. Maternal age, multiple birth, and extremely low birth weight infants. J Pediatr 2009;154(4):498–503.e2.
63. Adams-Chapman I, Hansen NI, Stoll BJ, et al. Neurodevelopmental outcome of extremely low birth weight infants with posthemorrhagic hydrocephalus requiring shunt insertion. Pediatrics 2008;121(5):e1167–77.

64. Synnes AR, Anson S, Baum J, et al. Incidence and pattern of hearing impairment in children with </= 800 g birthweight in British Columbia, Canada. Acta Paediatr 2012;101(2):e48–54.
65. Davis AS, Hintz SR, Van Meurs KP, et al. Seizures in extremely low birth weight infants are associated with adverse outcome. J Pediatr 2010;157(5):720–5.e2.
66. Hintz SR, Kendrick DE, Vohr BR, et al. Gender differences in neurodevelopmental outcomes among extremely preterm, extremely-low-birthweight infants. Acta Paediatr 2006;95(10):1239–48.
67. Doyle LW, Roberts G, Anderson PJ. Outcomes at age 2 years of infants <28 weeks' gestational age born in Victoria in 2005. J Pediatr 2010;156(1):49–53.e1.
68. Field DJ, Dorling JS, Manktelow BN, et al. Survival of extremely premature babies in a geographically defined population: prospective cohort study of 1994-9 compared with 2000-5. BMJ 2008;336(7655):1221–3.
69. Mercier CE, Dunn MS, Ferrelli KR, et al. Neurodevelopmental outcome of extremely low birth weight infants from the Vermont Oxford network: 1998-2003. Neonatology 2010;97(4):329–38.
70. Fellman V, Hellstrom-Westas L, Norman M, et al. One-year survival of extremely preterm infants after active perinatal care in Sweden. JAMA 2009;301(21):2225–33.
71. Costeloe KL, Hennessy EM, Haider S, et al. Short term outcomes after extreme preterm birth in England: comparison of two birth cohorts in 1995 and 2006 (the EPICure studies). BMJ 2012;345:e7976.
72. Manktelow BN, Seaton SE, Field DJ, et al. Population-based estimates of in-unit survival for very preterm infants. Pediatrics 2013;131(2):e425–32.

The Role of Neuroimaging in Predicting Neurodevelopmental Outcomes of Preterm Neonates

Soo Hyun Kwon, MD[a,1], Lana Vasung, MD, PhD[b,1], Laura R. Ment, MD[a,c], Petra S. Huppi, MD, PhD[b,*]

KEYWORDS

- MRI • DTI • fMRI • Preterm brain injury • Periventricular leukomalacia
- Neurodevelopmental outcome • White matter injury • DEHSI

KEY POINTS

- Neurodevelopmental outcomes of prematurely born children can be predicted using the conventional and sophisticated magnetic resonance imaging (MRI) techniques at birth and at term-equivalent age.
- Neurodevelopmental disabilities observed in preterm infants encompass a wide spectrum of deficits, ranging from motor and cognitive deficits, to behavioral and psychological problems.
- MRI is a noninvasive mode of neuroimaging that is superior to ultrasound and currently the best imaging tool available for outcome prediction of children born prematurely.

INTRODUCTION

One of the greatest concerns regarding preterm birth is the association between prematurity and impaired neurodevelopmental outcomes. Despite advances in both obstetric and neonatal strategies to prevent adverse health outcomes in those born prematurely, neurodevelopmental outcomes have changed little over time.[1–3] The multifactorial nature of neurodevelopment has posed a major challenge to predicting

This work was supported by NIH, NS053865 and NS074022 (L.R. Ment), T32 NIH HD07094 (S.H. Kwon), SNF33CM30_140334 (P.S. Huppi and L. Vasung), and 32473B_135817 (P.S. Huppi).
[a] Department of Pediatrics, Yale University School of Medicine, 1 Park Street, West Pavilion, New Haven, CT 06510, USA; [b] The Division of Development and Growth, Department of Paediatrics, Children's Hospital Geneva, 6 rue Willy Donzé, 1211 Geneva, Switzerland; [c] Department of Pediatric Neurology, Yale University School of Medicine, 1 Park Street, West Pavilion, New Haven, CT 06510, USA
[1] These authors contributed equally to this work.
* Corresponding author. Service du développement et de la croissance, Department de l'enfant et de l'adolesecent, Hopitaux Universitaires de Genève, 6 rue Willy Donzé, 1211 Genève, Switzerland.
E-mail address: petra.huppi@hcuge.ch

Clin Perinatol 41 (2014) 257–283
http://dx.doi.org/10.1016/j.clp.2013.10.003

long-term cognitive and behavioral outcomes in this population.[1,4] Cranial ultrasonography (cUS) is used widely in neonatal intensive care units to detect abnormalities in an effort to make predictions regarding neurodevelopmental outcomes, but this imaging modality has proved to be limited in its predictive value for both clinicians and families.[5] Given that survival of those who are at greatest risk of adverse neurodevelopmental outcomes have markedly increased through the years,[1,3] physicians and scientists must continually strive to improve the assessment of those at greatest risk and the ability to predict long-term neurodevelopmental outcomes at school age and in young adulthood.

Neurodevelopmental disabilities observed in preterm infants encompass a wide spectrum of deficits, ranging from motor and cognitive deficits to behavioral and psychological problems.[1] These morbidities have important public health, economic, and societal implications worldwide. In addition, the emotional burden to parents and families with preterm children in the immediate neonatal period and their overall quality of life through childhood, adolescence, and adulthood are more difficult to measure, but are nonetheless present.[6–8]

In order to best target interventions to prevent and/or treat these adverse neurodevelopmental sequelae in those at risk and most vulnerable, clinicians must be able to better identify high-risk preterm infants and better prognosticate neurodevelopmental outcomes using the clinical tools available. This article addresses the role of magnetic resonance (MR) imaging (MRI) in the prediction of neurodevelopmental outcomes in preterm infants and explores the usefulness of state-of-the-art MR strategies to better prognosticate these critical data.

STANDARD OF CARE: CRANIAL ULTRASONOGRAPHY

The most prevalent imaging technique in the neonatal intensive care unit is cranial ultrasonography.[9–11] Compared with MRI scans, there are many advantages to the use of cUS in neonates, including ease of use at the bedside, ability to perform serial studies, as well as cost.[10] cUS is sensitive in detecting intraventricular hemorrhage (IVH), ventriculomegaly, and focal cystic periventricular leukomalacia (PVL), but has significantly lower sensitivity in detecting white matter injury, especially compared with MRI.[12–17] For this reason, the results of studies assessing the value of cUS to predict both short-term and long-term neurodevelopmental outcomes have been widely variable.[5]

CONVENTIONAL MRI

MRI is a noninvasive neuroimaging modality that is able to provide anatomic detail of the developing brain without radiation. There have been significant advances in MRI technology but, even with improvements in neuroimaging with MR, there have been many challenges to its use in the neonatal population. Some of the practical barriers to its use in neonates have been the cost of MRI, equipment compatibility with the magnet, perception of the need for sedation, as well as general accessibility issues compared with bedside cUS, including transport to MRI and the overall stability of critically ill neonates to leave the neonatal intensive care unit.[15] However, with the development of MR-compatible incubators, imaging of the more critical neonates can be done in a safe, thermoregulated, and appropriate environment with continuous cardiorespiratory monitoring.[18,19] In addition, the use of neonatal head coils, neonate-specific MR protocols, and motion artifact correction have improved contrast and resulted in decreased scan times, improved image resolution and quality,[19–21] and obviated sedation during the MRI scan.[19,22,23]

With growing demand and increased usefulness in antenatal diagnosis and the acute neonatal setting, neonatal brain MRI is becoming standard clinical care in tertiary medical centers.[21,24] For neonates with hypoxic-ischemic encephalopathy who receive therapeutic hypothermia, MRI to delineate patterns of injury and predict neurodevelopmental outcomes has recently been recommended as standard of care.[25]

The usefulness of MRI in assessing preterm brain development and injury and predicting long-term neurodevelopmental outcomes for the very preterm population is less well proved. Nonetheless, as advancements in technology and continued research has shown that MRI in the neonatal population is feasible, the use at term-equivalent age to predict neurodevelopmental outcomes in the preterm population may soon become better defined.

MRI Sequences

Conventional MRI provides high-resolution images of the neonatal brain, offering greater anatomic details of the macrostructure and differentiation of gray and white matter than cUS. Neonatal MRI sequences and protocols vary with institutions, but typically include T1-weighted and T2-weighted images, diffusion-weighted imaging (DWI), susceptibility-weighted imaging (SWI), and less commonly fluid attenuated inversion recovery (FLAIR).[26–29] Quick brain MRI is an additional type of imaging protocol that was initially introduced for use in children with shunt-dependent hydrocephalus because of the short acquisition times,[30] but, given its poor contrast resolution and its limited ability to provide detailed images of preterm patterns of brain injury, it should not be used when imaging preterm neonates.

T1-weighted and T2-weighted images provide information on macrostructure of the brain, including anatomy, morphology, and volume. FLAIR images are T2-weighted with suppression of the cerebrospinal fluid (CSF) signal. This pulse sequence is used to null signal from fluids.[31] DWI images provide evidence for acute injury. In addition, SWI images reveal earlier hemorrhage, which may not be routinely seen on T1 and T2 studies of developing brain. For a summary of common MRI sequences used for neonates, refer to **Table 1**.

MRI and Neurodevelopmental Outcomes

Although it has been shown that MRI provides more comprehensive information of the neonatal brain structure, including more subtle abnormalities unable to be detected on cUS, the clinical implications of these findings require standardization, validation, and long-term follow-up. There have been numerous studies that have evaluated the ability of MRI at term-equivalent age to predict neurodevelopmental outcomes at 12 months to 9 years.[13,14,32–50] The studies with more recent cohorts, large sample sizes, and quantitative predictive data are summarized in **Table 2**.

White matter abnormalities

The most extensively studied MRI abnormalities shown to predict neurodevelopmental outcomes are white matter lesions. Types of white matter abnormalities have included periventricular leukomalacia, punctate white matter lesions (PWML), and diffuse excessive high signal intensities (DEHSI). The cause of these entities has yet to be completely understood. With regard to PVL and PWML, it is unclear whether they represent a spectrum of 1 disorder or separate entities with different causes, but they both correlate with long-term neurodevelopmental outcomes. In contrast, DEHSI (**Fig. 1**) have been shown in recent studies to not correlate with long-term outcomes[32–35,44,51,52] despite earlier studies associating it with neurodevelopmental

Table 1
MRI strategies

Standard MR Techniques	Description	Clinical Uses
T1-weighted and T2-weighted images	Used for qualitative image assessment. T1-weighted and T2-weighted images are MRI images that are designed to distinguish tissues with differing T1/T2 relaxation times and evaluate macroscopic changes in lesions and tissues, including sulci, ventricles, cysts	Detects brain malformations, intracranial hemorrhage, ischemic-hypoxic injury, GM and WM changes, ventriculomegaly, or atrophy.[123,124] T1 is best for evaluation of basal ganglia, thalamus, and posterior limb of internal capsule.[29] T2 can evaluate myelination and detect early ischemic change and focal WM injury.[123,124] Can also evaluate tissue volumes
SWI	Detects blood, iron, and calcifications within the brain[125]	Evaluates traumatic brain injury, coagulopathies, or other hemorrhagic disorders, vascular malformations, infarction, neoplasms, and neurodegenerative disorders[26]
DWI and ADC	Measures random motion of water in tissue and quantified as ADC[126]	Useful for early identification of arterial infarction[29,127]

Research MR Techniques	Description	Clinical Uses
Three-dimensional volumetric	Allows measurement of whole-brain volume as well as volumes of specific structures, ventricles, and cerebellum	Used for absolute quantification of brain structures and detection of deviations in normal volumes of tissues
DTI	Measures water diffusion along axis that coincides with fiber tracts and quantified as FA. Used to identify and map WM tracts[128]	Used to generate tractography data to evaluate fiber tracts. Color-coded FA map shows directionality of fibers. Can reveal premyelination[129]
fMRI	Detects changes in signals in spatially distinct regions that are correlated with task-related functional activity or resting state[130]	Can relate functional connectivity to neurodevelopmental outcomes
MRS	Measures concentrations of metabolites in regions of the brain	Used to study brain cellular metabolism, including metabolic disorders

Abbreviations: ADC, apparent diffusion coefficient; DTI, diffusion tensor imaging; FA, fractional anisotropy; fMRI, functional MRI; GM, gray matter; MRS, MR spectroscopy; WM, white matter.

delay.[52] Furthermore, there is increasing evidence from postmortem human studies showing that DEHSI might represent transient features of developing white matter.[53]

Classic periventricular leukomalacia is a form of white matter injury that is focal and cystic. It usually appears in the zone of periventricular crossroads of pathways,[54] an important anatomic localization relevant for proper ingrowth, outgrowth, and path selection of axonal fibers.[54] It is characterized histologically by coagulative necrosis within the subventricular lamina of the periventricular white matter, leading to the destruction of cellular elements, the formation of cysts (**Fig. 2**), and possibly secondary ventriculomegaly.[55] Possible mechanisms of injury include hypoxia-ischemia or inflammation secondary to infection leading to necrosis.[56]

PWML are nonspecific focal lesions in the white matter on MRI that are also commonly found in preterm infants. They are represented as increased signal on T1-weighted imaging and decreased signal on T2-weighted imaging (**Figs. 3** and **4**), and may histologically reflect petechial hemorrhages, gliotic scarring, mineralization, and more recently foci of activated microglia.[57–60]

The most common outcome measure in studies that try to correlate MRI findings and neurodevelopment outcomes is motor dysfunction, ranging from mild motor delay to severe cerebral palsy. Although the ability of MRI to predict cerebral palsy can be variable, one of the most important observations from past studies is that preterm children without white matter abnormalities on term MRI did not show significant neurodevelopmental deficits compared with full-term controls, specifically with regard to motor[14,35,36,38,40,49] or executive functioning,[46] showing that MRI has a high negative predictive value (NPV). Additional findings from many of these studies are that severity of white matter abnormalities is proportionally related to the severity of impairment.[35,36,40,48]

Compared with infants born term, preterm infants have been shown to have cognitive impairments, requiring special assistance at school.[61–63] White matter abnormalities have been shown in studies to be associated with lower cognition, language abilities, and executive functioning.[13,34–37,41,43,44,46,49]

DEHSI
DEHSI are a frequent finding on T2-weighted MR images (see **Fig. 1**) near term in children born prematurely,[64] seen in up to 80% of preterm infants at term-equivalent age.[33,52] They are hyperintense white matter signal abnormalities in the periventricular and subcortical white matter regions compared with the signal intensity of normal unmyelinated white matter. The cause of DEHSI remains unclear, but, after the finding was initially described by Maalouf and colleagues,[64] there have been theories that it may represent white matter injury in the developing brain and/or signify a maturational delay[53] in the white matter. Although Dyet and colleagues[52] showed that the presence of DEHSI predicted mild developmental delay at up to 36 months, subsequent studies have shown that, in the absence of the other lesions, DEHSI did not correlate with the neurodevelopmental abnormalities measured at 18 months, up to 9 years of age.[13,32–35,44,51]

Gray matter abnormalities
Gray matter (GM) can be assessed for morphology, including cortical folding and surface area, as well as signal abnormalities. GM abnormalities (assessed by size of the subarachnoid space, quality of gyral maturation, and presence of GM cortical signal abnormality) are also associated with poorer neurodevelopmental outcome.[13,42,47,65]

Cerebellar abnormalities
Cerebellar abnormalities have been categorized as destructive lesions versus those representing impaired development. Destructive lesions include cerebellar hemorrhage

Table 2
Prediction of neurodevelopmental outcomes with structural MRI

Study (Birth Years of Cohort)	Subjects (N)	Age at Birth (wk)	Age at Scan (wk)	Follow-up Age	MRI Findings and Outcomes	Odds Ratio	Diagnostic Value					
							CP or Motor Impairment		MDI or FSIQ		NDI	
							PPV	NPV	PPV	NPV	PPV	NPV
GM and WM												
Jeon et al[33] (2004–2008)	126	<32	34–43	18–24 mo	Cystic PVL and PWML were associated with CP	19.6 (CPVL) 90.9 (PWML)	—	—	—	—	—	—
de Bruine et al[34] (2006–2007)	110	<32	40–44	24 mo	PWML and VD predicted motor delay PWML was associated with MDI scores[a]	18.38 (PWML) 4.57 (VD)	0.63§	0.97§	0.25†	0.95†	—	—
Skiold et al[35] (2004–2007)	107	<27	38–41	30 mo	Moderate-severe WM abnormalities associated with CP, lower cognitive and language scores[a]	—	0.5§	0.98§	—	—	—	—
Setanen et al[36] (2001–2006)	217	<32	Term	5 y	Extent of MRI abnormalities predicted neurodevelopmental impairment[b]	—	0.44§	0.99§	0.44	0.92	0.75	0.91
Munck et al[37] (2001–2006)	180	≤1500 g and <37	Term	24 mo	Major abnormalities on MRI were associated with lower MDI and NDI scores[a]	—	0.23¶	0.98¶	0.13	1	—	—

Study	N	GA		Age	Findings						
Spittle et al[40] (2001–2003)	227	<30	38–42	5 y	Severity of WM abnormalities was proportionally related to severity of motor impairment	19.4	0.34§,¶	0.91§,¶	—	—	—	—
Miller et al[78] (1998–2003)	86	<34	31–33	12–18 mo	Moderate-severe abnormalities associated with lower MDI scores[a]	—	—	—	0.31	0.94	—	—
Woodward et al[13] (1998–2000, 2001–2002)	167	<30	38–42	24 mo	WM and GM abnormalities were associated with adverse neurodevelopmental outcomes[a]	3.6 (cognitive delay) 10.3 (motor delay) 9.6 (CP)	0.31§	0.95§	0.31	0.89	—	—
Iwata et al[44] (1995–2001)	76	≤32	38–42	9 y	WM injury predicted low FSIQ,[c] CP, and requirements for special assistance at school GM abnormalities were not associated with any impaired outcome	8.3 (lower IQ) 7.0 (CP)	—	—	—	—	—	—

Abbreviations: CP, cerebral palsy; CPVL, cystic periventricular leukomalacia; CR-CSp, periventricular corona radiate related to corticospinal tract; FSIQ, full-scale intelligence quotient; MDI, mental development index; NDI, neurodevelopmental impairment; NPV, negative predictive value; PPV, positive predictive value; PWML, punctate white matter lesions; VD, ventricular dilatation.

[a] Bayley Scales of Infant and Toddler Development.
[b] Wechsler Preschool and Primary Scale of Intelligence.
[c] Wechsler Intelligence Scale for Children.
§ PPV/NPV for the prediction of outcome of outcome of CP.
¶ Refers to PPV/NPV for the prediction of outcome of outcome of Motor impairment.
† Refers to PPV/NPV of PWML only for the prediction of outcome.

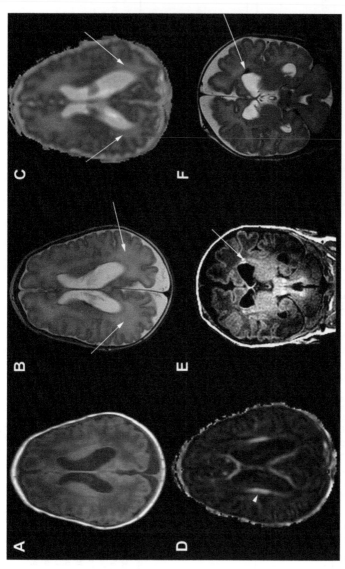

Fig. 1. T1 (*A, E*), T2 (*B, F*), fractional anisotropy (FA) (*D*), and apparent diffusion coefficient (ADC) (C) MRI images of a prematurely born infant (29 GW) at term-equivalent age. Note the DEHSI (*B, arrows*) of centrum semiovale at term-equivalent age. ADC map (C) of corresponding T2 slice (*B*) shows increased ADC values (C, *arrows*) often seen in newborns with moderate WM injury. FA map (*D*) of corresponding slice shows high FA values (*D, arrowhead*) in white matter corresponding with pyramidal tract often correlated with gross and fine motor performance. Moderate to severe white matter injury was defined using the criteria described by Woodward and colleagues[13] taking into account extent of white matter signal abnormality (*B, C, arrows; E, arrow*), periventricular leukomalacia (*E, F, arrows*) with periventricular white matter volume loss and dilatation of ventricles (*E,* asymmetric size of ventricles).

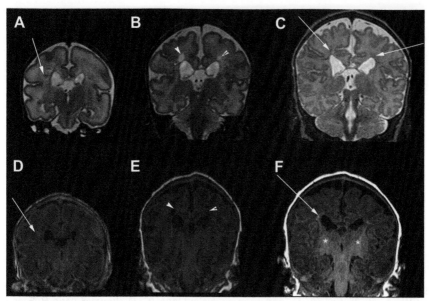

Fig. 2. Longitudinal T1 (*A–C*) and T2 (*D–F*) MRI images of prematurely born infant at birth to 29 GW (*A, E*), 33 GW (*B, E*), and term-equivalent age (*C, F*) showing typical evolution of periventricular leukomalacia. Note the low signal T2 MRI intensity (*A, arrow*) and areas of high T1 MRI signal intensity (*D, arrow*) at birth. Follow-up scan revealed formation of periventricular cysts (*B, E, arrowheads*) hyperintense on T2 (*B, arrowhead*) and hypointense on T1 (*E, arrowhead*) MRI images. At term-equivalent age (*C, F*), periventricular cysts were no longer identifiable, whereas injury of periventricular white matter persisted (low signal T2 MRI intensity (*A, C, arrows*) and areas of high T1 MRI signal intensity (*D, F, arrows*). Note the myelinization (hyperintense T1 MRI signal) of capsula interna (*F, stars*) on T1 MRI images. Clinical follow-up revealed delayed motor development with spastic tetraparesis. At 29 GW, MRI images (*A, D*) were acquired using the Siemens Avanto 1.5-T MRI scanner. T1 MRI images (*A*) were acquired using the following parameters: TR, 2000 milliseconds; TE, 3,12 milliseconds, FA, 15, field of view (FOV), 217 × 217; acquisition matrix, 256 × 230; slice thickness, 1.5 mm. T2 MRI images were acquired using the following parameters: recovery time (TR), 6130 milliseconds; echo time (TE), 125 milliseconds; FA, 150; FOV, 185 × 220; acquisition matrix, 448 × 265; slice thickness, 3.5 mm. At 33 GW and term-equivalent age, MRI images were acquired using 3.0-T Siemens Tim Trio human MRI scanner. T1 MRI images (*B, E*) were acquired using the following parameters: TR, 2200 milliseconds; TE, 2.49 milliseconds; FA, 8; FOV, 137 × 200; acquisition matrix, 256 × 176; slice thickness, 1.2 mm. The acquisition of T2 MRI images used the following parameters: TR, 4600 milliseconds; TE, 150 milliseconds; FA, 150; FOV, 128 × 200; acquisition matrix, 256 × 164; slice thickness, 1.2 mm; GW, weeks of gestation.

and infarction. Cerebellar hemorrhage is usually unilateral and associated with supratentorial lesions, leading to possible cerebellar atrophy with time. Cerebellar infarction is thought be secondary to general ischemia or to a vaso-occlusive event again leading to parenchymal destruction. In contrast, cerebellar underdevelopment has been depicted on MRI as deficits in cerebellar hemispheric volumes that occur bilaterally and symmetrically, often as a consequence of cerebral hemispheric lesions.[66,67]

The incidence and long-term implications of cerebellar injuries were previously under-recognized among premature infants, but, with the increased in use of MRI, cerebellar hemorrhage is increasingly recognized as a preterm pattern of injury.[68,69]

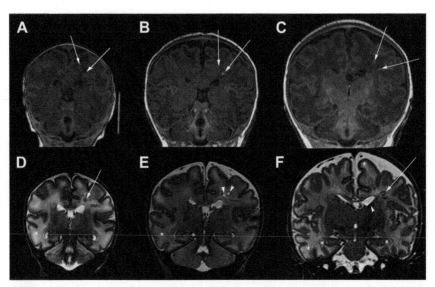

Fig. 3. Longitudinal T1 (*A–C*) and T2 (*D–F*) MRI images of prematurely born infant at birth to 31 GW (*A, E*), 35 GW (*B, E*), and term-equivalent age (*C, F*) showing various signs of moderate-severe white matter injury. Note the different imaging characteristics of white matter injury located in proximity of ventricles. White matter injury with high signal intensity on T1 MRI images (punctate lesions; *A–C, arrows*) and low signal intensity (*D, F, arrowheads*) on T2 MRI images. Because of the substantial destruction of tissue, white matter injury or PVL occasionally leads to formation of periventricular cysts (*E, arrowhead*; high T2 MRI signal intensity). At term-equivalent scan, areas of low T2 signal intensity (*F, arrowhead*) indicate hemorrhage in the ventricular zone and ganglionic eminence (germinal matrix). (*D–F*) Stars show the persistent high T2 signal intensity of the white matter often seen in children born prematurely at term-equivalent age. The clinical examinations in infancy, early childhood, and at school age revealed persistent right-sided hemiplegia. At 31 GW, MRI images (*A, D*) were acquired using the Siemens Avanto 1.5-T MRI scanner. T1 MRI images (*A*) were acquired using the following parameters: TR, 2000 milliseconds; TE, 3.12 milliseconds; FA, 15; FOV, 217 × 217; acquisition matrix, 256 × 230; slice thickness, 1.5 mm. T2 MRI images were acquired using the following parameters: TR, 6130 milliseconds; TE, 125 milliseconds; FA, 150; FOV, 185 × 220; acquisition matrix, 448 × 265; slice thickness, 3,5 mm. At 35 GW and term-equivalent age, MRI images were acquired using 3.0-T Siemens Tim Trio human MRI scanner. T1 MRI images (*B, E*) were acquired using the following parameters: TR, 2200 milliseconds; TE, 2.49 milliseconds; FA, 8; FOV, 137 × 200; acquisition matrix, 256 × 176; slice thickness, 1.2 mm. T2 MRI images were acquired using the following parameters: TR, 4600 milliseconds; TE, 150 milliseconds; FA, 150; FOV, 128 × 200; acquisition matrix, 256 × 164; slice thickness, 1.2 mm; GW, weeks of gestation.

In addition to motor function, the cerebellum is purported to play a role in a range of other important functions in children, such as cognition, learning, and behavior,[70–73] and is related to neurodevelopmental sequelae.[33,74] Because of the recent advent of these findings, there are as yet few follow-up studies of MRI-detected cerebellar injury.[75]

Interpretation of MRI Findings: A Systematic Methodology

Unlike the Papile and colleagues[76] or Volpe[77] classifications, which describe the severity of IVH, there are no uniformly accepted methods to classify the extent of

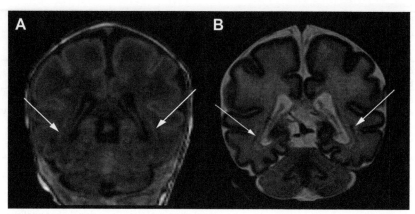

Fig. 4. T1 (*A*) and T2 (*B*) MRI images of infant born at 31 GW and scanned at 33 GW (*A, B*). Note the PWML in the periventricular crossroad of pathways[54] that show high T1 signal intensity (*A, arrows*) and low T2 MRI signal intensity (*B, arrows*). Clinical report at 13 months after birth (corrected age) revealed delayed psychomotor development. At 33 GW, MRI images (*A, B*) were acquired using the Siemens Avanto 1.5-T MRI scanner. T1 MRI images (*A*) were acquired using the following parameters: TR, 2000 milliseconds; TE, 3.12 milliseconds; FA, 15; FOV, 217 × 217; acquisition matrix, 256 × 230; slice thickness, 1.8 mm. T2 MRI images were acquired using the following parameters: TR, 600 milliseconds; TE, 127 milliseconds; FA, 150; FOV, 185 × 220; acquisition matrix, 448 × 227; slice thickness, 2.5 mm; GW, weeks of gestation.

different types of abnormalities on MRI, making interpretation of these findings difficult and subjective. Most importantly, this can impede the prognostic usefulness of MRI. However, with ongoing studies, there have been different classification systems proposed and used for the interpretation of MRI data (refer to **Table 3**).

One of the first evaluation scales to define severity of MR abnormalities and use them to predict long-term neurodevelopmental outcomes was developed by Miller and colleagues.[78] This study graded white matter abnormalities as minimal, moderate, or severe using more objective, predefined criteria of number and size of white matter signal abnormalities, and correlated them with adverse neurodevelopmental outcomes. After defining moderate to severe MRI abnormalities as moderate to severe white matter injury using the white matter abnormality severity scale, any ventriculomegaly (see **Fig. 1**), and/or severe IVH, and adjusting for gestational age at birth, the relative risk of having an abnormal outcome associate with moderate-severe MRI abnormality was 5.3.

Sie and colleagues[49] used a scoring system to compare neonatal MRI findings before 42 weeks' postconceptual age to follow up MRI findings at 18 months of age and relate them to neurodevelopmental outcomes. The study assessed for white matter signal intensity changes, hemorrhagic lesions, and cystic lesions in its score of severity. Severe abnormalities on MRI predicted Psychomotor Developmental Index (PDI) less than 70 with a positive predictive value (PPV) ranging from 0.85 to 1 and cerebral palsy (CP) with a PPV of 1. NPVs for normal PDI (>70) ranged from 0.94 to 1 and near-normal motor development was 1.

Woodward and colleagues[13] described and used a more comprehensive scoring system to define brain abnormalities in preterm infants near term age and related them to neurodevelopmental outcomes. The group used a scoring system to define extent of white matter injuries, which consisted of 5 components (extent of white

Table 3
Scoring systems for preterm MRI

Miller et al,[78] 2005				
Scoring System for WM	Normal	Minimal	Moderate	Severe
WM signal abnormalities	None	≤3 areas (<2 mm) of signal abnormality	>3 areas of signal abnormality or areas <2 mm, but >5% of the hemisphere involved	>5% of the hemisphere involved

Woodward et al,[13] 2006			
Scoring System for WM	Grade 1	Grade 2	Grade 3
WM signal abnormalities	None	≤2 focal regions of signal abnormalities (per hemisphere)	>2 focal regions of signal abnormalities (per hemisphere)
Periventricular WM volume loss	None	Mildly decreased WM volume and mild to moderately dilated ventricles	Markedly decreased WM volume with significantly dilated ventricles and/or extra-axial space
Cystic abnormalities	None	<2-mm single focal cyst	Multiple cysts or single ≥2-mm focal cyst
Ventricular dilatation	None	Moderate enlargement	Global enlargement
Thinning of corpus callosum	None	Focal thinning	Global thinning
Scoring System for GM	**Grade 1**	**Grade 2**	**Grade 3**
GM cortical signal abnormality	Normal	Focal	Extensive
Quality of gyral maturation	Normal for 40 wk	Delay of 2–4 wk in gyral development	Delay of >4 wk in gyral development
Size of the subarachnoid space	Small	Mildly enlarged	Significantly enlarged globally

Overall WM abnormality scores: (1) no abnormality, total score 5 to 6; (2) mild abnormality, total score 7 to 9; (3) moderate abnormality, total score 10 to 12; (4) severe abnormality, total score 13 to 15.
Overall GM abnormality scores: (1) normal, total score 3 to 5; (2) abnormal, total score 6 to 9.

matter signal abnormality including DEHSI, periventricular white matter volume loss, extent of cystic abnormalities, dilatation of ventricles, and thinning of the corpus callosum) that classified the injuries as mild, moderate, or severe.[13,79] A separate scoring system was used to define the extent of GM injuries, which looked at 3 components (extent of GM cortical signal abnormality, quality of gyral maturation, and size of the subarachnoid space). Moderate to severe cerebral white matter abnormalities predicted cognitive delay with an odds ratio (OR) of 3.6, motor delay with an OR of 10.3, and CP with an OR of 9.6. The OR of GM abnormalities in association with severe cognitive delay or CP ranged from 2 to 3.[13]

The scoring systems described earlier have included only assessments of white matter and GM.[13,49,78,79] More recently, Kidokoro and colleagues[80] developed the most comprehensive classification system to assess preterm brain injury and impaired brain growth, but it needs validation in a larger cohort. Although white matter injury has been the most commonly described pattern of injury in MRI, contributing to adverse neurodevelopmental outcomes, more recent studies have investigated the role of cortical GM, deep GM, and cerebellum in MR patterns of preterm brain injury as well as predictors of outcome.[69,81,82] However, the validity of this MRI assessment tool is still uncertain because the cohort used to develop this classification system has yet to complete the neurodevelopmental assessment at 2 years of age.[80]

These scoring systems offer a more objective and comprehensive method to classify magnitude of brain injury in the preterm population, given the wide range of complex MRI abnormalities associated with prematurity, as well as to predict neurodevelopmental outcomes. The development and use of more comprehensive and standardized evaluation criteria will likely lead to improvements in the predictive value of neurodevelopmental outcomes.

Timing of MRI

Both qualitative and quantitative MR techniques have been used to assess the preterm brain at different stages in development, including in the perinatal period, at term-equivalent age, and through childhood into adolescence. Compared with the MRI at the time of birth, the MRI at term-equivalent age remains the optimal scanning time for children born prematurely in the prediction of neurodevelopmental outcomes, given the greater clinical stability of the population at term as well as the success of feed and wrap protocols in obviating sedation. In addition, the most commonly studied timing of MRI scans in the preterm population to predict neurodevelopmental outcomes is term-equivalent age. However, there have been some studies investigating the correlation between serial MRI and neurodevelopmental outcomes, assessing changes in findings over time.

Dyet and colleagues[52] performed early and term MRI scans on infants born at less than 30 weeks' gestation (GW). Early MRIs were performed soon after birth, depending on clinical stability, and term MRIs were done at 36 weeks or later. Major destructive lesions, including cerebellar hemorrhage, were related to poorer neurodevelopmental outcomes in early scans. Findings on MRI at term age including posthemorrhagic ventricular dilatation and white matter injury also correlated with reduced developmental quotients.[52]

Miller and colleagues[78] performed MRI scans on infants at less than 34 weeks' gestation and correlated MRI findings at 31 to 33 weeks' gestation (when stable for transport to MRI) with 18-month neurodevelopmental outcomes. An MRI was repeated in a proportion of the same cohort at 35 to 38 weeks' corrected gestational age. This study showed that the degree of severity of adverse outcomes was related to the extent of white matter injury, ventriculomegaly, and IVH, and the risk of abnormal outcome was significantly associated with moderate to severe abnormalities on the early MRI with a relative risk (RR) of 5.6 and term MRI with an RR of 5.3.

COMPARISON OF CUS AND MR STRATEGIES

Compared with cUS, brain MRI provides more information regarding the full spectrum of injury to the developing brain. Although excellent for the detection of IVH, ventriculomegaly and cystic PVL, cUS is less able to detect cortical abnormalities, posterior fossa lesions, and more subtle white matter injury.[5,12–15,68] For these reasons, most studies that compare cranial ultrasound with MRI in the prediction of neurodevelopmental outcomes have shown that MRI is superior to cranial ultrasound in the detection of white matter injury.[5,12–15]

Review of those studies directly comparing cUS with MRI in the same cohort with CP as the outcome shows that both the PPV and NPV of MRI tend to be similar or higher compared with cUS.[83] Abnormalities on MRI were better able to predict CP in some studies with PPV of 0.9 versus 0.57 (for cUS),[50] 0.44 versus 0.73,[84] and 0.33 versus 0.6.[14] These studies showed increase in sensitivities for detection of future CP when using MRI compared with cUS: from 0.67 (using cUS) to 0.82 (using MRI),[50] 0.18 to 0.65,[13] and 0.43 to 0.86.[14]

In contrast, when comparing predictive values of cUS with MRI in the same cohort for cognitive outcomes, Woodward and colleagues[13] predicted severe cognitive delay with similar PPV and NPV with the two imaging modalities, but MRI had a higher sensitivity (0.41 vs 0.15) for severe cognitive delay on cUS but slightly lower specificities of 0.84 on MRI versus 0.95 on cUS.

PROMISING NEW MRI STRATEGIES

The development of sophisticated new MRI strategies has permitted a better understanding of corticogenesis in the prematurely born. Furthermore, data from many of these strategies, including volumetric imaging, diffusion tensor imaging, MR spectroscopy (MRS) and functional connectivity, has been shown to correlate with cognitive measures in preterm subjects at school age, adolescence, and young adulthood.

These strategies are described later, and the published neonatal outcome data are available. Although these studies do not represent the predictive usefulness of volumetric MRI in terms of PPV/NPV or sensitivity/specificity, the outcome data generated from each are presented in **Table 4**.

Volumetric Imaging

Volumetric analysis uses two-dimensional or three-dimensional MR images to quantitatively characterize alterations of brain development associated with prematurity and brain injury. It allows the measurement of the volume of specific brain structures, including the cortical and subcortical regions, cerebellum, and hippocampus.[85,86] Automated segmentation techniques can be used to differentiate GM and white matter as well as unmyelinated and myelinated tissue.[86–89]

Volume reductions in the whole brain, anatomic structures in the brain, and regions within white matter and cortical GM have been reported in preterm infants.[8,90–104] In addition, simple brain metric measurements using MRI as a method to assess brain growth and atrophy in neonates has been shown to correlate with outcome,[102] whereas more sophisticated methods, like surface reconstruction and sulcation index, allow more detailed insight into longitudinal maturation. Appearance of cortical convolutions follows the spatiotemporal schedule and is indirect marker of spatiotemporal and gender differences in brain maturation.[105] Dubois and colleagues[105] reported that sulcation of the cortex of preterm-born children starts in central regions and progresses in occipitorostral direction with frontal cortical regions being the last ones to convolute. The discrepancies in sulcation index between boys and girls, relative to the white matter and GM volume, seem to be early markers of gender dimorphism, whereas hemispheric differences (right hemisphere having greater cortical complexity earlier then left) is in agreement with the assumption that the left hemisphere is less under genetic control and more influenced by the in utero environment.[105] Furthermore, although the sulcation of the cortex depends on factors such as gender or region, there is recent evidence that mild white matter injury also influences the cortical complexity during early development. Dubois and colleagues[105] calculated the sulcation index at birth in 2 groups: children born prematurely with moderate white matter injury and prematurely born children without signs of white matter injury. Their results showed that children born prematurely with evidence of moderate white matter injury at birth have increased sulcation in the areas of the central sulcus and frontal lobe indicating an alteration of subsequent cortical development, probably caused by similar mechanisms involved in fetal white matter lesion–associated polymicrogyria.[63,105]

Although the volume estimation at term-equivalent age of various anatomic tissues has been shown to be a useful predictor of long-term outcome, measurements of volume and cortical surface or sulcation index at birth were recently shown to be correlated with early functional outcome at term.[62] For equivalent time interval, larger surfaces at birth implied more mature neurofunctional scores at term.[62]

Decreased volumes, either within whole brain, within anatomic structures, or within GM or white matter, have been associated with markers of outcome. Smaller brain volume at term-equivalent age, when correcting for effects of white matter injury, is correlated with subsequent performance on object working memory tasks in infancy.[104] Subsequent working memory performance in infancy was also shown to be associated with reductions in volumes of dorsolateral prefrontal, sensory, motor, parieto-occipital, and premotor cortex.[104] Tan and colleagues[95] showed that brain volume is closely related to the mental outcome in the first year. Total white matter volumes in sensory, motor, and midtemporal regions at term-equivalent age are strong predictors of neurodevelopmental outcome in the first year of life.[106] Both Inder and colleagues[107] and Gadin and colleagues[90] showed that the overall GM volume at term predicts neurodevelopmental outcome, whereas Boardman and colleagues[99] showed association between decreased volumes of deep GM and neurocognitive outcome. The volume at term-equivalent age of cerebellum,[97,108] the size of ventricles[109] with presence of white matter injury and volume of brain stem[103] are also good predictors of poorer neurodevelopmental outcome in first years of life.

Diffusion Tensor Imaging

Assessing the microstructural development of the white matter and GM in prematurely born infants has become feasible with the recent advances in diffusion tensor imaging. Diffusion tensor imaging (DTI) relies on water motion providing the useful parameters for describing the underlying microstructure. Measure of fractional anisotropy (FA) describes the degree to which water diffusion is restricted in one direction relative to all others, whereas the measure of apparent diffusion coefficient (ADC) describes overall magnitude of diffusion with the single scalar value. During normal development, FA values of the white matter increase and ADC values decrease. Thus, white matter injury is often marked at term-equivalent age by high T2 signal intensities (see **Fig. 1**B) in areas that additionally show persistently high values of ADC (see **Fig. 1**C) and lower values of FA.

FA values of major white matter tracts were correlated with gross and fine motor performance. Lower FA in regions of corpus callosum, at term-equivalent age, was shown to correlate with the psychomotor developmental index.[110,111] Furthermore, the lower values of FA at term in the posterior limb of the internal capsule were associated with neurodevelopmental outcomes in the first year of life. Follow-up of children with abnormal neurologic examinations in the first year of life showed decreased FA values in the posterior limb of the internal capsule at term age when measured retrospectively.[112] In addition, FA of the optic radiation correlated with visual function.[113,114]

Functional MRI

Functional MRI (fMRI) uses deoxygenated hemoglobin in the body as an endogenous contrast agent to produce a blood oxygenation level–dependent (BOLD) signal. This

Table 4
Prediction of neurodevelopmental outcomes with advanced MRI

Study (y)	Subjects (No)	Age at Birth (wk)	Age at Scan (wk)	Follow-up Age	MRI Findings and Outcomes
Volumetric					
Gadin et al[90] (2007–2009)	20	<30	36 to discharge	6 mo	Decreased subcortical GM volume was associated with low PDI[a] (P = .03)
van Kooij et al[97] (2007–2008)	112	<31	39–45	24 mo	Cerebellar volume was positively correlated with cognition (β = 8.6, P = .009, R² model = 0.23)
Tan et al[95] (2004–2007)	65	<29	40–43	9 mo	Total brain volume was correlated with MDI[a] (R = 0.48; P = .002)
Maunu et al[131] (2001–2006)	≤1500 g or <31	Term		24 mo	Ventricular dilatation with additional brain disorder was associated with CP (P = .009), MDI[a] <70 (P = .03), and NDI[a] (P<.05)
Lind et al[92] (2001–2006)	164	<1500 g	Term	24 mo	Lower volumes of total brain tissue, cerebrum, frontal lobes, basal ganglia, thalami, and cerebellum, and larger ventricles were associated with neurodevelopmental impairment[a] (P<.005)
Shah et al[108] (2006)	83	<33	38–43	24 mo	Lower cerebellar volumes were correlated with WM injury and neurodevelopmental outcomes[a] (P = .02)
Jary et al[91] (2003–2006)	25	<30	38–47	25 mo	In infants with posthemorrhagic ventricular dilatation: • Total cerebral volume correlated with MDI[a] (R = 0.4, P = .02) and PDI[a] (R = 0.7; P<.0001) • Thalamic (R = 0.7, P = .0002) and cerebellar (R = 0.6; P = .002) volumes correlated with PDI[a]
Thompson et al[96] (2001–2003)	184	<30	38–42	24 mo	Smaller hippocampal volumes were correlated with MDI[a] (P<.001) and PDI[a] (P<.003)
Tich et al[102] (2001–2003)	182	<30	40	24 mo	Biparietal diameter was correlated with MDI[a] and PDI[a] (P<.01)
Beauchamp et al[98] (2001–2003)	156	<30	38–42	24 mo	Decrease in hippocampal volume was associated with working memory deficits (P<.01)

Lind et al[100] (2001–2003)	97	<1500 g and <37	Term	5 y	Cerebellar volume was associate with poorer executive function ($P = .05$; b = 0.77) and motor skills ($P = .05$; b = 0.87)
Boardman et al[99] (2001–2003)	80	≤34	37–44	24–31 mo	Volume reduction of WM basal ganglia (dorsomedial complex of the thalami and the globus pallidi) were associated with decreased DQ[b] (H = 18.825; $P<.001$)
Woodward et al[104] (1998–2000)	92	<32	39–41	24 mo	Total brain volume was associated with working memory performance ($P = .02$)
Inder et al[107] (1998–2000)	119	≤32	39–41	12 mo	Reductions in cortical and deep GM along with increased CSF volumes were associated with neurodevelopmental impairment[c] ($P<.05$)
Peterson et al[106] (1998–2000)	10	<37	35	18–20 mo	Decreased volumes in sensorimotor and midtemporal regions were correlated with cognitive outcome[a] ($\beta = 0.94$; $P = .003$)
DWI/DTI					
van Kooij et al[111] (2006–2007)	67	<31	Term	24 mo	In girls, volume ($\beta = 0.03$; $P = .056$) and length of CC ($\beta = 14.13$; $P = .005$) and R PLIC ($\beta = 0.1$; $P<.001$) was associated with cognition[a] In boys, volume ($\beta = 0.05$; $P = .055$) length ($\beta = 13.13$; $P = .012$) and FA ($\beta = 21.11$; $P = .053$) of the left PLIC was associated with fine motor performance[a]
van Kooij et al[110] (2006–2007)	63	<31	Term	24 mo	FA of WM was associated with cognitive ($R^2 = 0.31$), fine motor ($R^2 = 0.26$), and gross motor ($R^2 = 0.26$) performance[a]
Drobyshevsky et al[132] (2002–2004)	24	<32	30 and 36	18–24 mo	FA at 30 wk GA was correlated with PD[a] (R = 0.55; $P<.05$)
Rogers et al[133] (2001–2003)	111	<30	37–43	5 y	Higher ADC in the orbitofrontal cortex was associated with social-emotional problems ($\beta = 0.29$; $P≤.01$)
Krishnan et al[134] (2001–2003)	38	<34	38–44	24 mo	Lower ADC in the WM without overt lesions was associated with poorer DQ[b] ($P = .014$)

(continued on next page)

Table 4
(continued)

Study (y)	Subjects (No)	Age at Birth (wk)	Age at Scan (wk)	Follow-up Age	MRI Findings and Outcomes
Kaukola et al[135] (1998–2002)	30	<32	38–42	24 mo	Higher ADC in the corona radiata was associated with poorer gross motor outcome[b] (P = .004)
Als et al[136] (2000–2002)	30	28–33	42	9 mo	Higher FA in the L internal capsule was associated with better neurobehavioral functioning[a] (P = .03)
Rose et al[112] (1999–2001)	78	<32	33–42	18 mo	FA of the right PLIC was correlated with neurodevelopment[a] (ρ = 0.371, P = .002)
Rose et al[137] (1999–2001)	24	<1800 g	37	4 y	FA in the L and R PLIC was correlated with gross motor function (R = −0.65; P = .04) and gait deficits (R = −0.89; P = .001)
Arzoumanian et al[138] (1998–2000)	63	≤33	34–42	18–24 mo	FA in the PLIC was associated with abnormal neurologic examinations (P = .005)
MRS					
Gadin et al[90] (2007–2009)	20	<30	36 to discharge	6 mo	MRS measurements did not correlate with neurodevelopmental outcome[a]
van Kooij et al[97] (2007–2008)	112	<31	39–45	24 mo	Cerebellar NAA/Cho ratio were associated with cognition[a] (P = .007)
Augustine et al[122] (2000–2003)	36	≤32	35–43	18–24 mo	Metabolite ratios from MRS were not associated with neurodevelopmental outcome[a]

Abbreviations: DQ, developmental quotient; GA, gestational age in weeks; L, left; PLIC, posterior limb of the internal capsule; R, right.
[a] Bayley Scales of Infant Development.
[b] Griffith Mental Development Scales.
[c] Denver Developmental Screening Tool.

signal detects regional changes in hemodynamics of the brain that are correlated with functional activity (**Fig. 5**).[115] By using these BOLD signals in neonates, it is possible to identify networks with synchronous neuronal activity in sleeping neonates to study resting-state functional connectivity throughout development.

Born and colleagues[116] were the first to use fMRI to show brain activation using visual stimulation in healthy newborns and since then multiple studies have investigated the correlation between passive functions with fMRI as a clinical tool to evaluate the sensorimotor, visual, and auditory systems in infants with brain injury.[117] The prognostic implications of these findings have yet to be determined and further research in the use of fMRI in the preterm population may contribute to the predictive abilities of long-term neurodevelopmental outcomes in the preterm population.

MRS

MRS is a noninvasive measure of brain biochemistry. MRS provides information about common metabolites found in the brain, such as N-acetyl-aspartate (NAA), choline (Cho)-containing compounds, creatine, and lactate, which are involved in cellular metabolic pathways.[118] NAA is present in axons and considered to be a marker for neurons. It has been found to increase with advancing gestational age and maturity.[119] Cho-containing compounds are involved in ATP synthesis. Creatine is thought to be related to membrane metabolism. Lactate may be a marker for impaired metabolism from decreased cerebral blood flow in term neonates with hypoxic-ischemic injury,[120] but increases may be normal in preterm infants because of differences in metabolism.[121]

Thus far, there have been few studies examining the role of MRS in the prediction of neurodevelopmental outcomes in preterm infants. One study showed that cognitive scores were correlated with NAA/Cho ratio in the cerebellum,[97] but 2 studies did not find metabolite measurement on MRS to be a good predictor of neurodevelopmental outcome at 6 months[90] and 18 months to 24 months of age.[122]

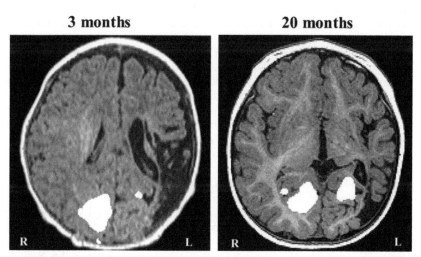

3 months   **20 months**

Fig. 5. fMRI activation map during the visual stimulation in an event-related fMRI paradigm in a infant with a perinatal stroke, showing the absence of cortical response at 3 months and recovery of cortical activation at 20 months. (*From* Seghier ML, Huppi PS. The role of functional magnetic resonance imaging in the study of brain development, injury, and recovery in the newborn. Semin Perinatol 2010;34:83; with permission.)

SUMMARY

MRI is a noninvasive mode of neuroimaging that is superior to ultrasound and is currently the best imaging tool available. It has great potential for clinical use in characterizing the extent of preterm brain injury in neonates and predicting neurodevelopmental outcomes. Although current studies have reported a wide range of PPVs of MRI as a diagnostic tool for long-term outcome prediction, there is consistent reporting of high NPV in predicting neurodevelopmental impairment. With regard to advanced MRI modalities, additional research is needed to prove clinical usefulness, but they hold promise. With the combination of conventional and advanced MRI techniques, it is hoped to be able to attain a more comprehensive view of the preterm brain, including both macrostructural and microstructural changes, to better predict those at highest risk of impairment, as well as to precisely define the type and extent of deficits likely to develop in the future. The goal is to find new ways to prevent, predict, and treat adverse outcomes and improve the function and quality of life of the preterm population as they age into adulthood.

REFERENCES

1. Behrman RE, Butler AS. Preterm birth: causes, consequences, and prevention. Washington, DC: National Academy of Sciences; 2007.
2. Hintz SR, Kendrick DE, Wilson-Costello DE, et al. Early-childhood neurodevelopmental outcomes are not improving for infants born at <25 weeks' gestational age. Pediatrics 2011;127:62–70.
3. Stoll BJ, Hansen NI, Bell EF, et al. Neonatal outcomes of extremely preterm infants from the NICHD Neonatal Research Network. Pediatrics 2010;126:443–56.
4. Hack M. Dilemmas in the measurement of developmental outcomes of preterm children. J Pediatr 2012;160:537–8.
5. Nongena P, Ederies A, Azzopardi DV, et al. Confidence in the prediction of neurodevelopmental outcome by cranial ultrasound and MRI in preterm infants. Arch Dis Child Fetal Neonatal Ed 2010;95:F388–90.
6. Harvey ME, Nongena P, Gonzalez-Cinca N, et al. Parents' experiences of information and communication in the neonatal unit about brain imaging and neurological prognosis: a qualitative study. Acta Paediatr 2013;102(4):360–5.
7. Hodek JM, von der Schulenburg JM, Mittendorf T. Measuring economic consequences of preterm birth – Methodological recommendations for the evaluation of personal burden on children and their caregivers. Health Econ Rev 2011;1:6.
8. Maunu J, Parkkola R, Rikalainen H, et al. Brain and ventricles in very low birth weight infants at term: a comparison among head circumference, ultrasound, and magnetic resonance imaging. Pediatrics 2009;123:617–26.
9. Austin T, O'Reilly H. Advances in imaging the neonatal brain. Expert Opin Med Diagn 2011;5:95–107.
10. van Wezel-Meijler G, Steggerda SJ, Leijser LM. Cranial ultrasonography in neonates: role and limitations. Semin Perinatol 2010;34:28–38.
11. Panigrahy A, Wisnowski JL, Furtado A, et al. Neuroimaging biomarkers of preterm brain injury: toward developing the preterm connectome. Pediatr Radiol 2012;42(Suppl 1):S33–61.
12. Inder TE, Anderson NJ, Spencer C, et al. White matter injury in the premature infant: a comparison between serial cranial sonographic and MR findings at term. AJNR Am J Neuroradiol 2003;24:805–9.
13. Woodward LJ, Anderson PJ, Austin NC, et al. Neonatal MRI to predict neurodevelopmental outcomes in preterm infants. N Engl J Med 2006;355:685–94.

14. Mirmiran M, Barnes PD, Keller K, et al. Neonatal brain magnetic resonance imaging before discharge is better than serial cranial ultrasound in predicting cerebral palsy in very low birth weight preterm infants. Pediatrics 2004;114:992–8.
15. Leijser LM, Liauw L, Veen S, et al. Comparing brain white matter on sequential cranial ultrasound and MRI in very preterm infants. Neuroradiology 2008;50: 799–811.
16. Ciambra G, Arachi S, Protano C, et al. Accuracy of transcranial ultrasound in the detection of mild white matter lesions in newborns. Neuroradiol J 2013;26:284–9.
17. Leijser LM, de Bruine FT, Steggerda SJ, et al. Brain imaging findings in very preterm infants throughout the neonatal period: part I. Incidences and evolution of lesions, comparison between ultrasound and MRI. Early Hum Dev 2009;85:101–9.
18. Hillenbrand CM, Reykowski A. MR Imaging of the newborn: a technical perspective. Magn Reson Imaging Clin N Am 2012;20:63–79.
19. Mathur AM, Neil JJ, McKinstry RC, et al. Transport, monitoring, and successful brain MR imaging in unsedated neonates. Pediatr Radiol 2008;38:260–4.
20. Panigrahy A, Borzage M, Bluml S. Basic principles and concepts underlying recent advances in magnetic resonance imaging of the developing brain. Semin Perinatol 2010;34:3–19.
21. Arthurs OJ, Edwards A, Austin T, et al. The challenges of neonatal magnetic resonance imaging. Pediatr Radiol 2012;42:1183–94.
22. Neubauer V, Griesmaier E, Baumgartner K, et al. Feasibility of cerebral MRI in non-sedated preterm-born infants at term-equivalent age: report of a single centre. Acta Paediatr 2011;100:1544–7.
23. Haney B, Reavey D, Atchison L, et al. Magnetic resonance imaging studies without sedation in the neonatal intensive care unit: safe and efficient. J Perinat Neonatal Nurs 2010;24:256–66.
24. Hintz SR, O'Shea M. Neuroimaging and neurodevelopmental outcomes in preterm infants. Semin Perinatol 2008;32:11–9.
25. Ment LR, Bada HS, Barnes P, et al. Practice parameter: neuroimaging of the neonate: report of the Quality Standards Subcommittee of the American Academy of Neurology and the Practice Committee of the Child Neurology Society. Neurology 2002;58:1726–38.
26. Meoded A, Poretti A, Northington FJ, et al. Susceptibility weighted imaging of the neonatal brain. Clin Radiol 2012;67:793–801.
27. Simbrunner J, Riccabona M. Imaging of the neonatal CNS. Eur J Radiol 2006; 60:133–51.
28. van Wezel-Meijler G, Leijser LM, de Bruine FT, et al. Magnetic resonance imaging of the brain in newborn infants: practical aspects. Early Hum Dev 2009;85: 85–92.
29. Rutherford M, Srinivasan L, Dyet L, et al. Magnetic resonance imaging in perinatal brain injury: clinical presentation, lesions and outcome. Pediatr Radiol 2006;36:582–92.
30. Rozovsky K, Ventureyra EC, Miller E. Fast-brain MRI in children is quick, without sedation, and radiation-free, but beware of limitations. J Clin Neurosci 2013;20: 400–5.
31. Rutherford MA, Ward P, Malamatentiou C. Advanced MR techniques in the term-born neonate with perinatal brain injury. Semin Fetal Neonatal Med 2005;10: 445–60.
32. Hart A, Whitby E, Wilkinson S, et al. Neuro-developmental outcome at 18 months in premature infants with diffuse excessive high signal intensity on MR imaging of the brain. Pediatr Radiol 2011;41:1284–92.

33. Jeon TY, Kim JH, Yoo SY, et al. Neurodevelopmental outcomes in preterm infants: comparison of infants with and without diffuse excessive high signal intensity on MR images at near-term-equivalent age. Radiology 2012;263:518–26.

34. de Bruine FT, van den Berg-Huysmans AA, Leijser LM, et al. Clinical implications of MR imaging findings in the white matter in very preterm infants: a 2-year follow-up study. Radiology 2011;261:899–906.

35. Skiold B, Vollmer B, Bohm B, et al. Neonatal magnetic resonance imaging and outcome at age 30 months in extremely preterm infants. J Pediatr 2012;160: 559–66.e1.

36. Setanen S, Haataja L, Parkkola R, et al. Predictive value of neonatal brain MRI on the neurodevelopmental outcome of preterm infants by 5 years of age. Acta Paediatr 2013;102:492–7.

37. Munck P, Haataja L, Maunu J, et al. Cognitive outcome at 2 years of age in Finnish infants with very low birth weight born between 2001 and 2006. Acta Paediatr 2010;99:359–66.

38. Spittle AJ, Boyd RN, Inder TE, et al. Predicting motor development in very preterm infants at 12 months' corrected age: the role of qualitative magnetic resonance imaging and general movements assessments. Pediatrics 2009;123:512–7.

39. Spittle AJ, Treyvaud K, Doyle LW, et al. Early emergence of behavior and social-emotional problems in very preterm infants. J Am Acad Child Adolesc Psychiatry 2009;48:909–18.

40. Spittle AJ, Cheong J, Doyle LW, et al. Neonatal white matter abnormality predicts childhood motor impairment in very preterm children. Dev Med Child Neurol 2011;53:1000–6.

41. Reidy N, Morgan A, Thompson DK, et al. Impaired language abilities and white matter abnormalities in children born very preterm and/or very low birth weight. J Pediatr 2013;162:719–24.

42. Omizzolo C, Scratch SE, Stargatt R, et al. Neonatal brain abnormalities and memory and learning outcomes at 7 years in children born very preterm. Memory 2013. [Epub ahead of print]. http://dx.doi.org/10.1080/09658211.2013. 809765.

43. Iwata S, Iwata O, Bainbridge A, et al. Abnormal white matter appearance on term FLAIR predicts neuro-developmental outcome at 6 years old following preterm birth. Int J Dev Neurosci 2007;25:523–30.

44. Iwata S, Nakamura T, Hizume E, et al. Qualitative brain MRI at term and cognitive outcomes at 9 years after very preterm birth. Pediatrics 2012;129:e1138–47.

45. Nanba Y, Matsui K, Aida N, et al. Magnetic resonance imaging regional T1 abnormalities at term accurately predict motor outcome in preterm infants. Pediatrics 2007;120:e10–9.

46. Woodward LJ, Clark CA, Pritchard VE, et al. Neonatal white matter abnormalities predict global executive function impairment in children born very preterm. Dev Neuropsychol 2011;36:22–41.

47. Clark CA, Woodward LJ. Neonatal cerebral abnormalities and later verbal and visuospatial working memory abilities of children born very preterm. Dev Neuropsychol 2010;35:622–42.

48. Edgin JO, Inder TE, Anderson PJ, et al. Executive functioning in preschool children born very preterm: relationship with early white matter pathology. J Int Neuropsychol Soc 2008;14:90–101.

49. Sie LT, Hart AA, van Hof J, et al. Predictive value of neonatal MRI with respect to late MRI findings and clinical outcome. A study in infants with periventricular densities on neonatal ultrasound. Neuropediatrics 2005;36:78–89.

50. Valkama AM, Paakko EL, Vainionpaa LK, et al. Magnetic resonance imaging at term and neuromotor outcome in preterm infants. Acta Paediatr 2000;89:348–55.
51. Kidokoro H, Anderson PJ, Doyle LW, et al. High signal intensity on T2-weighted MR imaging at term-equivalent age in preterm infants does not predict 2-year neurodevelopmental outcomes. AJNR Am J Neuroradiol 2011;32:2005–10.
52. Dyet LE, Kennea N, Counsell SJ, et al. Natural history of brain lesions in extremely preterm infants studied with serial magnetic resonance imaging from birth and neurodevelopmental assessment. Pediatrics 2006;118:536–48.
53. Kostovic I, Jovanov-Milosevic N, Rados M, et al. Perinatal and early postnatal reorganization of the subplate and related cellular compartments in the human cerebral wall as revealed by histological and MRI approaches. Brain Struct Funct 2012. [Epub ahead of print]. http://dx.doi.org/10.1007/s00429-012-0496-0490.
54. Judas M, Rados M, Jovanov-Milosevic N, et al. Structural, immunocytochemical, and MR imaging properties of periventricular crossroads of growing cortical pathways in preterm infants. AJNR Am J Neuroradiol 2005;26:2671–84.
55. Hart AR, Whitby EW, Griffiths PD, et al. Magnetic resonance imaging and developmental outcome following preterm birth: review of current evidence. Dev Med Child Neurol 2008;50:655–63.
56. Counsell SJ, Rutherford MA, Cowan FM, et al. Magnetic resonance imaging of preterm brain injury. Arch Dis Child Fetal Neonatal Ed 2003;88:F269–74.
57. Niwa T, de Vries LS, Benders MJ, et al. Punctate white matter lesions in infants: new insights using susceptibility-weighted imaging. Neuroradiology 2011;53:669–79.
58. van de Looij Y, Lodygensky GA, Dean J, et al. High-field diffusion tensor imaging characterization of cerebral white matter injury in lipopolysaccharide-exposed fetal sheep. Pediatr Res 2012;72:285–92.
59. Dean JM, van de Looij Y, Sizonenko SV, et al. Delayed cortical impairment following lipopolysaccharide exposure in preterm fetal sheep. Ann Neurol 2011;70:846–56.
60. Kinney HC, Volpe JJ. Modeling the encephalopathy of prematurity in animals: the important role of translational research. Neurol Res Int 2012;2012:295389.
61. Graf WD, Nagel SK, Epstein LG, et al. Pediatric neuroenhancement: ethical, legal, social, and neurodevelopmental implications. Neurology 2013;80:1251–60.
62. Dubois J, Benders M, Borradori-Tolsa C, et al. Primary cortical folding in the human newborn: an early marker of later functional development. Brain 2008;131:2028–41.
63. Inder TE, Huppi PS, Zientara GP, et al. The postmigrational development of polymicrogyria documented by magnetic resonance imaging from 31 weeks' postconceptional age. Ann Neurol 1999;45:798–801.
64. Maalouf EF, Duggan PJ, Rutherford MA, et al. Magnetic resonance imaging of the brain in a cohort of extremely preterm infants. J Pediatr 1999;135:351–7.
65. Brown NC, Inder TE, Bear MJ, et al. Neurobehavior at term and white and gray matter abnormalities in very preterm infants. J Pediatr 2009;155:32–8, 38.e1.
66. Volpe JJ. Cerebellum of the premature infant: rapidly developing, vulnerable, clinically important. J Child Neurol 2009;24:1085–104.
67. Limperopoulos C, Bassan H, Gauvreau K, et al. Does cerebellar injury in premature infants contribute to the high prevalence of long-term cognitive, learning, and behavioral disability in survivors? Pediatrics 2007;120:584–93.

68. Steggerda SJ, Leijser LM, Wiggers-de Bruine FT, et al. Cerebellar injury in preterm infants: incidence and findings on US and MR images. Radiology 2009; 252:190–9.
69. Merrill JD, Piecuch RE, Fell SC, et al. A new pattern of cerebellar hemorrhages in preterm infants. Pediatrics 1998;102:E62.
70. Levisohn L, Cronin-Golomb A, Schmahmann JD. Neuropsychological consequences of cerebellar tumour resection in children: cerebellar cognitive affective syndrome in a paediatric population. Brain 2000;123(Pt 5):1041–50.
71. Ris MD, Beebe DW, Armstrong FD, et al. Cognitive and adaptive outcome in extracerebellar low-grade brain tumors in children: a report from the Children's Oncology Group. J Clin Oncol 2008;26:4765–70.
72. Nagel BJ, Delis DC, Palmer SL, et al. Early patterns of verbal memory impairment in children treated for medulloblastoma. Neuropsychology 2006;20: 105–12.
73. Robertson PL, Muraszko KM, Holmes EJ, et al. Incidence and severity of postoperative cerebellar mutism syndrome in children with medulloblastoma: a prospective study by the Children's Oncology Group. J Neurosurg 2006;105: 444–51.
74. Limperopoulos C, Robertson RL, Sullivan NR, et al. Cerebellar injury in term infants: clinical characteristics, magnetic resonance imaging findings, and outcome. Pediatr Neurol 2009;41:1–8.
75. Limperopoulos C, Chilingaryan G, Sullivan N, et al. Injury to the premature cerebellum: outcome is related to remote cortical development. Cereb Cortex 2012. [Epub ahead of print]. http://dx.doi.org/10.1093/cercor/bhs354.
76. Papile LA, Burstein J, Burstein R, et al. Incidence and evolution of subependymal and intraventricular hemorrhage: a study of infants with birth weights less than 1,500 gm. J Pediatr 1978;92:529–34.
77. Volpe JJ. Neurology of the newborn. 5th edition. Philadelphia: Saunders/Elsevier; 2008. 1 online resource (xiv, 1094 p).
78. Miller SP, Ferriero DM, Leonard C, et al. Early brain injury in premature newborns detected with magnetic resonance imaging is associated with adverse early neurodevelopmental outcome. J Pediatr 2005;147:609–16.
79. Inder TE, Wells SJ, Mogridge NB, et al. Defining the nature of the cerebral abnormalities in the premature infant: a qualitative magnetic resonance imaging study. J Pediatr 2003;143:171–9.
80. Kidokoro H, Neil JJ, Inder TE. New MR imaging assessment tool to define brain abnormalities in very preterm infants at term. AJNR Am J Neuroradiol 2013. [Epub ahead of print]. http://dx.doi.org/10.3174/ajnr.A3521.
81. Messerschmidt A, Brugger PC, Boltshauser E, et al. Disruption of cerebellar development: potential complication of extreme prematurity. AJNR Am J Neuroradiol 2005;26:1659–67.
82. Pierson CR, Folkerth RD, Billiards SS, et al. Gray matter injury associated with periventricular leukomalacia in the premature infant. Acta Neuropathol 2007; 114:619–31.
83. de Vries LS, Benders MJ, Groenendaal F. Imaging the premature brain: ultrasound or MRI? Neuroradiology 2013;55(Suppl 2):13–22.
84. de Vries LS, van Haastert IC, Benders MJ, et al. Myth: cerebral palsy cannot be predicted by neonatal brain imaging. Semin Fetal Neonatal Med 2011;16: 279–87.
85. El-Dib M, Massaro AN, Bulas D, et al. Neuroimaging and neurodevelopmental outcome of premature infants. Am J Perinatol 2010;27:803–18.

86. Gui L, Lisowski R, Faundez T, et al. Morphology-driven automatic segmentation of MR images of the neonatal brain. Med Image Anal 2012;16:1565–79.

87. Huppi PS, Warfield S, Kikinis R, et al. Quantitative magnetic resonance imaging of brain development in premature and mature newborns. Ann Neurol 1998;43: 224–35.

88. Weisenfeld NI, Warfield SK. Automatic segmentation of newborn brain MRI. Neuroimage 2009;47:564–72.

89. Prastawa M, Gilmore JH, Lin W, et al. Automatic segmentation of MR images of the developing newborn brain. Med Image Anal 2005;9:457–66.

90. Gadin E, Lobo M, Paul DA, et al. Volumetric MRI and MRS and early motor development of infants born preterm. Pediatr Phys Ther 2012;24:38–44.

91. Jary S, De Carli A, Ramenghi LA, et al. Impaired brain growth and neurodevelopment in preterm infants with posthaemorrhagic ventricular dilatation. Acta Paediatr 2012;101:743–8.

92. Lind A, Parkkola R, Lehtonen L, et al. Associations between regional brain volumes at term-equivalent age and development at 2 years of age in preterm children. Pediatr Radiol 2011;41:953–61.

93. Shah DK, Guinane C, August P, et al. Reduced occipital regional volumes at term predict impaired visual function in early childhood in very low birth weight infants. Invest Ophthalmol Vis Sci 2006;47:3366–73.

94. Spittle AJ, Doyle LW, Anderson PJ, et al. Reduced cerebellar diameter in very preterm infants with abnormal general movements. Early Hum Dev 2010;86:1–5.

95. Tan M, Abernethy L, Cooke R. Improving head growth in preterm infants–a randomised controlled trial II: MRI and developmental outcomes in the first year. Arch Dis Child Fetal Neonatal Ed 2008;93:F342–6.

96. Thompson DK, Wood SJ, Doyle LW, et al. Neonate hippocampal volumes: prematurity, perinatal predictors, and 2-year outcome. Ann Neurol 2008;63:642–51.

97. Van Kooij BJ, Benders MJ, Anbeek P, et al. Cerebellar volume and proton magnetic resonance spectroscopy at term, and neurodevelopment at 2 years of age in preterm infants. Dev Med Child Neurol 2012;54:260–6.

98. Beauchamp MH, Thompson DK, Howard K, et al. Preterm infant hippocampal volumes correlate with later working memory deficits. Brain 2008;131:2986–94.

99. Boardman JP, Craven C, Valappil S, et al. A common neonatal image phenotype predicts adverse neurodevelopmental outcome in children born preterm. Neuroimage 2010;52:409–14.

100. Lind A, Haataja L, Rautava L, et al. Relations between brain volumes, neuropsychological assessment and parental questionnaire in prematurely born children. Eur Child Adolesc Psychiatry 2010;19:407–17.

101. Peterson BS, Vohr B, Staib LH, et al. Regional brain volume abnormalities and long-term cognitive outcome in preterm infants. JAMA 2000;284:1939–47.

102. Tich SN, Anderson PJ, Hunt RW, et al. Neurodevelopmental and perinatal correlates of simple brain metrics in very preterm infants. Arch Pediatr Adolesc Med 2011;165:216–22.

103. Valkama AM, Tolonen EU, Kerttul LI, et al. Brainstem size and function at term age in relation to later neurosensory disability in high-risk, preterm infants. Acta Paediatr 2001;90:909–15.

104. Woodward LJ, Edgin JO, Thompson D, et al. Object working memory deficits predicted by early brain injury and development in the preterm infant. Brain 2005;128:2578–87.

105. Dubois J, Benders M, Cachia A, et al. Mapping the early cortical folding process in the preterm newborn brain. Cereb Cortex 2008;18:1444–54.

106. Peterson BS, Anderson AW, Ehrenkranz R, et al. Regional brain volumes and their later neurodevelopmental correlates in term and preterm infants. Pediatrics 2003;111:939–48.

107. Inder TE, Warfield SK, Wang H, et al. Abnormal cerebral structure is present at term in premature infants. Pediatrics 2005;115:286–94.

108. Shah DK, Anderson PJ, Carlin JB, et al. Reduction in cerebellar volumes in preterm infants: relationship to white matter injury and neurodevelopment at two years of age. Pediatr Res 2006;60:97–102.

109. Inder TE, Huppi PS, Warfield S, et al. Periventricular white matter injury in the premature infant is followed by reduced cerebral cortical gray matter volume at term. Ann Neurol 1999;46:755–60.

110. van Kooij BJ, de Vries LS, Ball G, et al. Neonatal tract-based spatial statistics findings and outcome in preterm infants. AJNR Am J Neuroradiol 2012;33:188–94.

111. van Kooij BJ, van Pul C, Benders MJ, et al. Fiber tracking at term displays gender differences regarding cognitive and motor outcome at 2 years of age in preterm infants. Pediatr Res 2011;70:626–32.

112. Rose J, Butler EE, Lamont LE, et al. Neonatal brain structure on MRI and diffusion tensor imaging, sex, and neurodevelopment in very-low-birthweight preterm children. Dev Med Child Neurol 2009;51:526–35.

113. Bassi L, Ricci D, Volzone A, et al. Probabilistic diffusion tractography of the optic radiations and visual function in preterm infants at term equivalent age. Brain 2008;131:573–82.

114. Berman JI, Glass HC, Miller SP, et al. Quantitative fiber tracking analysis of the optic radiation correlated with visual performance in premature newborns. AJNR Am J Neuroradiol 2009;30:120–4.

115. Ogawa S, Menon RS, Tank DW, et al. Functional brain mapping by blood oxygenation level-dependent contrast magnetic resonance imaging. A comparison of signal characteristics with a biophysical model. Biophys J 1993;64:803–12.

116. Born P, Rostrup E, Leth H, et al. Change of visually induced cortical activation patterns during development. Lancet 1996;347:543.

117. Seghier ML, Huppi PS. The role of functional magnetic resonance imaging in the study of brain development, injury, and recovery in the newborn. Semin Perinatol 2010;34:79–86.

118. Michaelis T, Merboldt KD, Bruhn H, et al. Absolute concentrations of metabolites in the adult human brain in vivo: quantification of localized proton MR spectra. Radiology 1993;187:219–27.

119. Kreis R, Hofmann L, Kuhlmann B, et al. Brain metabolite composition during early human brain development as measured by quantitative in vivo 1H magnetic resonance spectroscopy. Magn Reson Med 2002;48:949–58.

120. Miller SP, Newton N, Ferriero DM, et al. Predictors of 30-month outcome after perinatal depression: role of proton MRS and socioeconomic factors. Pediatr Res 2002;52:71–7.

121. Leth H, Toft PB, Pryds O, et al. Brain lactate in preterm and growth-retarded neonates. Acta Paediatr 1995;84:495–9.

122. Augustine EM, Spielman DM, Barnes PD, et al. Can magnetic resonance spectroscopy predict neurodevelopmental outcome in very low birth weight preterm infants? J Perinatol 2008;28:611–8.

123. Mathur AM, Neil JJ, Inder TE. Understanding brain injury and neurodevelopmental disabilities in the preterm infant: the evolving role of advanced magnetic resonance imaging. Semin Perinatol 2010;34:57–66.

124. Oishi K, Faria AV, Mori S. Advanced neonatal NeuroMRI. Magn Reson Imaging Clin N Am 2012;20:81–91.
125. Griffiths ST, Elgen IB, Chong WK, et al. Cerebral magnetic resonance imaging findings in children born extremely preterm, very preterm, and at term. Pediatr Neurol 2013;49:113–8.
126. Beaulieu C. The basis of anisotropic water diffusion in the nervous system – a technical review. NMR Biomed 2002;15:435–55.
127. Lequin MH, Dudink J, Tong KA, et al. Magnetic resonance imaging in neonatal stroke. Semin Fetal Neonatal Med 2009;14:299–310.
128. Mukherjee P, McKinstry RC. Diffusion tensor imaging and tractography of human brain development. Neuroimaging Clin N Am 2006;16:19–43, vii.
129. Wimberger DM, Roberts TP, Barkovich AJ, et al. Identification of "premyelination" by diffusion-weighted MRI. J Comput Assist Tomogr 1995;19:28–33.
130. Ment LR, Hirtz D, Huppi PS. Imaging biomarkers of outcome in the developing preterm brain. Lancet Neurol 2009;8:1042–55.
131. Maunu J, Lehtonen L, Lapinleimu H, et al. Ventricular dilatation in relation to outcome at 2 years of age in very preterm infants: a prospective Finnish cohort study. Dev Med Child Neurol 2011;53:48–54.
132. Drobyshevsky A, Bregman J, Storey P, et al. Serial diffusion tensor imaging detects white matter changes that correlate with motor outcome in premature infants. Dev Neurosci 2007;29:289–301.
133. Rogers CE, Anderson PJ, Thompson DK, et al. Regional cerebral development at term relates to school-age social-emotional development in very preterm children. J Am Acad Child Adolesc Psychiatry 2012;51:181–91.
134. Krishnan ML, Dyet LE, Boardman JP, et al. Relationship between white matter apparent diffusion coefficients in preterm infants at term-equivalent age and developmental outcome at 2 years. Pediatrics 2007;120:e604–9.
135. Kaukola T, Perhomaa M, Vainionpaa L, et al. Apparent diffusion coefficient on magnetic resonance imaging in pons and in corona radiata and relation with the neurophysiologic measurement and the outcome in very preterm infants. Neonatology 2010;97:15–21.
136. Als H, Duffy FH, McAnulty GB, et al. Early experience alters brain function and structure. Pediatrics 2004;113:846–57.
137. Rose J, Mirmiran M, Butler EE, et al. Neonatal microstructural development of the internal capsule on diffusion tensor imaging correlates with severity of gait and motor deficits. Dev Med Child Neurol 2007;49:745–50.
138. Arzoumanian Y, Mirmiran M, Barnes PD, et al. Diffusion tensor brain imaging findings at term-equivalent age may predict neurologic abnormalities in low birth weight preterm infants. AJNR Am J Neuroradiol 2003;24:1646–53.

Index

Note: Page numbers of article titles are in **boldface** type.

Clin Perinatol 41 (2014) 285–294
http://dx.doi.org/10.1016/S0095-5108(13)00157-7
0095-5108/14/$ – see front matter © 2014 Elsevier Inc. All rights reserved.

Moving?

Make sure your subscription moves with you!

To notify us of your new address, find your **Clinics Account Number** (located on your mailing label above your name), and contact customer service at:

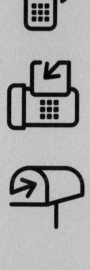

Email: **journalscustomerservice-usa@elsevier.com**

800-654-2452 (subscribers in the U.S. & Canada)
314-447-8871 (subscribers outside of the U.S. & Canada)

Fax number: **314-447-8029**

Elsevier Health Sciences Division
Subscription Customer Service
3251 Riverport Lane
Maryland Heights, MO 63043

*To ensure uninterrupted delivery of your subscription, please notify us at least 4 weeks in advance of move.

Printed and bound by CPI Group (UK) Ltd, Croydon, CR0 4YY

03/10/2024

01040487-0013